Integrating Clinical and Translational Research Networks

Integrating Clinical and Translational Research Networks—Building Team Medicine

Editors

Ravi Salgia
Prakash Kulkarni

MDPI • Basel • Beijing • Wuhan • Barcelona • Belgrade • Manchester • Tokyo • Cluj • Tianjin

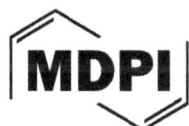

Editors
Ravi Salgia
City of Hope National Medical Center
USA

Prakash Kulkarni
City of Hope National Medical Center
US

Editorial Office
MDPI
St. Alban-Anlage 66
4052 Basel, Switzerland

This is a reprint of articles from the Special Issue published online in the open access journal *Journal of Clinical Medicine* (ISSN 2077-0383) (available at: https://www.mdpi.com/journal/jcm/special_issues/Team_Medicine).

For citation purposes, cite each article independently as indicated on the article page online and as indicated below:

LastName, A.A.; LastName, B.B.; LastName, C.C. Article Title. *Journal Name* **Year**, *Volume Number*, Page Range.

ISBN 978-3-0365-0396-7 (Hbk)
ISBN 978-3-0365-0397-4 (PDF)

© 2021 by the authors. Articles in this book are Open Access and distributed under the Creative Commons Attribution (CC BY) license, which allows users to download, copy and build upon published articles, as long as the author and publisher are properly credited, which ensures maximum dissemination and a wider impact of our publications.

The book as a whole is distributed by MDPI under the terms and conditions of the Creative Commons license CC BY-NC-ND.

Contents

About the Editors vii

Ravi Salgia and Prakash Kulkarni
Integrating Clinical and Translational Research Networks—Building Team Medicine
Reprinted from: *J. Clin. Med.* **2020**, *9*, 2975, doi:10.3390/jcm9092975 1

**Rebecca Pharaon, Samuel Chung, Arya Amini, Ellie Maghami, Arnab Chowdhury,
Nayana Vora, Sue Chang, Robert Kang, Thomas Gernon, Kelly Hansen, Christina Kelly,
Denise Ackerman, Lalit Vora, Sagus Sampath and Erminia Massarelli**
An Analysis and Comparison of Survival and Functional Outcomes in Oropharyngeal
Squamous Cell Carcinoma Patients Treated with Concurrent Chemoradiation Therapy within
City of Hope Cancer Center Sites
Reprinted from: *J. Clin. Med.* **2020**, *9*, 3083, doi:10.3390/jcm9103083 3

**Joanne E. Mortimer, Laura Kruper, Mary Cianfrocca, Sayeh Lavasani, Sariah Liu,
Niki Tank-Patel, Mina Sedrak, Wade Smith, Daphne Stewart, James Waisman,
Christina Yeon, Tina Wang and Yuan Yuan**
Use of HER2-Directed Therapy in Metastatic Breast Cancer and How Community Physicians
Collaborate to Improve Care
Reprinted from: *J. Clin. Med.* **2020**, *9*, 1984, doi:10.3390/jcm9061984 15

Daniel J. Kim, Dan Otap, Nora Ruel, Naveen Gupta, Naveed Khan and Tanya Dorff
NCI–Clinical Trial Accrual in a Community Network Affiliated with a Designated
Cancer Center
Reprinted from: *J. Clin. Med.* **2020**, *9*, 1970, doi:10.3390/jcm9061970 25

**Ravi Salgia, Isa Mambetsariev, Tingting Tan, Amanda Schwer, Daryl P. Pearlstein,
Hazem Chehabi, Angel Baroz, Jeremy Fricke, Rebecca Pharaon, Hannah Romo,
Thomas Waddington, Razmig Babikian, Linda Buck, Prakash Kulkarni, Mary Cianfrocca,
Benjamin Djulbegovic and Sumanta K. Pal**
Complex Oncological Decision-Making Utilizing Fast-and-Frugal Trees in a Community
Setting—Role of Academic and Hybrid Modeling
Reprinted from: *J. Clin. Med.* **2020**, *9*, 1884, doi:10.3390/jcm9061884 33

**Cary A. Presant, Ravi Salgia, Prakash Kulkarni, Brian L. Tiep, Shamel Sanani,
Benjamin Leach, Kimlin Ashing, Jossie Sandoval, Mina S. Sedrak, Shana Landau,
Sophia Yeung, Dan Raz and Shanmugga Subbiah**
Implementing Lung Cancer Screening and Prevention in Academic Centers, Affiliated Network
Offices and Collaborating Care Sites
Reprinted from: *J. Clin. Med.* **2020**, *9*, 1820, doi:10.3390/jcm9061820 57

**Nicholas J. Salgia, Errol J. Philip, Mohammadbagher Ziari, Kelly Yap
and Sumanta Kumar Pal**
Advancing the Science and Management of Renal Cell Carcinoma: Bridging the Divide between
Academic and Community Practices
Reprinted from: *J. Clin. Med.* **2020**, *9*, 1508, doi:10.3390/jcm9051508 69

Linda D. Bosserman, Mary Cianfrocca, Bertram Yuh, Christina Yeon, Helen Chen, Stephen Sentovich, Amy Polverini, Finly Zachariah, Debbie Deaville, Ashley B. Lee, Mina S. Sedrak, Elisabeth King, Stacy Gray, Denise Morse, Scott Glaser, Geetika Bhatt, Camille Adeimy, TingTing Tan, Joseph Chao, Arin Nam, Isaac B. Paz, Laura Kruper, Poornima Rao, Karen Sokolov, Prakash Kulkarni, Ravi Salgia, Jonathan Yamzon and Deron Johnson
Integrating Academic and Community Cancer Care and Research through Multidisciplinary Oncology Pathways for Value-Based Care: A Review and the City of Hope Experience
Reprinted from: *J. Clin. Med.* **2021**, *10*, 188, doi:10.3390/jcm10020188 . . . . **87**

Edward Wenge Wang, Christina Hsiao Wei, Sariah Liu, Stephen Jae-Jin Lee, Susan Shehayeb, Scott Glaser, Richard Li, Siamak Saadat, James Shen, Thanh Dellinger, Ernest Soyoung Han, Daphne Stewart, Sharon Wilczynski, Mihaela Cristea and Lorna Rodriguez-Rodriguez
Frontline Management of Epithelial Ovarian Cancer—Combining Clinical Expertise with Community Practice Collaboration and Cutting-Edge Research
Reprinted from: *J. Clin. Med.* **2020**, *9*, 2830, doi:10.3390/jcm9092830 . . . . **127**

Shanmuga Subbiah, Arin Nam, Natasha Garg, Amita Behal, Prakash Kulkarni and Ravi Salgia
Small Cell Lung Cancer from Traditional to Innovative Therapeutics: Building a Comprehensive Network to Optimize Clinical and Translational Research
Reprinted from: *J. Clin. Med.* **2020**, *9*, 2433, doi:10.3390/jcm9082433 . . . . **143**

Marilena Melas, Shanmuga Subbiah, Siamak Saadat, Swapnil Rajurkar and Kevin J. McDonnell
The Community Oncology and Academic Medical Center Alliance in the Age of Precision Medicine: Cancer Genetics and Genomics Considerations
Reprinted from: *J. Clin. Med.* **2020**, *9*, 2125, doi:10.3390/jcm9072125 . . . . **163**

Swapnil Rajurkar, Isa Mambetsariev, Rebecca Pharaon, Benjamin Leach, TingTing Tan, Prakash Kulkarni and Ravi Salgia
Non-Small Cell Lung Cancer from Genomics to Therapeutics: A Framework for Community Practice Integration to Arrive at Personalized Therapy Strategies
Reprinted from: *J. Clin. Med.* **2020**, *9*, 1870, doi:10.3390/jcm9061870 . . . . **189**

Misagh Karimi, Chongkai Wang, Bahareh Bahadini, George Hajjar and Marwan Fakih
Integrating Academic and Community Practices in the Management of Colorectal Cancer: The City of Hope Model
Reprinted from: *J. Clin. Med.* **2020**, *9*, 1687, doi:10.3390/jcm9061687 . . . . **215**

Tina Wang, Sariah Liu, Thomas Joseph and Yung Lyou
Managing Bladder Cancer Care during the COVID-19 Pandemic Using a Team-Based Approach
Reprinted from: *J. Clin. Med.* **2020**, *9*, 1574, doi:10.3390/jcm9051574 . . . . **223**

Jennifer Liu, Eutiquio Gutierrez, Abhay Tiwari, Simran Padam, Daneng Li, William Dale, Sumanta K. Pal, Daphne Stewart, Shanmugga Subbiah, Linda D. Bosserman, Cary Presant, Tanyanika Phillips, Kelly Yap, Addie Hill, Geetika Bhatt, Christina Yeon, Mary Cianfrocca, Yuan Yuan, Joanne Mortimer and Mina S. Sedrak
Strategies to Improve Participation of Older Adults in Cancer Research
Reprinted from: *J. Clin. Med.* **2020**, *9*, 1571, doi:10.3390/jcm9051571 . . . . **229**

About the Editors

Ravi Salgia, MD, Ph.D., is Chair of Medical Oncology & Therapeutics Research at City of Hope National Medical Center, in Duarte, California. Dr. Salgia also holds the Arthur and Rosalie Kaplan Chair in Medical Oncology, and is the Associate Director for Clinical Sciences Research in the City of Hope's Comprehensive Cancer Center. Previously, Dr. Salgia was Professor of Medicine, Pathology and Dermatology, and the Director of the Thoracic Oncology Program, and Aerodigestive Tract Program Translational Research at the University of Chicago. His research interests focus on novel therapeutics against lung cancer. Dr. Salgia has been honored with numerous awards, including being named one of the Top Doctors in America. He is a member of the editorial board for several top Journals and has authored or coauthored ~300 peer-reviewed publications and book chapters and is the sole Editor of two books that are currently under publication. Prior to his tenure at the University of Chicago School of Medicine, Dr. Salgia was faculty at the Dana-Farber Cancer Institute and Harvard Medical School. Dr. Salgia earned his undergraduate summa cum laude in mathematics, biology, and chemistry, and then his MD and Ph.D. degrees from Loyola University in Chicago, IL, where he also completed fellowships in neurochemistry and physiology. He continued his postgraduate training with an internship and residency in internal medicine at The Johns Hopkins University School of Medicine in Baltimore, MD, followed by a fellowship in medical oncology at Dana-Farber Cancer Institute in Boston, MA, during which time he also served as a clinical fellow at Harvard Medical School in Boston.

Prakash Kulkarni, Ph.D., is currently a Research Professor at the Department of Medical Oncology & Therapeutics Research at the City of Hope National Medical Center, Duarte, California. Dr. Kulkarni obtained a Ph.D. in biochemistry from India and did his postdoctoral training in cell biology at New York University. Subsequently, he held Staff Scientist positions in the Division of Chemistry & Chemical Engineering as well as in the Division of Biology at the California Institute of Technology, and later, in the Department of Genetics at Yale University. Dr. Kulkarni began his independent academic career as an Assistant Professor of Urology and Oncology in the Brady Urological Institute at Johns Hopkins University where he was named the Irene and Bernard L. Schwartz Scholar of the Patrick C Walsh Prostate Research Fund. He then moved as Research Associate Professor to the Institute of Bioscience & Biotechnology Research at the University of Maryland before he moved to City of Hope. Dr. Kulkarni is an Editorial Board Member of several Journals and also is the Associate Editor-in-Chief of Biomolecules. In addition, he is a member of the Organizing Committee of International Meetings, and serves as a Scientific Expert to various government and philanthropic organizations in the US, Europe, and Australia. In addition to cancer biology, he maintains a strong interest in prostate cancer as well as other solid tumors.

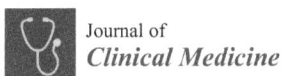

Editorial

Integrating Clinical and Translational Research Networks—Building Team Medicine

Ravi Salgia * and Prakash Kulkarni

City of Hope National Medical Center, Duarte, CA 91010, USA; pkulkarni@coh.org
* Correspondence: rsalgia@coh.org; Tel.: +1-626-471-9200

Received: 7 September 2020; Accepted: 14 September 2020; Published: 15 September 2020

In the United States (US), medical centers are widely recognized as vital components of the health care system. In general, however, the academic medical centers are differentiated from their community counterparts by their mission which typically focuses on clinical care, education, and research. Nonetheless, community clinics/hospitals fill a critical need and play a complementary role serving as the primary sites for health care in most communities. Furthermore, new health care reform initiatives in the US and economic pressures have created opportunities and incentives for hospitals and health systems to integrate, resulting in a nationwide trend toward consolidation. As a result, academic medical centers are leveraging their substantial assets to merge, acquire, or establish partnerships with their community peers with the ultimate goal of ensuring that all patients, regardless of their physical proximity to major medical institutions, can benefit from recent clinical advances.

This trend is highly pervasive across medical specialties, and as these alliances accelerate, they will continue to affect the oncology groups providing services at these institutions in particular. Thus, we believe a deeper understanding of the new landscape, changing relationships, and marketplace dynamics will help both academic and private practice oncologists adapt to this ongoing change. At the City of Hope, a United States National Cancer Institute (NCI)-designated Comprehensive Cancer Center, the leadership, working closing with the Chair of Medical Oncology and others, was swift in recognizing this challenge and executing a game plan to ensure that the best medical care developed and practiced by its academic center can be accessed by cancer patients throughout the enterprise, especially within the community centers. With >75 faculties in the Department of Medical Oncology, and 27 community centers in Southern California, we believe this is a sizeable enterprise in which we implemented this approach to integrate the academic and community centers. Thus, we trust that it would be valuable to share our experience with other healthcare providers and organizations in the US and other parts of the world so that they can benefit from our experience.

It is now increasingly recognized that in addition to physicians, physician-scientists, and other healthcare-related professionals, basic research scientists also contribute significantly to the emerging inter- and cross-disciplinary, team-oriented culture of translational science. Therefore, approaches that combine the knowledge, skills, experience, expertise, and visions of clinicians in academic medical centers and their affiliated community centers and hospitals, together with basic research scientists, are critical in shaping the emerging culture of translational research so that patients from the urban as well as suburban settings can avail the benefits of the latest developments in science and medicine.

This Special Issue is an embodiment of this ethos. It includes a series of papers authored by teams of leading clinicians, basic research scientists, and translational researchers. The authors discuss how engaging and collaborating with community-based practices, where the majority of older patients with cancer receive their care, can ensure that these patients receive the highest-quality, evidence-based care. Based on our collective experience, we would like to stress that the success of academic-community collaborative programs not only depends on the good will and vision of the participants but also on the medical administration, academic leadership, policy makers who define the principles and rules by which cooperation within the health care industry occurs. We refer to this cooperation and collaboration as 'Team Medicine'.

We take this opportunity to thank the City of Hope leadership for the support and encouragement; the authors for taking time from their hectic schedules, especially during this unprecedented pandemic to share their unique experience, vision, and ideas; and the patients and their families for their participation and enduring spirit. We trust that our experience embodied in this singular compendium will serve as a 'Rosetta Stone' for other institutions and practitioners.

Funding: This research received no external funding.

Conflicts of Interest: The authors declare no conflict of interest.

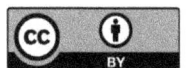
© 2020 by the authors. Licensee MDPI, Basel, Switzerland. This article is an open access article distributed under the terms and conditions of the Creative Commons Attribution (CC BY) license (http://creativecommons.org/licenses/by/4.0/).

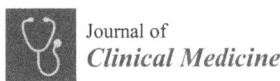

Article

An Analysis and Comparison of Survival and Functional Outcomes in Oropharyngeal Squamous Cell Carcinoma Patients Treated with Concurrent Chemoradiation Therapy within City of Hope Cancer Center Sites

Rebecca Pharaon [1,†], Samuel Chung [1,†], Arya Amini [2], Ellie Maghami [3], Arnab Chowdhury [4], Nayana Vora [2], Sue Chang [5], Robert Kang [3], Thomas Gernon [3], Kelly Hansen [6], Christina Kelly [6], Denise Ackerman [7], Lalit Vora [8], Sagus Sampath [2] and Erminia Massarelli [1,*]

1. Department of Medical Oncology and Therapeutics Research, City of Hope National Medical Center, Duarte, CA 91010, USA; rpharaon@coh.org (R.P.); schung@coh.org (S.C.)
2. Department of Radiation Oncology, City of Hope National Medical Center, Duarte, CA 91010, USA; aamini@coh.org (A.A.); NVora@coh.org (N.V.); ssampath@coh.org (S.S.)
3. Department of Head and Neck Surgery, City of Hope National Medical Center, Duarte, CA 91010, USA; emaghami@coh.org (E.M.); rkang@coh.org (R.K.); tgernon@coh.org (T.G.)
4. Department of Computational and Quantitative Medicine, City of Hope National Medical Center, Duarte, CA 91010, USA; achowdhury@coh.org
5. Department of Pathology, City of Hope National Medical Center, Duarte, CA 91010, USA; suchang@coh.org
6. Department of Speech and Language Pathology, City of Hope National Medical Center, Duarte, CA 91010, USA; kehansen@coh.org (K.H.); chrikelly@coh.org (C.K.)
7. Department of Clinical Nutrition, City of Hope National Medical Center, Duarte, CA 91010, USA; dackerma@coh.org
8. Department of Diagnostic Radiology, City of Hope National Medical Center, Duarte, CA 91010, USA; LVora@coh.org
* Correspondence: emassarelli@coh.org; Tel.: +1-626-256-4673
† These authors contributed equally to this work and should be considered co-first authors.

Received: 8 July 2020; Accepted: 22 September 2020; Published: 24 September 2020

Abstract: Oropharyngeal squamous cell carcinoma (OPSCC) is a subset of head and neck cancers that can arise due to human papillomavirus (HPV) infection. We designed a retrospective analysis to determine differences in outcomes of OPSCC patients treated at City of Hope (COH) Cancer Center's main campus versus selected satellite sites with COH-associated faculty and facilities. Patients diagnosed with OPSCC and treated with concurrent chemoradiation therapy ($n = 94$) were identified and included in the study. Patients underwent treatment at the COH main campus site ($n = 50$) or satellite sites ($n = 44$). The majority of patients were Caucasian, male, and diagnosed with p16 positive stage IV locally advanced OPSCC by AJCC 7th edition. Most patients completed their prescribed cumulative radiation therapy dose and had a complete response to treatment. No significant difference in overall survival and progression-free survival was observed between the main campus and the satellite sites. Our study demonstrates successful treatment completion rates as well as comparable recurrence rates between the main campus and COH-associated satellite sites. A trend toward significant difference in feeding tube dependency at 6-months was observed. Differences in feeding tube placement and dependency rates could be addressed by the establishment of on-site supportive services in satellite sites.

Keywords: oropharyngeal cancer; concurrent chemoradiation therapy; human papillomavirus; feeding tube dependency

1. Introduction

Head and neck cancers, a heterogenous group of cancers originating in the head and neck region, are strongly linked to risk factors such as tobacco use, alcohol consumption, and human papillomavirus (HPV) infection. Oropharyngeal squamous cell carcinomas (OPSCC) are one of the most common head and neck cancers; however, HPV-associated OPSCCs denote a distinct subtype of oropharyngeal cancer with rising incidence compared to the smoking-associated counterpart [1,2]. It has been shown that HPV-associated OPSCC has better prognosis [3–7] and is less likely to have a second primary site [8], but the occurrence of distant metastases is not significantly different than HPV-negative cancer [7,9].

Due to the association between OPSCC and HPV-mediated oncogenesis, the 8th edition of the American Joint Committee on Cancer (AJCC) denoted specific staging criteria and standard treatment for HPV-associated OPSCC, as well as emphasized the importance of extranodal extension (ENE) when determining staging and treatment for patients [10]. Standard treatment generally includes a multimodality approach consisting of transoral robotic surgery (TORS) for early stages or resectable tumors, and radiation therapy with or without concurrent chemotherapy as adjuvant or definitive treatment depending on tumor (T) and nodal (N) disease or high-risk pathologic features such as ENE or carcinoma-involved margins. In the incurable recurrent or metastatic (R/M) OPSCC setting, systemic treatment options include immune checkpoint inhibitors plus or minus chemotherapy with platinum/5-fluorouracil depending on PD-L1 expression, and novel approaches in immunotherapy combinations and HPV vaccines are currently undergoing investigation [11,12].

Cancer patient outcomes after treatment at academic versus satellite sites have been previously explored in esophageal cancer, soft tissue sarcoma, and laryngeal cancer, reporting a trend of improved survival for patients treated at high-volume teaching facilities [13–15]. In choosing their treatment center, patients have to account for the geographical location, financial cost, and insurance-approved providers, which can greatly limit their options. Previous studies have examined head and neck cancer outcomes in patients treated at academic centers versus community sites with controversial results [16–18]. Currently, academic center and community clinic affiliations have increased to allow patients to have access to high quality and standardized care. However, outcomes analysis has not been studied in partnered academic and satellite sites operating under the same umbrella.

At our institution, City of Hope (COH) Comprehensive Cancer Center, we have established various satellite sites distributed throughout the Southern California region in order to accommodate geographic restrictions and traffic limitations for our patients. Due to the complex nature of treating head and neck cancers, the coordination of various treatments and providers requires precise and effective medical practice. Functional and survival outcomes are dependent on the timing of adjuvant or definitive treatment as well as dedicated follow-up of patients with adequate supportive service such as speech pathology, nutrition specialists, and physical and occupational therapy. Several quality assurance measures are in place at COH, including reviews of satellite site radiation treatment plans performed at the main campus prior to treatment start.

We designed a retrospective study to analyze and compare survival and functional outcomes in patients treated at COH's main campus versus selected satellite sites with COH-associated faculty and radiation therapy facilities.

2. Materials and Methods

2.1. Patient and Study Criteria

A retrospective analysis of patients diagnosed with OPSCC and treated with concurrent chemoradiation therapy (CRT) was conducted at COH main campus and selected satellite sites. Main eligibility criteria included a diagnosis of OPSCC, age 18 years or older, definitive/adjuvant treatment including concurrent CRT at a COH site between February 2009 to February 2017, available demographic, treatment, and survival data, functional outcomes, and recent follow-up at a COH site within a year. We utilized our institutional electronic medical record (EMR) to analyze 400 consecutive head and neck cancer patients from various COH sites to enroll in our study. Of the initial 400 patients reviewed, only 94 met the inclusion criteria including OPSCC diagnosis, recent follow-up, and history of CRT treatment at a COH site. Confounding factors considered were age, gender, and T stage. The study was conducted in accordance with the Declaration of Helsinki, and the protocol was approved by the COH institutional review board (#19010).

The primary endpoint was overall survival (OS) of patients treated at the main COH campus versus patients treated at selected COH satellite sites, including South Pasadena, Rancho Cucamonga, Antelope Valley, and Santa Clarita. Secondary endpoints included treatment responses, feeding tube dependency, weight loss, and narcotic use.

2.2. Statistical Considerations

The primary analysis of this retrospective study design is to determine the differences in outcomes of OPSCC patients treated at COH Cancer Center main campus versus selected COH-associated satellite sites. Before carrying out inferential statistical procedures, exploratory data analysis was performed. Patient characteristics, including age, gender, race, smoking status, stage at diagnosis, cancer site, and p16 status by immunohistochemistry (IHC), and treatment variables, including chemotherapy agent selected, and dose reduction or interruption, and treatment responses were summarized using descriptive statistics. For continuous variables, means/medians, standard deviations, range and for categorical variables, patient counts, and percentages were provided by cancer center sites (Tables 1 and 2). Two sample mean/proportion tests (one-sided/two-sided) were performed for quantitative variables. To test homogeneity (equivalent to testing independence) between the main campus and the COH-associated satellite cancer center sites grouped by categorical patient characteristics and treatment outcomes, Pearson's chi-square test was performed. Fisher's exact test was performed as an alternative where the expected cell counts were small (less than 5). PEG Tube replacement and feeding tube dependency were also compared between two groups (sites).

Table 1. Patient Characteristics by Treatment Site.

		Main Campus ($n = 50$) n, %	Satellite Sites ($n = 44$) n, %	p-Value
Age median		58	61	
Gender	Female	10 (20)	5 (11)	$p = 0.25$
	Male	40 (80)	39 (89)	
Vital Status	Alive	44 (88)	43 (98)	$p = 0.12$
	Deceased	6 (12)	1 (2)	
Race	Caucasian	38 (76)	32 (73)	$p = 0.08$
	African American	1 (2)	1 (2)	
	Asian	8 (16)	3 (7)	
	Native American	1 (2)	0 (0)	
	Other/Unknown	2 (4)	8 (18)	
Smoking status	Never	25 (50)	22 (50)	$p = 1.00$
	Former/Current	25 (50)	22 (5)	
AJCC 7th Edition Stage	I	0 (0)	0 (0)	$p = 0.24$
	II	2 (4)	2 (5)	
	III	5 (10)	9 (20)	
	IV	43 (86)	33 (75)	
T stage	T0–2	31 (62)	38 (86)	$p = 0.008$
	T3–4	19 (38)	6 (14)	
N stage	N0–2a	14 (28)	19 (43)	$p = 0.124$
	N2b-N3	36 (72)	25 (57)	
M stage	M0	50 (100)	44 (100)	—
	M1	0 (0)	0 (0)	
Cancer site	Tonsil	17 (34)	25 (57)	$p = 0.06$
	Base of Tongue	29 (58)	15 (34)	
	Oropharynx, NOS	4 (8)	4 (9)	
P16 status	Positive	42 (84)	30 (68)	$p = 0.18$
	Negative	4 (8)	6 (14)	
	Unknown	4 (8)	8 (18)	

Table 2. Treatment and functional outcomes.

		Main Campus n, %	Satellite Sites n, %	p-Value
Chemotherapy agent	Cisplatin	39 (78)	21 (48)	p = 0.001
	Carboplatin	4 (8)	1 (2)	
	Cetuximab	6 (12)	21 (48)	
	Platinum/Paclitaxel	1 (2)	1 (2)	
Chemotherapy drug change		5 (10)	2 (5)	p = 0.31
Chemotherapy interruption/missed dose		11 (22)	9 (20)	p = 0.86
Chemotherapy dose reduction		4 (8)	3 (7)	p = 0.83
Radiation therapy interruption		7 (14)	6 (14)	p = 0.96
PEG tube placement	Yes	12 (24)	24 (55)	p = 0.002
	No	38 (76)	20 (45)	
Prophylactic PEG tube placement		4 (33)	20 (83)	p = 0.003
PEG tube dependency	>6 months	2 (17)	11 (46)	p = 0.08
Weight loss during treatment	≤10%	37 (74)	26 (59)	p = 0.12
	>10%	13 (26)	18 (41)	
Weight loss baseline to 6 months post-treatment	≤10%	24 (48)	14 (32)	p = 0.11
	>10%	26 (52)	30 (68)	
Hospitalizations during treatment		6 (12)	4 (9)	p = 0.65
Treatment Response	Complete response	35 (70)	37 (84)	p = 0.24
	Partial response	13 (26)	5 (11)	
	Progressive/persistent disease	2 (4)	2 (5)	
Recurrent disease		5 (10)	7 (16)	p = 0.39
3-month narcotic use	Yes	16 (32)	13 (30)	p = 0.98
	No	34 (68)	25 (57)	
	Unknown	8 (16)	6 (13)	
6-month narcotic use	Yes	9 (18)	10 (23)	p = 0.83
	No	33 (66)	28 (64)	
	Unknown	8 (16)	6 (13)	
Progression-free survival	2-year	47 (94)	37 (84)	p = 0.12
	5-year	46 (92%)	37 (84)	p = 0.23

Survival estimates were calculated based on the Kaplan-Meier product-limit method, and 95% confidence intervals were calculated using the "exponential" Greenwood variance (log-log transformation) estimate. Differences between Kaplan-Meier curves were assessed by the log-rank test. OS was measured from the date of diagnosis to death from any cause. Patients who were alive at the last contact date were censored. Progression-free survival (PFS) was measured from the date of diagnosis to disease progression or death, whichever occurred first. All calculations were performed using RStudio 1.2.5033; study data were locked for analysis on 15 January 2020.

3. Results

3.1. Patient Characteristics

94 patients met the inclusion criteria and were included in this retrospective analysis of patients treated between 2009 and 2017 (50 patients at the main COH site and 44 at the satellite sites). Clinicopathologic patient characteristics are presented in Table 1. Majority of patients were p16 positive ($n = 72$, 77%) with primary sites including base of tongue, tonsil, or oropharynx not otherwise specified (Figure 1A). The variables were well-balanced between the two groups, except for T stage demonstrating a significantly higher rate of T3/4 disease treated at the main campus and T0/T2 disease treated at the satellite sites ($p = 0.008$, Table 1 and Figure 1B).

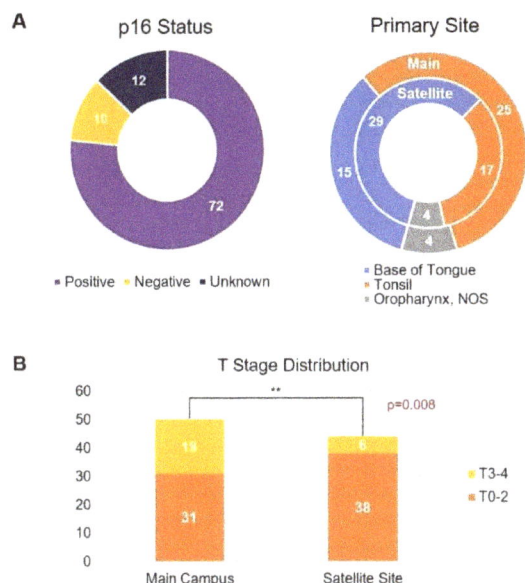

Figure 1. (**A**) P16 breakdown and oropharynx primary site breakdown in patient population and (**B**) T stage disease distribution by treatment site.

3.2. Treatment

All patients were treated with CRT either as definitive or adjuvant therapy. Concurrent chemotherapy agents included cisplatin 40 milligrams per meter squared (mg/m^2) weekly, high dose cisplatin 100 mg/m^2 every 3 weeks, carboplatin AUC 2 weekly, cetuximab 400 mg/m^2 loading dose followed by 250 mg/m^2 weekly, and platinum/paclitaxel (carboplatin AUC 2 with paclitaxel 50 mg/m^2 weekly or cisplatin 20 mg/m^2 with paclitaxel 30 mg/m^2) (Table 2). A small subset of patients (5 [10%] at the main campus vs. 2 [5%] at the satellite sites) were initially treated with induction chemotherapy (TPF—docetaxel, cisplatin, and fluorouracil) followed by CRT with cisplatin, carboplatin, or cetuximab. Cisplatin was highly favored at the main campus ($n = 39$, 78%) with the rest receiving cetuximab ($n = 6$, 12%), carboplatin ($n = 4$, 8%), and carboplatin/paclitaxel ($n = 1$, 2%). In contrast, cisplatin and cetuximab use was equally distributed at the satellite sites ($n = 21$, 48% each), while the remaining two patients either received carboplatin or cisplatin/paclitaxel. Of the 60 cisplatin-treated patients, 58 (98%) received the recommended total minimum dose of 200 mg/m^2 with two patients (2%) receiving less due to prior surgical resection/physician's choice.

All patients were treated with intensity modulated radiotherapy (IMRT) and the median radiation therapy dose was 68.8 Gray (Gy) (50 to 70 Gy) given at 2 Gy per fraction. A subset of patients at both sites ($n = 23$, 25%) underwent surgical resection with TORS prior to concurrent CRT. This subset of patients was subsequently treated with adjuvant CRT and given an average radiation dose of 65.3 Gy (50 to 66 Gy), as determined by pathologic risk features and performance status. Average length of radiotherapy treatment was 48 days at the main campus and 50 days at the satellite sites. Forty-nine (98%) patients at the main campus and 43 (98%) patients at the satellite sites completed their prescribed radiation therapy dose. Patients experienced common CRT effects as reported by the treating physician including mucositis, skin toxicities, hearing loss, neuropathy, nausea/vomiting, consistent with typical acute toxicities from CRT; however, proper grading of toxicity was not available except for weight loss (Table 2).

Five patients at the main campus switched chemotherapy drugs from high-dose cisplatin to carboplatin or cetuximab, and two patients at the satellite sites switched from high dose cisplatin to carboplatin and from cetuximab to weekly cisplatin due to adverse symptoms secondary to the original chemotherapy. The reasons for chemotherapy drug switch included tinnitus, elevated creatinine, and azotemia. Overall, the chemotherapy dose was reduced by at least 20% in seven patients (four at the main campus vs. three at the satellite sites, $p = 0.83$) treated with high-dose cisplatin (100 mg/m^2) due to adverse symptoms. The number of patients who missed a therapy dose(s) or had chemotherapy treatment interruptions because of significant treatment-related adverse events (i.e., azotemia, leukopenia, neutropenia, thrombocytopenia), unplanned hospitalizations, or patient decisions were similar among the COH main campus and satellite groups (11 vs. nine patients, $p = 0.86$). During the course of radiation therapy treatment, seven patients in the main campus and six patients in the satellite sites had treatment interruptions/breaks of at least two days. The reasons for treatment interruptions were related to severe weight loss ($n = 2$), thus requiring another radiotherapy treatment planning computed tomography scan, toxicities secondary to treatment ($n = 7$), insurance issues ($n = 1$), patient's choice ($n = 1$), and unplanned hospitalizations ($n = 2$). Reasons for unexpected hospitalization (six at the main campus vs. four at the satellite sites) were related to significant treatment-related adverse events such as severe dehydration, severe adverse infusion reaction to cetuximab, aspiration pneumonia, G-tube cellulitis, or pulmonary embolism.

The percentage of patients who completed the prescribed full treatment dose of both chemotherapy and radiation therapy without interruptions of radiation therapy was 86% ($n = 43$) at the main campus and 82% ($n = 36$) at the satellite locations.

3.3. Survival Outcomes

Patients underwent restaging imaging 12 weeks after completion of treatment to measure their response to treatment. Thirty-five (70%) patients achieved a complete response (CR) to treatment, 13 (26%) patients had a partial response (PR), and two (4%) patients had progression of disease (POD)/persistent disease at the main center site. Thirty-seven (84%) patients achieved a CR, five (11%) patients had a PR, and two (5%) patients had POD/persistent disease at the satellite sites. The patients with POD/persistent disease were subsequently treated with pembrolizumab at the main cancer site, or further lines of chemotherapy (carboplatin/paclitaxel, carboplatin/gemcitabine, cetuximab) followed by nivolumab or pembrolizumab at the satellite sites.

With a follow-up of 140 months (~12 years), median OS was not yet reached for both the main campus and the satellite sites (Figure 2A). Between both sites, there was no significant difference in OS ($p = 0.22$) and PFS ($p = 0.88$) (Figure 2A,B). No significant difference in two-year (47 [94%] vs. 37 [84%] patients, $p = 0.12$) and five-year (46 [92%] vs. 37 [84%] patients, $p = 0.23$) PFS was observed between the main campus and the satellite sites, respectively (Table 2).

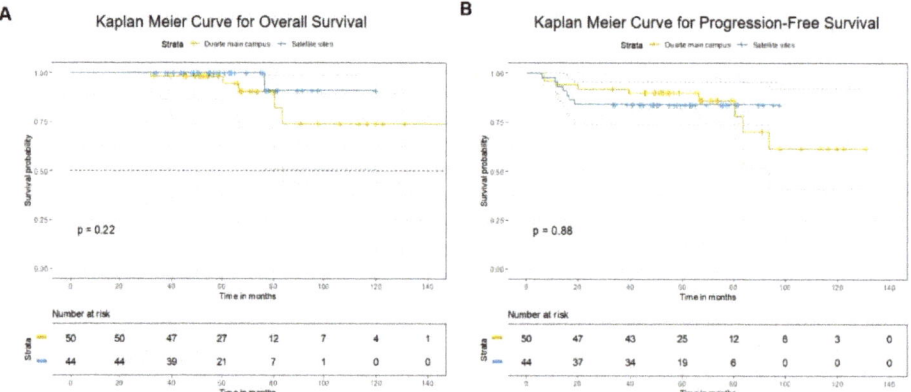

Figure 2. (**A**) Kaplan-Meier curve for overall survival by treatment site and (**B**) Kaplan-Meier curve for progression-free survival by treatment site.

3.4. Functional Outcomes

Modified Barium Swallow Studies (MBSS) were performed more frequently at the main cancer center than the satellite sites due to the presence of a comprehensive team of speech pathologists. 12 patients (24%) underwent feeding tube placement at the main campus, prophylactically ($n = 4$) or during treatment ($n = 8$). Two of the 12 patients continued to be feeding tube dependent after 6 months. Twenty-four patients (55%) underwent feeding tube placement at the satellite sites, prophylactically ($n = 20$) or during treatment ($n = 4$). Eleven of the 24 patients continued to be feeding tube-dependent at 6 months. Prophylactic feeding tube placement was associated with higher rates of 6-month feeding tube dependency ($n = 2$, 100% at main site, $n = 9$, 92% at satellite sites). Weight loss was recorded throughout CRT treatment and during the 6-month post-treatment follow-up. Thirty-seven patients (74%) lost ≤10% baseline weight during treatment while the remaining 13 (26%) lost >10% of their initial body weight at the main site. Twenty-six (59%) patients lost ≤10% baseline weight, while the remaining 18 (41%) lost >10% of their baseline weight during treatment at the satellite sites. Twenty-four patients (48%) lost ≤10% baseline weight at the 6-month post-treatment follow-up, while 26 (53%) lost >10% of their initial body weight at the main site. Fourteen patients (32%) and 30 patients (68%), respectively, lost ≤ and >10% of their initial body weight at the 6-month post-treatment follow-up at the satellite sites. Overall, at 6 months after completion of treatment, both sites noted an increased number of patients experiencing >10% baseline weight loss (13 to 26 patients at the main campus and 18 to 30 patients at the satellite sites). Of the 12 patients who underwent feeding tube placement at the main site, 4 (33%) and 7 (58%) patients lost >10% baseline weight during treatment and at 6 months post-treatment, respectively. Of the 24 patients who underwent feeding tube placement at the satellite sites, eight (33%) and 16 (66%) patients lost >10% baseline weight during treatment and at 6 months post-treatment, respectively.

Narcotic use was recorded at 3- and 6-month timepoints after completion of radiation therapy. At the main center, 16 (32%) patients had recorded persistent use of narcotics at a 3 months post-treatment interval and 9 (18%) patients required persistent narcotic use at the 6-month mark. At the satellite sites, a similar number of patients ($n = 13$, 30%) reported narcotic use 3 months post-treatment, and 10 (23%) patients registered persistent narcotic use at the 6-month mark.

4. Discussion

We conducted a retrospective analysis of HPV-positive OPSCC patients treated with definitive or postoperative CRT at a large NCI-designated comprehensive cancer center (COH) main campus and compared it to selected institutional satellite sites with availability of dedicated radiation therapy facilities staffed with COH faculty with primary endpoint of OS and secondary endpoints including treatment response, feeding tube dependency, and weight loss throughout treatment and 6 months post-treatment. Our analysis is the first to compare patient outcomes in a comprehensive NCI designated cancer center and its affiliated satellite sites. COH main site and satellite sites demonstrated OS rates consistent with already published favorable survival rates in OPSCC treated with multimodality therapy approach [7,19], while median OS at ~12 years was not reached (Figure 2A). No significant difference in two-year (94% vs. 84%, $p = 0.12$) and five-year (92% vs. 84%, $p = 0.23$) PFS was observed between the main campus and the satellite sites (Table 2). Our data did not align with previously reported analyses of head and neck cancer outcomes in academic centers versus community sites that demonstrated superior survival rates in patients treated at academic institutions [16,18]. One major difference between our study and the previously mentioned analyses [16,18] relates to the fact that our patients were treated under an umbrella institution, COH, regardless of treatment center location. Overall, our institution takes strides to standardize patient care across all sites by the longstanding establishment of weekly radiation oncology web rounds dedicated to reviewing all radiation treatment plans at any COH site. Our outcomes are possible because of these efforts of treatment compliance between main and satellite centers where there is some uniformity in dose delivery, nodal coverage based on primary site and nodal disease distribution, overall treatment volumes, and established guidelines for treatment planning. Furthermore, the medical oncologists at the COH satellites are part of the medical oncology main department and are required to attend quarterly retreats with the oncologists at main campus.

Regarding differences in the choice of concurrent systemic therapy, the oncologists at the main campus site strongly favored cisplatin as the chemotherapy agent of choice (78%), whereas satellite site medical oncologists equally favored cisplatin (48%) and cetuximab (48%) when treating their patients ($p = 0.001$). Considering the different distribution of tumor size between the two groups of patients with main campus seeing a higher number of T3–4 disease (19 [38%] vs. six [14%], $p = 0.008$) (Table 1 and Figure 1B), the choice of cisplatin-based therapy could have been influenced by the more advanced stage of disease at presentation. In addition, these patients were treated before the completion and publication of The Radiation Therapy Oncology Group (RTOG) 1016 clinical trial that compared systemic therapy agent cisplatin versus cetuximab, a monoclonal antibody against EGFR, in HPV-positive OPSCC, and reported superior PFS with cisplatin over cetuximab (78% vs. 67%, $p < 0.001$) [20]. A small subset of patients underwent treatment with induction chemotherapy followed by CRT in our analysis (five at the main campus vs. two patients at the satellite sites, $p = 0.31$). While the use of induction chemotherapy in head and neck cancers is controversial, a recent phase II trial demonstrated feasibility of different induction regimens stratified by disease risk in locally advanced head and neck squamous cell carcinoma [21].

In our study, chemotherapy dose reductions occurred among patients who were treated with high-dose cisplatin, underscoring the heavy burden of side effects that this treatment carries and the need for continuous monitoring by the medical oncologist to avoid permanent renal and neurological impairment effect on quality of life and survival outcomes. The majority of patients completed their prescribed cumulative radiation therapy dose ($n = 94$, 98%). The rate of treatment interruptions and hospitalizations were comparable between the two groups of patients when adjusted by systemic treatment choice (Table 2). Chronic narcotic use at 3 months did not differ between the two groups (32% at the main campus vs. 30% at the satellite sites, $p = 0.98$) (Table 2), demonstrating a significant number of patients persistently using narcotics after completing treatment. Chronic narcotic use was trending downwards at 6 months, and is in line with previously reported data in patients with OPSCC [22].

Our retrospective analysis demonstrated a significant difference in the rate of feeding tube placement between the main campus and satellite sites (24% vs. 55%, $p = 0.002$). Of those patients, four (33%) at the main campus and 20 (83%) at the satellite sites underwent prophylactic tube placement ($p = 0.003$). A trend towards significance in feeding tube persistence at 6 months was observed (17% vs. 46%, $p = 0.08$) (Table 2 and Figure 3).

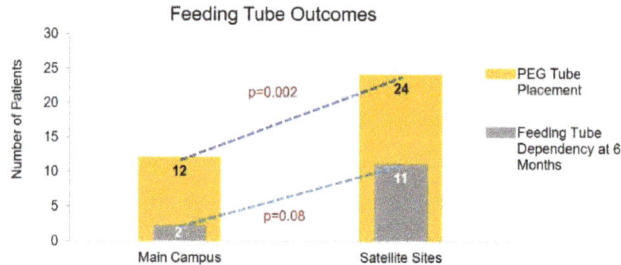

Figure 3. Feeding tube placement and 6-month dependency by treatment site.

MBSS were more likely to be performed at the main campus versus satellite sites given the availability of on-site speech pathology at the main campus. Multiple studies have been conducted to determine the advantage of prophylactic versus reactive PEG tube placement and the results are controversial [23–29]. However, studies have reported the significance of prophylactic PEG tube placement on enteral feed dependency rates [23,24,29], consistent with our feeding tube outcomes. This difference highlights the need for supportive service availability at satellite sites that could be potentially reached with remote consultation with institutional dedicated nutritionists and speech pathologists at our COH satellite centers. There was no significant difference in the degree of weight loss between the two groups of patients with the majority maintaining a ≤10% baseline weight loss (75% vs. 59%, $p = 0.12$); however, this could be the result of a higher prophylactic feeding tube rate in the satellite centers than main campus (Table 2).

Overall, patients who are at a higher risk of recurrence due to poor pathologic features, comorbidities, and nutritional status should be identified earlier during treatment so that they can have access to supportive services. At our institution, we are working on directing those patients earlier on to speech pathologists and nutritionists to eventually identify ones who might benefit from treatment modifications or early implementation of dietary needs. Furthermore, we are exploring the feasibility of implementing a program that allows for an initial comprehensive speech and nutrition evaluation at the main campus with continued telehealth follow-ups in the satellite sites and return to the main campus for repeat instrumental testing when necessary. This would reduce the need of in-person visits with speech pathologists and nutritionists and we plan to understand if this initiative could be effective in improving the 6 months feeding tube persistence rate. Due to the COVID-19 pandemic, numerous institutions have implemented telehealth services in order to accommodate patients and decrease needless exposure. Our institution offers outpatient telemedicine consults and follow-up visits via telephone or video call, and this service has been extended to our satellite sites. In the future, this implementation will greatly benefit patients undergoing treatment at satellite sites that need speech pathology and nutritionist oversight but do not have access to the main academic center, in order to minimize unnecessary feeding tube placements and ensure good functional outcomes.

Precision medicine in oropharyngeal cancers is difficult to accomplish as we do not select treatment based on molecular targets other than HPV status. Currently, HPV status is the only biological feature on which we establish disease risk and prognosis. We clearly understand that there is a need for molecular-driven treatment selection in the future. Due to EMR integration between the main campus and satellite sites, a wide range of patient information is readily accessible, thus allowing for academic and community physicians to efficiently collaborate on research studies. Based on this joint retrospective analysis, we are conducting and examining the molecular status of these academic and community patients to try to understand if we can translate meaningful results.

We recognize that our study contains limitations including intrinsic bias of patient selection in a retrospective analysis and limitations of our EMR search which identified our cohort of patients. We designated the HPV-associated OPSCC according to p16 IHC status, based on the evidence of concordance between p16 IHC staining and HPV in situ hybridization in HPV-associated oropharyngeal carcinomas that makes p16 IHC a surrogate marker for HPV infection [30]. The discrepancies between our study in OPSCC and those who observed improved survival in head and neck cancer patients treated at an academic institution could be attributed to the excellent prognosis of HPV-positive OPSCC. Disparities in disease stage, socioeconomic factors, patient location, and insurance play a role in the different characteristics of patients treated at the main campus compared to the satellite sites. Worse prognosis primary sites such as oral cavity and larynx could potentially demonstrate differences in survival.

In conclusion, our study highlights the importance of the necessity to treat OPSCC in tertiary cancer centers and their associated satellite network with availability of dedicated and experienced radiation and medical oncologists and up-to-date facilities that allow continuous communication between physicians and supportive services including speech pathology and nutrition. We are currently designing a prospective study to assess the implementation of telemedicine for supportive services in the satellite sites. This is of great importance as poor functional outcomes represent a heavy burden for our current HPV-positive OPSCC population that is young, very functional, and deserves high standards of post-treatment quality of life.

Author Contributions: Conceptualization, R.P., S.C. (Samuel Chung), and E.M. (Erminia Massarelli); Methodology, R.P., S.C. (Samuel Chung), and E.M. (Erminia Massarelli); Validation, R.P., S.C. (Samuel Chung), E.M. (Ellie Maghami), A.A., A.C., S.S., and E.M. (Erminia Massarelli); Formal Analysis, R.P., S.C. (Samuel Chung), A.A., A.C., and E.M. (Erminia Massarelli); Data Curation, R.P., S.C. (Samuel Chung), A.A., S.C (Samuel Chung), S.S., and E.M. (Erminia Massarelli); Writing—Original Draft Preparation, R.P., S.C. (Samuel Chung), and E.M. (Erminia Massarelli); Writing—Review and Editing, R.P., S.C. (Samuel Chung), E.M. (Ellie Maghami), A.A., A.C., N.V., S.C. (Sue Chang), T.G., R.K., K.H., C.K., D.A., L.V., S.S., and E.M. (Erminia Massarelli). All authors have read and agreed to the manuscript.

Funding: This research received no external funding.

Acknowledgments: We would like to thank the City of Hope head and neck cancer medical, surgical, and radiation oncologists, nurses, and supportive teams for their dedication to their patients. The authors have no funding to disclose.

Conflicts of Interest: The authors declare no conflict of interest.

References

1. Gillison, M.L.; D'Souza, G.; Westra, W.; Sugar, E.; Xiao, W.; Begum, S.; Viscidi, R. Distinct Risk Factor Profiles for Human Papillomavirus Type 16–Positive and Human Papillomavirus Type 16–Negative Head and Neck Cancers. *JNCI J. Natl. Cancer Inst.* **2008**, *100*, 407–420. [CrossRef]
2. Applebaum, K.M.; Furniss, C.S.; Zeka, A.; Posner, M.R.; Smith, J.F.; Bryan, J.; Eisen, E.A.; Peters, E.S.; McClean, M.D.; Kelsey, K.T. Lack of Association of Alcohol and Tobacco with HPV16-Associated Head and Neck Cancer. *JNCI J. Natl. Cancer Inst.* **2007**, *99*, 1801–1810. [CrossRef]
3. Benson, E.; Li, R.; Eisele, D.; Fakhry, C. The clinical impact of HPV tumor status upon head and neck squamous cell carcinomas. *Oral Oncol.* **2014**, *50*, 565–574. [CrossRef] [PubMed]
4. Chaturvedi, A.K. Epidemiology and clinical aspects of HPV in head and neck cancers. *Head Neck Pathol.* **2012**, *6* (Suppl. 1), S16–S24. [CrossRef] [PubMed]
5. Chung, C.H.; Gillison, M.L. Human papillomavirus in head and neck cancer: Its role in pathogenesis and clinical implications. *Clin. Cancer Res.* **2009**, *15*, 6758–6762. [CrossRef] [PubMed]
6. Fakhry, C.; Westra, W.H.; Li, S.; Cmelak, A.; Ridge, J.A.; Pinto, H.; Forastiere, A.; Gillison, M.L. Improved survival of patients with human papillomavirus-positive head and neck squamous cell carcinoma in a prospective clinical trial. *J. Natl. Cancer Inst.* **2008**, *100*, 261–269. [CrossRef] [PubMed]
7. Ang, K.K.; Harris, J.; Wheeler, R.; Weber, R.; Rosenthal, D.I.; Nguyen-Tan, P.F.; Westra, W.H.; Chung, C.H.; Jordan, R.C.; Lu, C.; et al. Human papillomavirus and survival of patients with oropharyngeal cancer. *N. Engl. J. Med.* **2010**, *363*, 24–35. [CrossRef]
8. Morris, L.G.; Sikora, A.G.; Patel, S.G.; Hayes, R.B.; Ganly, I. Second primary cancers after an index head and neck cancer: Subsite-specific trends in the era of human papillomavirus-associated oropharyngeal cancer. *J. Clin. Oncol.* **2011**, *29*, 739–746. [CrossRef]
9. O'Sullivan, B.; Huang, S.H.; Siu, L.L.; Waldron, J.; Zhao, H.; Perez-Ordonez, B.; Weinreb, I.; Kim, J.; Ringash, J.; Bayley, A.; et al. Deintensification candidate subgroups in human papillomavirus-related oropharyngeal cancer according to minimal risk of distant metastasis. *J. Clin. Oncol.* **2013**, *31*, 543–550. [CrossRef]
10. Lydiatt, W.M.; Patel, S.G.; O'Sullivan, B.; Brandwein, M.S.; Ridge, J.A.; Migliacci, J.C.; Loomis, A.M.; Shah, J.P. Head and Neck cancers-major changes in the American Joint Committee on cancer eighth edition cancer staging manual. *CA Cancer J. Clin.* **2017**, *67*, 122–137. [CrossRef]
11. Burtness, B.; Harrington, K.J.; Greil, R.; Soulières, D.; Tahara, M.; De Castro, G., Jr.; Psyrri, A.; Rotlan, N.B.; Neupane, P.C.; Bratland, A. KEYNOTE-048: Phase 3 study of first-line pembrolizumab (P) for recurrent/metastatic head and neck squamous cell carcinoma (R/M HNSCC). In Proceedings of the ESMO 2018 Congress, Munich, Germany, 19–23 October 2018.

12. Massarelli, E.; William, W.; Johnson, F.; Kies, M.; Ferrarotto, R.; Guo, M.; Feng, L.; Lee, J.J.; Tran, H.; Kim, Y.U.; et al. Combining Immune Checkpoint Blockade and Tumor-Specific Vaccine for Patients With Incurable Human Papillomavirus 16-Related Cancer: A Phase 2 Clinical Trial. *JAMA Oncol.* **2018**, *5*, 67–73. [CrossRef] [PubMed]
13. Verhoef, C.; van de Weyer, R.; Schaapveld, M.; Bastiaannet, E.; Plukker, J.T. Better survival in patients with esophageal cancer after surgical treatment in university hospitals: A plea for performance by surgical oncologists. *Ann. Surg. Oncol.* **2007**, *14*, 1678–1687. [CrossRef] [PubMed]
14. Gutierrez, J.C.; Perez, E.A.; Moffat, F.L.; Livingstone, A.S.; Franceschi, D.; Koniaris, L.G. Should soft tissue sarcomas be treated at high-volume centers? An analysis of 4205 patients. *Ann. Surg.* **2007**, *245*, 952–958. [CrossRef] [PubMed]
15. Chen, A.Y.; Fedewa, S.; Pavluck, A.; Ward, E.M. Improved survival is associated with treatment at high-volume teaching facilities for patients with advanced stage laryngeal cancer. *Cancer* **2010**, *116*, 4744–4752. [CrossRef] [PubMed]
16. Lassig, A.A.D.; Joseph, A.M.; Lindgren, B.R.; Fernandes, P.; Cooper, S.; Schotzko, C.; Khariwala, S.; Reynolds, M.; Yueh, B. The effect of treating institution on outcomes in head and neck cancer. *Otolaryngol. Head Neck Surg.* **2012**, *147*, 1083–1092. [CrossRef]
17. Kubicek, G.J.; Wang, F.; Reddy, E.; Shnayder, Y.; Cabrera, C.E.; Girod, D.A. Importance of treatment institution in head and neck cancer radiotherapy. *Otolaryngol. Head Neck Surg.* **2009**, *141*, 172–176. [CrossRef]
18. Benasso, M.; Lionetto, R.; Corvò, R.; Ponzanelli, A.; Vitale, V.; Rosso, R. Impact of the treating institution on the survival of patients with head and neck cancer treated with concomitant alternating chemotherapy and radiation. *Eur. J. Cancer* **2003**, *39*, 1895–1898. [CrossRef]
19. Patel, M.A.; Blackford, A.L.; Rettig, E.M.; Richmon, J.D.; Eisele, D.W.; Fakhry, C. Rising population of survivors of oral squamous cell cancer in the United States. *Cancer* **2016**, *122*, 1380–1387. [CrossRef]
20. Trotti, A.; Harris, J.; Gillison, M.; Eisbruch, A.; Harari, P.M.; Adelstein, D.J.; Sturgis, E.M.; Galvin, J.M.; Koyfman, S.; Blakaj, D.; et al. NRG-RTOG 1016: Phase III Trial Comparing Radiation/Cetuximab to Radiation/Cisplatin in HPV-related Cancer of the Oropharynx. *Int. J. Radiat. Oncol. Biol. Phys.* **2018**, *102*, 1604–1605. [CrossRef]
21. Haddad, R.I.; Massarelli, E.; Lee, J.J.; Lin, H.Y.; Hutcheson, K.; Lewis, J.; Garden, A.S.; Blumenschein, G.R., Jr.; William, W.N., Jr.; Pharaon, R.R.; et al. Weekly paclitaxel, carboplatin, cetuximab, and cetuximab, docetaxel, cisplatin, and fluorouracil, followed by local therapy in previously untreated, locally advanced head and neck squamous cell carcinoma. *Ann. Oncol.* **2019**, *30*, 471–477. [CrossRef]
22. McDermott, J.D.; Eguchi, M.; Stokes, W.A.; Amini, A.; Hararah, M.; Ding, D.; Valentine, A.; Bradley, C.J.; Karam, S.D. Short- and Long-term Opioid Use in Patients with Oral and Oropharynx Cancer. *Otolaryngol. Head Neck Surg.* **2019**, *160*, 409–419. [CrossRef] [PubMed]
23. Koyfman, S.A.; Adelstein, D.J. Enteral Feeding Tubes in Patients Undergoing Definitive Chemoradiation Therapy for Head-and-Neck Cancer: A Critical Review. *Int. J. Radiat. Oncol. Biol. Phys.* **2012**, *84*, 581–589. [CrossRef] [PubMed]
24. Chen, A.M.; Li, B.-Q.; Lau, D.H.; Farwell, D.G.; Luu, Q.; Stuart, K.; Newman, K.; Purdy, J.A.; Vijayakumar, S. Evaluating the Role of Prophylactic Gastrostomy Tube Placement Prior to Definitive Chemoradiotherapy for Head and Neck Cancer. *Int. J. Radiat. Oncol. Biol. Phys.* **2010**, *78*, 1026–1032. [CrossRef] [PubMed]
25. Lee, J.H.; Machtay, M.; Unger, L.D.; Weinstein, G.S.; Weber, R.S.; Chalian, A.A.; Rosenthal, D.I. Prophylactic gastrostomy tubes in patients undergoing intensive irradiation for cancer of the head and neck. *Arch. Otolaryngol. Head Neck Surg.* **1998**, *124*, 871–875. [CrossRef]
26. Kramer, S.; Newcomb, M.; Hessler, J.; Siddiqui, F. Prophylactic versus reactive PEG tube placement in head and neck cancer. *Otolaryngol. Head Neck Surg.* **2014**, *150*, 407–412. [CrossRef]
27. Silander, E.; Nyman, J.; Bove, M.; Johansson, L.; Larsson, S.; Hammerlid, E. Impact of prophylactic percutaneous endoscopic gastrostomy on malnutrition and quality of life in patients with head and neck cancer: A randomized study. *Head Neck* **2012**, *34*, 1–9. [CrossRef]
28. Olson, R.; Karam, I.; Wilson, G.; Bowman, A.; Lee, C.; Wong, F. Population-based comparison of two feeding tube approaches for head and neck cancer patients receiving concurrent systemic-radiation therapy: Is a prophylactic feeding tube approach harmful or helpful? *Support. Care Cancer* **2013**, *21*, 3433–3439. [CrossRef]

29. Williams, G.F.; Teo, M.T.; Sen, M.; Dyker, K.E.; Coyle, C.; Prestwich, R.J. Enteral feeding outcomes after chemoradiotherapy for oropharynx cancer: A role for a prophylactic gastrostomy? *Oral Oncol.* **2012**, *48*, 434–440. [CrossRef]
30. Lewis, J.S., Jr.; Thorstad, W.L.; Chernock, R.D.; Haughey, B.H.; Yip, J.H.; Zhang, Q.; El-Mofty, S.K. p16 positive oropharyngeal squamous cell carcinoma:an entity with a favorable prognosis regardless of tumor HPV status. *Am. J. Surg. Pathol.* **2010**, *34*, 1088–1096. [CrossRef]

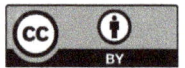

© 2020 by the authors. Licensee MDPI, Basel, Switzerland. This article is an open access article distributed under the terms and conditions of the Creative Commons Attribution (CC BY) license (http://creativecommons.org/licenses/by/4.0/).

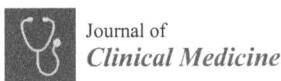

Article

Use of HER2-Directed Therapy in Metastatic Breast Cancer and How Community Physicians Collaborate to Improve Care

Joanne E. Mortimer [1,*], Laura Kruper [2], Mary Cianfrocca [1], Sayeh Lavasani [1], Sariah Liu [1], Niki Tank-Patel [1], Mina Sedrak [1], Wade Smith [1], Daphne Stewart [1], James Waisman [1], Christina Yeon [1], Tina Wang [1] and Yuan Yuan [1]

[1] Department of Medical Oncology and Therapeutics Research, City of Hope Comprehensive Cancer Center, Duarte, CA 91010, USA; mcianfrocca@coh.org (M.C.); slavasani@coh.org (S.L.); sarliu@coh.org (S.L.); nikpatel@coh.org (N.T.-P.); msedrak@coh.org (M.S.); wsmith@coh.org (W.S.); dapstewart@coh.org (D.S.); jwaisman@coh.org (J.W.); cyeon@coh.org (C.Y.); tinawang@coh.org (T.W.); yuyuan@coh.org (Y.Y.)
[2] Department of Surgery, Division of Breast Surgery, City of Hope Comprehensive Cancer Center, Duarte, CA 91010, USA; lkruper@coh.org
* Correspondence: jmortimer@coh.org; Tel.: +626-471-9200

Received: 6 May 2020; Accepted: 18 June 2020; Published: 24 June 2020

Abstract: The development of new HER2-directed therapies has resulted in a significant prolongation of survival for women with metastatic HER2-positive breast cancer. Discoveries in the laboratory inform clinical trials which are the basis for improving the standard of care and are also the backbone for quality improvement. Clinical trials can be completed more rapidly by expanding trial enrollment to community sites. In this article we review some of the challenges in treating metastatic breast cancer with HER2-directed therapies and our strategies for incorporating our community partners into the research network.

Keywords: breast cancer; community; research; HER2-directed therapy

1. Introduction

Although breast cancers arise from a single organ, the biology and natural history of the disease can be extremely variable. Gene expression profiling allows us to subcategorize breast cancer into four "intrinsic subtypes", each with a unique natural history and response to therapy—Luminal A, Luminal B, Basal-like, and HER2 (human epidermal growth factor receptor 2) "enriched" [1,2]. However, until uniform genomic profiling becomes feasible, clinical decision making is based on tumor histology, stage, hormone receptor status, and HER2 status. This paper focuses on the use of HER2-targeted therapies in metastatic breast cancer and the importance of clinical trials and community practice collaboration in understanding the biology of this disease and advancing therapy.

2. HER2 and Breast Cancer

Four membrane tyrosine kinase receptors constitute the HER family. HER1 (also known as EGFR; epidermal growth factor receptor), HER3, and HER4 bind to almost a dozen different ligands, while HER2 has no known ligands. Rather, HER2 is activated through homo- and heterodimerization with other HER family members, and these complexes activate intracellular signaling pathways such as MAPK (mitogen-activated protein kinase) and PI3K (phosphoinositide 3-kinase) that results in tumor growth, invasion, migration, and survival [3]. The different receptors, ligands, and intracellular signaling pathways provide opportunities for drug development with agents used alone, in combination with each other, and with chemotherapy. The gene that encodes HER2 is amplified in 15–20% of all breast cancers and defines a uniquely aggressive natural history with high grade histologies, greater likelihood to metastasize to visceral sites, and shortened survivals [4,5]. Gene amplification or protein over expression identifies patients who are candidates for HER2-directed therapies.

The humanized IgG monoclonal antibody, trastuzumab, targets the extracellular domain of HER2 effectively preventing intracellular signaling. While trastuzumab has minimal activity as a single agent, when combined with chemotherapy there is a prolongation in survival for women with metastatic breast cancer [6–8]. Trastuzumab has been shown to improve disease outcomes in all stages of HER2-amplified breast cancer [9]. The development of HER2-directed therapies, and trastuzumab in particular, is one of the greatest success stories in the treatment of breast cancer and is as important as hormone receptor status in its clinical impact.

3. Assessment of HER2 Status

Candidacy for HER2-directed therapies is based on a pathologic determination from the primary tumor or metastatic focus of disease. It is generally agreed that HER2 positivity is defined as 3+ staining by immunohistochemical staining (IHC) of the protein or gene amplification of HER2 by fluorescence in situ hybridization (FISH). Recently, companion studies described using in situ hybridization to report gene copy number per cell. This resulted in a HER2 "equivocal" status and required modification of the ASCO/CAP (American Society of Clinical Oncology/College of American Pathologists) guidelines for HER2 assessment [10].

The standard of care dictates that a tumor biopsy be performed on all patients suspected of having recurrent or metastatic breast cancer in order to document the disease as well as to determine the hormone receptor and HER2 status, which guide the choice of systemic therapy. The estrogen receptor (ER), progesterone receptor (PR), or HER2 status on a recurrence may differ from the original primary in 20–30% of instances. Furthermore, although it is not feasible to biopsy all sites of metastatic disease, discordance of receptors within an individual patient occurs in 15–20% of lesions [11–13]. Ultimately, the choice of systemic therapy is determined on a small sample of tumor obtained on a larger site of disease and thus may not reflect the tumor status at all sites.

HER2-directed therapies are effective only in patients whose cancers are HER2-positive. The NSABP B47 randomized over 3000 women with early stage breast cancer whose HER2 status was negative (1+, and 2+ by IHC of FISH< 2.0) to receive conventional adjuvant chemotherapy with or without 12 months of trastuzumab. No benefit was seen with the addition of trastuzumab and cardiac toxicity was observed in 2.3% receiving trastuzumab [14]. It is probably not realistic to assume that all HER2-positive patients benefit from HER2-directed therapies. Given a predictable incidence of cardiac toxicity, it would be ideal to treat only women who are likely to benefit from these treatments. The goal of precision medicine is to identify which patients benefit from HER2-directed therapies.

4. Functional Imaging to Predict Response to HER2 Therapies

We have developed ^{64}Cu-labeled trastuzumab as a PET imaging agent to study women with recurrent/metastatic breast cancer. In our experience uptake on ^{64}Cu-trastuzumab PET/CT correlates with the qualitative assessment of HER2 by IHC. Higher uptake of ^{64}Cu-trastuzumab is seen in women with IHC levels of 3+ compared to 1+ [15,16]. Functional imaging with ^{64}Cu-trastuzumab PET/CT does not assess HER2 status, but demonstrates that trastuzumab is effectively delivered to the cancer. This pharmacodynamics data is clinically more relevant than knowing the intensity of uptake by IHC or degree of gene amplification. The current standard of care for patients with newly diagnosed metastatic HER2-positive cancer utilizes a combination of chemotherapy, trastuzumab, and pertuzumab. It is, therefore, not possible for functional imaging with radiolabeled trastuzumab to predict impact of trastuzumab on treatment efficacy when response to therapy is confounded by the concurrent administration of chemotherapy.

Ado-trastuzumab emtansine (TDM1) binds to the extracellular domain of HER2 and undergoes receptor-mediated internalization inhibiting intracellular signaling pathways [17]. Because its activity is dependent upon trastuzumab binding to the HER2 protein, it is the ideal drug to test whether functional imaging with ^{64}Cu-trastuzumab PET/CT is able to predict for response to therapy. In our experience, pretreatment ^{64}Cu-trastuzumab PET/CT in women with recurrent/metastatic disease is able to identify which individuals are unlikely to benefit from TDM1. Additionally, ^{64}Cu-trastuzumab PET/CT has identified disease within the CNS and has also demonstrated that uptake of ^{64}Cu-trastuzumab can be heterogeneous within a single patient. If that uptake in individual sites falls below a certain level, TDM1 is not effective in those areas and the response is mixed [18].

5. Current Treatment for Metastatic HER2-Positive Breast Cancer

Like trastuzumab, pertuzumab is also a monoclonal antibody that binds to the extracellular domain of HER2, but at a different epitope from that bound by trastuzumab. Pertuzumab prevents dimerization with other HER family members (HER1, HER3, and HER4) [19]. Neither trastuzumab or pertuzumab are very active as single agents, but the combination is synergistic. In women with metastatic HER2-positive breast cancer that has progressed on a trastuzumab-containing regimen, the combination of pertuzumab with trastuzumab produces clinical benefit in more than half of patients [20]. The CLEOPATRA study demonstrated that the addition of pertuzumab to trastuzumab and docetaxel improved overall survival and established this three-drug combination as first-line therapy in metastatic disease. With more than 8 years of follow up, 37% of women who started treatment with pertuzumab, trastuzumab, and docetaxel are still alive. The study was designed to administer at least 6 cycles of docetaxel or until toxicity, and the duration of docetaxel was left to the discretion of the treating oncologist. Pertuzumab and trastuzumab were continued until disease progression. The median number of treatment cycles containing docetaxel was 8 (range 6–10) and the median total cycles was 24 with a maximum of 167 [21,22]. The prolonged survival in this population is also related to the efficacy of subsequent treatment.

Two antibody drug conjugates (ADC) have utilized trastuzumab to deliver a cytotoxic payload. Ado-trastuzumab emtansine (TDM1) utilizes maytansine as the cytotoxic component and has been found to be superior to other regimens containing chemotherapy and HER2-directed agents. It is currently considered second or third line therapy [17,23]. Fam-trastuzumab-deruxtecan uses the topoisomerase I inhibitor, deruxtecan as its payload. In the DESTINY 01 trial, 184 women with HER2-positive metastatic breast cancer who had received a median of six prior therapies were treated with fam-trastuzumab-deruxtecan. Objective responses were observed in 112 (60.9%) women with a median duration of response of 14.8 months [24]. Fam-trastuzumab-deruxtecan is used as third-line therapy.

The two ADCs differ in other ways. Fam-trastuzumab-deruxtecan has a higher drug-to-antibody ratio than TDM1 (DAR = 8 vs. DAR = 3.4, respectively) and fam-trastuzumab-deruxtecan is selectively cleaved by cathepsins that are up regulated in tumor cells. Deruxtecan is also highly cell-membrane permeable and is readily released across cell membranes. A potential benefit for this mechanism is that release of the cytotoxic component may have cytotoxic effects on adjacent tumor cells regardless of the tumor's HER2 dependency [25]. Since the majority of breast cancers (~60%) express HER2 to some degree, fam-trastuzumab-deruxtecan has the potential to benefit many patients [26,27]. Currently the drug is considered for 3rd line and beyond [28].

The oral tyrosine kinase inhibitor, tucatinib, is a selective inhibitor of HER2. In combination with capecitabine and trastuzumab, objective tumor responses have been demonstrated in heavily pretreated patients with metastatic HER2-positive breast cancer including women with brain metastases. The HER2CLIMB study randomized women with metastatic HER2-positive breast cancer who had received prior trastuzumab, pertuzumab, and TDM1 to receive trastuzumab and capecitabine with or without tucatinib. Progression-free survival (PFS) favored the addition of tucatinib (7.8 months compared with 5.4 months). The overall survival also favored the tucatinib arm with a survival prolongation of 4.5 months; 21.9 months vs. 17.4 months. For the 291 women with brain metastases, the median PFS was 7.6 months in the tucatinib arm and 5.4 months in the control arm ($p < 0.001$) [29].

Tucatinib was recently approved by the FDA. Tucatinib + trastuzumab + capecitabine is currently considered as a treatment for advanced unresectable or metastatic HER2-positive breast cancer, including patients with brain metastases, who have received one or more lines of prior HER2-targeted therapy in the metastatic setting [30]. In the HER2CLIMB study, 291 patients were enrolled who had brain metastases—48% in the tucatinib arm and 46% in the control arm. The CNS (central nervous system) progression-free survival and median overall survival favored the tucatinib arm making this an important therapy in patients with HER2+ breast cancer metastatic to brain [31].

There are additional active agents that also deserve mention. Lapatinib was the first dual inhibitor of HER2 and HER1. Until the development of TDM1, lapatinib and capecitabine were considered to be second-line therapy [32]. Currently, lapatinib is combined with trastuzumab as a "next-line" of therapy [33]. The NALA trial randomized patients who had received at least two prior treatments for metastatic disease to receive either neratinib or lapatinib in combination with capecitabine. At 6 and 12 months, the progression-free survival was significantly longer with neratinib as well as a significant increase in the time to intervention for symptomatic CNS. Neratinib provides another treatment option for treating metastatic disease [34]. Even after disease progression on trastuzumab, additional chemotherapy with trastuzumab has been shown to be more effective than chemotherapy alone [35].

The explosion in new and highly effective therapies has transformed metastatic HER2-positive breast cancer into a chronic disease. Conventional chemotherapy still has a role as salvage treatment and is more effective when combined with trastuzumab [35]. New drug development and combining the currently available HER2-directed agents with drugs that modulate intracellular signaling are currently on-going in the clinic.

6. HER2 Activating Mutations—A Unique Clinical Entity

Bose used DNA sequencing on samples obtained from ACOSOG (American College of Surgeons Oncology Groupz) 1031 and data from other sequencing studies to identify somatic mutations in tumors that were pathologically determined to be HER2-negative. Seven of the 13 mutations were classified as activating mutations. Cell line studies showed a unique dependence on EGFR phosphorylation and led to an assessment of the therapeutic efficacy of the dual kinase inhibitors of HER2 and EGFR, lapatinib and neratinib. Neratinib demonstrated a stronger inhibition of cell growth than lapatinib and was effective in all activating mutations [36]. It is estimated that HER2-activating mutations occur in 1.6–2.5% of invasive ductal carcinomas and 7.5% of invasive lobular cancers [36,37]. Clinical trials of neratinib in this population have demonstrated efficacy and have identified another way of targeting HER2 [38,39]. This unique genotype demonstrates the potential use of next generation sequencing in breast cancer.

7. Engaging the Community in Clinical Research

City of Hope recently acquired 30 community practice sites and in doing so dramatically expanded the number of colleagues in surgical, medical, and radiation oncology and almost tripled the number of new breast patients. With such a rapid expansion, our goal was to develop a common culture of research and quality clinical care that is at the heart of City of Hope's values. This initiative was led by a steering committee of interdisciplinary subspecialty physicians and business leaders who met regularly. This team identified the individual community physicians who had an interest in treating breast cancer and in conducting clinical research and worked with all the stakeholders to define quality of care. We convened a meeting of all clinical faculty with an interest in breast cancer, compiled a brief resource inventory (systematic identification and access to any potential contributions to this program), and identified barriers to achieving our predefined quality of care. The sharing of our unique differences in practice and the challenges that each individual experienced, resulted in a respect for what each partner brought to the program and how we could work together to solve these problems. Through a culture of respect and trust we were able to define quality metrics for the clinical care of patients with breast cancer and created treatment guidelines which included eligibility for clinical trial participation (see Table 1). Clinical research requires physicians who are interested in conducting clinical trials and a practice site that has a patient population interested in study participation. It is also critical to have competent clinical research coordinators, a research pharmacy, and radiologists who support serial radiologic interpretation of x-rays using RECIST and PERCIST.

Table 1. City of Hope Institutional guidelines HER2+ metastatic disease.

HR− and HER2+ Breast Cancer	HR+ and HER2+ Breast Cancer
FIRST: Biopsy confirmation of Diagnosis and Receptor Status ALL Pt should have BRCA tested	
1st line #19339 NRG Trial pertuzumab, trastuzumab, taxane +/− atezolizumab	**1st line #19339 NRG Trial** pertuzumab, trastuzumab, taxane +/− atezolizumab
1st Line* pertuzumab, trastuzumab and taxane	1st Line* pertuzumab, trastuzumab and taxane
* #20048 Alpelisib in maintenance alpelisib combination in PIK3CA mutation	*** #20048 Alpelisib in maintenance** alpelisib combination in PIK3CA mutation
2nd Line #19599 (HER2CLIMB-02) tucatinib or placebo in combination with TDM1 for unresectable locally-advanced or metastatic disease	**2nd Line #19599 (HER2CLIMB-02)** tucatinib or placebo in combination with TDM1 for unresectable locally-advanced or metastatic disease
2nd Line TDM1 or tucatinib/capecitabine/trastuzumab	2nd Line TDM1 or tucatinib/capecitabine/trastuzumab
3rd Line tucatinib/capecitabine/trastuzumab or fam-trastuzumab-deruxtecan	3rd Line tucatinib/capecitabine/trastuzumab or or fam-trastuzumab-deruxtecan
4th or + Line Prior pertuzumab, trastuzumab, TDM1 consider fam-trastuzumab-deruxtecan or neratinib/capecitabine, lapatinib/trastuzumab Chemo + trastuzumab	4th or + Line Prior pertuzumab, trastuzumab, TDM1 consider fam-trastuzumab-deruxtecan or neratinib/capecitabine, lapatinib/trastuzumab or Chemo + trastuzumab or an AI or LHRH agonist + Tamoxifen/trastuzumab
Bone Directed Therapy— Zometa q1 month x 9, then q3 months until Hospice or Xgeva q1 month until Hospice (Xgeva is 2x more expensive)	

All research decision-making is made by the breast cancer research team (Breast Disease Team), composed of medical, surgical, and radiation oncologists, basic scientists, statisticians, pharmacists, research nurses, clinical research associates, and the Executive Director for Affiliate sites. Breast Disease Team meetings are available on a remote platform so that our community partners can participate, and meeting minutes are submitted to all. The Breast Disease Team meets on a weekly basis to review proposed study concepts, endorse the written protocols developed from an approved concept, troubleshoot operational problems, and review active patients on study. Our current clinical research portfolio in HER2-positive breast cancer focuses on two main areas: 1. Defining new therapies and new roles for these systemic therapies (an area largely driven by the cooperative groups and Pharma), and 2. Identifying which patients are likely to benefit from HER2-directed therapies using functional imaging, which is a City of Hope research initiative.

The Executive Director for Affiliates oversees research at the community sites and is aware of the physicians' interests, patient population, and clinical trial infrastructure at the individual offices. The full clinical trial portfolio is not activated at every site and phase I clinical trials are generally restricted to the main campus. The most successful clinical trials to conduct in the community are those therapeutic trials that focus on improving disease outcomes through the use of new agents or testing approved agents used in different settings. For example, mutations in PIK3A have been associated with worse outcomes in adjuvant therapy trials and in CLEOPATRA [21,40]. A phase III NRG trial builds on the positive results of CLEOPATRA in women with metastatic HER2-positive disease and tests the benefit of adding the immune checkpoint inhibitor, atezolizumab, as first line therapy. A Novartis sponsored trial randomizes women with metastatic disease and a PIK3A mutation to a placebo controlled double blind trial of alpelisib added during the patients' maintenance of trastuzumab and pertuzumab. We are currently enrolling patients with documented HER2-activating mutations to a phase II trial sponsored by PUMA of neratinib, trastuzumab, (and fulvestrant if also ER-positive).

Our radiolabeled trastuzumab imaging studies require a radiopharmacy and expertise by a committed team of radiologists and physicist who interpret the images. Our community oncologists play an important role in these studies by referring patients, thereby allowing us to complete accrual expeditiously. They are authors on our publications and are recognized by their local communities as true experts who participate in innovative research.

8. Optimizing Partnerships

The Breast Disease Team has a number of initiatives to ensure inclusion of our community partners in research, and the weekly Breast Disease Team meeting is at the heart of these collaborations. Discussions at weekly Tumor Boards and a bi-weekly treatment planning meeting frequently highlight on-going studies and identify study candidates. City of Hope is a founding member of the NCCN (national comprehensive cancer network) and has a long history of participating in guideline panels. While some of the guidelines for treating breast cancer are definitive, others offer acceptable treatment options. The breast cancer team on the main campus meets on an annual basis to compile our guideline preferences for treatment, including, not only standard of care but the open studies for clinical trial participation as well (see Table 1).

9. Future Directions

We continue to activate investigator-initiated, cooperative group, and Pharma trials in the community that focus on improving the outcomes for women with metastatic HER2-positive disease. Our imaging research will utilize radiolabeled trastuzumab to predict for response to new agents such as fam-trastuzumab-deruxtecan and tucatinib [24,29]. These studies will rely on our community partners to refer interested patients for study participation.

National Cancer Institute-designated Comprehensive Cancer Centers (NCI-CCC) such as City of Hope strive to provide expert interdisciplinary clinical care and cutting-edge treatments and technologies. Between 1998 and 2008, 6.4% of adults between 22 and 65 years of age who were diagnosed with cancer in Los Angeles County received treatment at an NCI-CCC. For all primary tumor sites, the survival of patients treated at an NCI-CCC was superior to patients treated at a non-NCI-CCC. In this study, 6.5% of the 31,764 breast cancer patients included in the analysis were treated at an NCI-CCC and their survival was superior to those treated at non NCI-CCC sites [41]. Realistically, the majority of cancer patients will receive their care in community sites, and it is an important part of the mission of a Comprehensive Cancer Center to ensure that the standard of care in the community is comparable to the care that is delivered in these large research centers. Clinical research is at the heart of improving quality care.

Author Contributions: Conceptualization and writing, J.E.M., L.K. and Y.Y.; writing, review and editing, M.C., S.L. (Sayeh Lavasani), S.L. (Sariah Liu), N.T.-P., M.S., W.S., D.S., J.W., C.Y. and T.W. All authors have read and agreed to the published version of the manuscript.

Funding: This research received no external funding.

Acknowledgments: The authors thank Nicola Welch, CMPP for editorial assistance and critical review of the manuscript.

Conflicts of Interest: The authors declare no conflict of interest.

References

1. Prat, A.; Pineda, E.; Adamo, B.; Galván, P.; Fernández, A.; Gaba, L.; Díez, M.; Viladot, M.; Arance, A.; Muñoz, M. Clinical implications of the intrinsic molecular subtypes of breast cancer. *Breast* **2015**, *24*, S26–S35. [CrossRef]
2. Prat, A.; Pascual, T.; Adamo, B. Intrinsic molecular subtypes of HER2+ breast cancer. *Oncotarget* **2017**, *8*, 73362–73363. [CrossRef]
3. Hayes, D.F. HER2 and Breast Cancer—A Phenomenal Success Story. *N. Engl. J. Med.* **2019**, *381*, 1284–1286. [CrossRef]
4. Slamon, D.; Clark, G.; Wong, S.; Levin, W.; Ullrich, A.; McGuire, W. Human breast cancer: Correlation of relapse and survival with amplification of the HER-2/neu oncogene. *Science* **1987**, *235*, 177–182. [CrossRef]
5. Press, M.F.; Pike, M.C.; Chazin, V.R.; Hung, G.; Udove, J.A.; Markowicz, M.; Danyluk, J.; Godolphin, W.; Sliwkowski, M.; Akita, R.; et al. Her-2/*neu* Expression in Node-negative Breast Cancer: Direct Tissue Quantitation by Computerized Image Analysis and Association of Overexpression with Increased Risk of Recurrent Disease. *Cancer Res.* **1993**, *53*, 4960–4970.
6. Cobleigh, M.A.; Vogel, C.L.; Tripathy, D.; Robert, N.J.; Scholl, S.; Fehrenbacher, L.; Wolter, J.M.; Paton, V.; Shak, S.; Lieberman, G.; et al. Multinational Study of the Efficacy and Safety of Humanized Anti-HER2 Monoclonal Antibody in Women Who Have HER2-Overexpressing Metastatic Breast Cancer That Has Progressed After Chemotherapy for Metastatic Disease. *J. Clin. Oncol.* **1999**, *17*, 2639. [CrossRef]
7. Vogel, C.; Cobleigh, M.; Tripathy, D.; Harris, L.; Fehrenbacher, L.; Slamon, D.; Ash, M.; Novotny, W.; Stewart, S.; Shak, S. First-line, non-hormonal, treatment of women with HER2 overexpressing metastatic breast cancer with herceptin (trastuzumab, humanised anti-HER2 antibody) [abstract 275]. *Proc. Am. Soc. Clin. Oncol.* **2001**, *20*, 71a.
8. Slamon, D.J.; Leyland-Jones, B.; Shak, S.; Fuchs, H.; Paton, V.; Bajamonde, A.; Fleming, T.; Eiermann, W.; Wolter, J.; Pegram, M.; et al. Use of Chemotherapy plus a Monoclonal Antibody against HER2 for Metastatic Breast Cancer That Overexpresses HER2. *N. Engl. J. Med.* **2001**, *344*, 783–792. [CrossRef]
9. Giordano, S.H.; Temin, S.; Chandarlapaty, S.; Crews, J.R.; Esteva, F.J.; Kirshner, J.J.; Krop, I.E.; Levinson, J.; Lin, N.U.; Modi, S.; et al. Systemic Therapy for Patients With Advanced Human Epidermal Growth Factor Receptor 2–Positive Breast Cancer: ASCO Clinical Practice Guideline Update. *J. Clin. Oncol.* **2018**, *36*, 2736–2740. [CrossRef]
10. Wolff, A.C.; Hammond, M.E.H.; Allison, K.H.; Harvey, B.E.; Mangu, P.B.; Bartlett, J.M.S.; Bilous, M.; Ellis, I.O.; Fitzgibbons, P.; Hanna, W.; et al. Human Epidermal Growth Factor Receptor 2 Testing in Breast Cancer: American Society of Clinical Oncology/College of American Pathologists Clinical Practice Guideline Focused Update. *J. Clin. Oncol.* **2018**, *36*, 2105–2122. [CrossRef]
11. Niehans, G.A.; Singleton, T.P.; Dykoski, D.; Kiang, D.T. Stability of HER-2/neu Expression Over Time and at Multiple Metastatic Sites. *J. Natl. Cancer Inst.* **1993**, *85*, 1230–1235. [CrossRef] [PubMed]
12. Bergh, J. Quo Vadis With Targeted Drugs in the 21st Century? *J. Clin. Oncol.* **2009**, *27*, 2–5. [CrossRef] [PubMed]
13. Blancas, I.; Muñoz-Serrano, A.J.; Legerén, M.; Ruiz-Ávila, I.; Jurado, J.M.; Delgado, M.T.; Garrido, J.M.; González Bayo, B.; Rodríguez-Serrano, F. Immunophenotypic Conversion between Primary and Relapse Breast Cancer and its Effects on Survival. *Gynecol. Obstet. Investig.* **2020**, in press. [CrossRef] [PubMed]
14. Fehrenbacher, L.; Cecchini, R.S.; Jr, C.E.G.; Rastogi, P.; Costantino, J.P.; Atkins, J.N.; Crown, J.P.; Polikoff, J.; Boileau, J.-F.; Provencher, L.; et al. NSABP B-47/NRG Oncology Phase III Randomized Trial Comparing Adjuvant Chemotherapy With or Without Trastuzumab in High-Risk Invasive Breast Cancer Negative for HER2 by FISH and With IHC 1+ or 2+. *J. Clin. Oncol.* **2020**, *38*, 444–453. [CrossRef] [PubMed]
15. Mortimer, J.; Conti, P.; Shan, T.; Carroll, M.; Kofi, P.; Colcher, D.; Raubitschek, A.; Bading, J. 64Cu-DOTA-trastuzumab positron emission tomography imaging of HER2 in women with advanced breast cancer. *Cancer Res.* **2012**, *72*, 229s.
16. Mortimer, J.E.; Bading, J.R.; Colcher, D.M.; Conti, P.S.; Frankel, P.H.; Carroll, M.I.; Tong, S.; Poku, E.; Miles, J.K.; Shively, J.E.; et al. Functional Imaging of Human Epidermal Growth Factor Receptor 2–Positive Metastatic Breast Cancer Using 64Cu-DOTA-Trastuzumab PET. *J. Nucl. Med.* **2014**, *55*, 23–29. [CrossRef]

17. Burris, H.A.; Rugo, H.S.; Vukelja, S.J.; Vogel, C.L.; Borson, R.A.; Limentani, S.; Tan-Chiu, E.; Krop, I.E.; Michaelson, R.A. Girish, S.; et al. Phase II Study of the Antibody Drug Conjugate Trastuzumab-DM1 for the Treatment of Human Epidermal Growth Factor Receptor 2 (HER2)–Positive Breast Cancer After Prior HER2-Directed Therapy. *J. Clin. Oncol.* **2011**, *29*, 398–405. [CrossRef]
18. Mortimer, J.E.; Shively, J.E. Functional Imaging of Human Epidermal Growth Factor Receptor 2–Positive Breast Cancers and a Note about NOTA. *J. Nucl. Med.* **2019**, *60*, 23–25. [CrossRef]
19. Barthélémy, P.; Leblanc, J.; Goldbarg, V.; Wendling, F.; Kurtz, J.-E. Pertuzumab: Development Beyond Breast Cancer. *Anticancer Res.* **2014**, *34*, 1483–1491.
20. Baselga, J.; Gelmon, K.A.; Verma, S.; Wardley, A.; Conte, P.; Miles, D.; Bianchi, G.; Cortes, J.; McNally, V.A.; Ross, G.A.; et al. Phase II Trial of Pertuzumab and Trastuzumab in Patients With Human Epidermal Growth Factor Receptor 2–Positive Metastatic Breast Cancer That Progressed During Prior Trastuzumab Therapy. *J. Clin. Oncol.* **2010**, *28*, 1138–1144. [CrossRef]
21. Swain, S.M.; Miles, D.; Kim, S.-B.; Im, Y.-H.; Im, S.-A.; Semiglazov, V.; Ciruelos, E.; Schneeweiss, A.; Loi, S.; Monturus, E.; et al. Pertuzumab, trastuzumab, and docetaxel for HER2-positive metastatic breast cancer (CLEOPATRA): End-of-study results from a double-blind, randomised, placebo-controlled, phase 3 study. *Lancet Oncol.* **2020**, *21*, 519–530. [CrossRef]
22. Swain, S.M.; Baselga, J.; Kim, S.-B.; Ro, J.; Semiglazov, V.; Campone, M.; Ciruelos, E.; Ferrero, J.-M.; Schneeweiss, A.; Heeson, S.; et al. Pertuzumab, Trastuzumab, and Docetaxel in HER2-Positive Metastatic Breast Cancer. *N. Engl. J. Med.* **2015**, *372*, 724–734. [CrossRef]
23. Yan, H.; Yu, K.; Zhang, K.; Liu, L.; Li, Y. Efficacy and safety of trastuzumab emtansine (T-DM1) in the treatment of HER2-positive metastatic breast cancer (MBC): A meta-analysis of randomized controlled trial. *Oncotarget.* **2017**, *8*, 102458. [CrossRef] [PubMed]
24. Modi, S.; Saura, C.; Yamashita, T.; Park, Y.H.; Kim, S.-B.; Tamura, K.; Andre, F.; Iwata, H.; Ito, Y.; Tsurutani, J.; et al. Trastuzumab Deruxtecan in Previously Treated HER2-Positive Breast Cancer. *N. Engl. J. Med.* **2020**, *382*, 610–621. [CrossRef] [PubMed]
25. Ogitani, Y.; Aida, T.; Hagihara, K.; Yamaguchi, J.; Ishii, C.; Harada, N.; Soma, M.; Okamoto, H.; Oitate, M.; Arakawa, S.; et al. DS-8201a, A Novel HER2-Targeting ADC with a Novel DNA Topoisomerase I Inhibitor, Demonstrates a Promising Antitumor Efficacy with Differentiation from T-DM1. *Clin. Cancer Res.* **2016**, *22*, 5097–5108. [CrossRef] [PubMed]
26. Cuadros, M.; Villegas, R. Systematic Review of HER2 Breast Cancer Testing. *Appl. Immunohistochem. Mol. Morphol.* **2009**, *17*, 1–7. [CrossRef] [PubMed]
27. Yau, T.K.; Sze, H.; Soong, I.S.; Hioe, F.; Khoo, U.S.; Lee, A.W.M. HER2 overexpression of breast cancers in Hong Kong: Prevalence and concordance between immunohistochemistry and in-situ hybridisation assays. *Hong Kong Med. J.* **2008**, *14*, 130–135. [PubMed]
28. NCCN. Clinical Practice Guidelines in Oncology: Prostate Cancer (v.3.2011). Available online: http://www.nccn.org (accessed on 9 June 2011).
29. Murthy, R.K.; Loi, S.; Okines, A.; Paplomata, E.; Hamilton, E.; Hurvitz, S.A.; Lin, N.U.; Borges, V.; Abramson, V.; Anders, C.; et al. Tucatinib, Trastuzumab, and Capecitabine for HER2-Positive Metastatic Breast Cancer. *N. Engl. J. Med.* **2019**, *382*, 597–609. [CrossRef]
30. Network, N.C.C. Breast Version 4. 2020. Available online: https://www.nccn.org/professionals/physician_gls/pdf/breast.pdf (accessed on 28 April 2020).
31. Lin, N.U.; Borges, V.; Anders, C.; Murthy, R.K.; Paplomata, E.; Hamilton, E.; Hurvitz, S.; Loi, S.; Okines, A.; Abramson, V.; et al. Intracranial Efficacy and Survival With Tucatinib Plus Trastuzumab and Capecitabine for Previously Treated HER2-Positive Breast Cancer With Brain Metastases in the HER2CLIMB Trial. *J. Clin. Oncol.* **2020**, in press. [CrossRef]
32. Geyer, C.E.; Forster, J.; Lindquist, D.; Chan, S.; Romieu, C.G.; Pienkowski, T.; Jagiello-Gruszfeld, A.; Crown, J.; Chan, A.; Kaufman, B.; et al. Lapatinib plus Capecitabine for HER2-Positive Advanced Breast Cancer. *N. Engl. J. Med.* **2006**, *355*, 2733–2743. [CrossRef]
33. Blackwell, K.L.; Burstein, H.J.; Storniolo, A.M.; Rugo, H.S.; Sledge, G.; Aktan, G.; Ellis, C.; Florance, A.; Vukelja, S.; Bischoff, J.; et al. Overall Survival Benefit With Lapatinib in Combination With Trastuzumab for Patients With Human Epidermal Growth Factor Receptor 2–Positive Metastatic Breast Cancer: Final Results From the EGF104900 Study. *J. Clin. Oncol.* **2012**, *30*, 2585–2592. [CrossRef] [PubMed]

34. Nasrazadani, A.; Brufsky, A. Neratinib: The emergence of a new player in the management of HER2+ breast cancer brain metastasis. *Future Oncol.* **2020**, *16*, 247–254. [CrossRef] [PubMed]
35. Tripathy, D.; Slamon, D.J.; Cobleigh, M.; Arnold, A.; Saleh, M.; Mortimer, J.E. Safety of treatment of metastatic breast cancer with trastuzumab beyond disease progression. *J. Clin. Oncol.* **2004**, *22*, 1063–1070. [CrossRef]
36. Bose, R.; Kavuri, S.M.; Searleman, A.C.; Shen, W.; Shen, D.; Koboldt, D.C.; Monsey, J.; Goel, N.; Aronson, A.B.; Li, S.; et al. Activating HER2 Mutations in HER2 Gene Amplification Negative Breast Cancer. *Cancer Discov.* **2013**, *3*, 224–237. [CrossRef]
37. Ma, C.X.; Bose, R.; Gao, F.; Freedman, R.A.; Telli, M.L.; Kimmick, G.; Winer, E.; Naughton, M.; Goetz, M.P.; Russell, C.; et al. Neratinib Efficacy and Circulating Tumor DNA Detection of *HER2* Mutations in *HER2* Nonamplified Metastatic Breast Cancer. *Clin. Cancer Res.* **2017**, *23*, 5687–5695. [CrossRef]
38. Ben-Baruch, N.E.; Bose, R.; Kavuri, S.M.; Ma, C.X.; Ellis, M.J. HER2-Mutated Breast Cancer Responds to Treatment With Single-Agent Neratinib, a Second-Generation HER2/EGFR Tyrosine Kinase Inhibitor. *J. Natl. Compr. Cancer Netw.* **2015**, *13*, 1061–1064. [CrossRef]
39. Hyman, D.M.; Piha-Paul, S.A.; Won, H.; Rodon, J.; Saura, C.; Shapiro, G.I.; Juric, D.; Quinn, D.I.; Moreno, V.; Doger, B.; et al. HER kinase inhibition in patients with HER2- and HER3-mutant cancers. *Nature* **2018**, *554*, 189–194. [CrossRef] [PubMed]
40. Pogue-Geile, K.L.; Kim, C.; Jeong, J.-H.; Tanaka, N.; Bandos, H.; Gavin, P.G.; Fumagalli, D.; Goldstein, L.C.; Sneige, N.; Burandt, E.; et al. Predicting Degree of Benefit From Adjuvant Trastuzumab in NSABP Trial B-31. *J. Natl. Cancer Inst.* **2013**, *105*, 1782–1788. [CrossRef]
41. Wolfson, J.A.; Sun, C.-L.; Wyatt, L.P.; Hurria, A.; Bhatia, S. Impact of care at comprehensive cancer centers on outcome: Results from a population-based study. *Cancer* **2015**, *121*, 3885–3893. [CrossRef] [PubMed]

© 2020 by the authors. Licensee MDPI, Basel, Switzerland. This article is an open access article distributed under the terms and conditions of the Creative Commons Attribution (CC BY) license (http://creativecommons.org/licenses/by/4.0/).

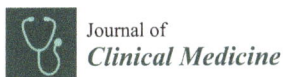

Article

NCI–Clinical Trial Accrual in a Community Network Affiliated with a Designated Cancer Center

Daniel J. Kim, Dan Otap, Nora Ruel, Naveen Gupta, Naveed Khan and Tanya Dorff *

City of Hope Comprehensive Cancer Center, Department of Medical Oncology and Developmental Therapeutics, Duarte, CA 91010, USA; danieljkim@coh.org (D.J.K.); dotap@coh.org (D.O.); nruel@coh.org (N.R.); ngupta@coh.org (N.G.); nakhan@coh.org (N.K.)
* Correspondence: tdorff@coh.org

Received: 29 April 2020; Accepted: 17 June 2020; Published: 24 June 2020

Abstract: Most cancer care is delivered in the community, while most clinical trials exist in academic centers. We analyzed clinical trial accrual of a tertiary care cancer center and its affiliated community sites to better understand what types of trials accrued at the community sites and whether community accrual increased ethnic diversity. The institutional clinical trial database was searched for solid tumor accruals during 2018–2019. Patient's race was abstracted, and trial's funding source, phase, and disease type/stage were tabulated. Of 3689 accruals, 133 were at community sites, representing 26 unique trials while the main campus accrued to 93 unique trials. Community site accruals were highest for breast and colorectal cancer, but patients with less common cancers such as renal, nasopharyngeal, and gastric cancer were also accrued at community sites. Accruals occurred to randomized trials, as well as phase Ib and translational biomarker studies. Minority patients constituted 20.0% and 32.5% of community site accruals for therapeutic and non-therapeutic trials respectively, compared to 20.6% and 29.8% of main campus accruals for therapeutic and non-therapeutic trials, respectively. We conclude that community sites affiliated with an academic cancer center can accrue to a broad spectrum of clinical trials while enhancing racial diversity in participation of clinical trials. Further expansion of access to clinical trials in community sites is necessary to broaden patient access to state-of-the-art and next-generation treatment options.

Keywords: clinical trials; community practice; minorities; ethnicity; race

---

1. Introduction

Community oncology practices provide approximately 55% of all care for cancer patients in the United States [1]. Providing access to clinical trials in community oncology practices has been a major initiative of the National Cancer Institute (NCI, Rockville, MD, USA), as evidenced by the creation of the National Community Oncology Research Program (NCORP, Bethesda, MD, USA) in 2014. The NCORP was created by consolidating the previous NCI supported networks of the CCOP–community clinical oncology program and the NCI Community Cancer Centers Program (NCCCP, Bethesda, MD, USA). Up to a third of clinical trial accrual in NCI studies is contributed by these community oncology practices [2], yet the overall clinical trial accrual remains lower than desirable: fewer than 5% of adult cancer patients enroll in clinical trials [3], despite 70% of cancer patients expressing interest in enrolling in a clinical trial [4].

Aside from increasing treatment options and providing access to the latest innovations in cancer care, participation in clinical trials has been shown to improve overall treatment quality vis-à-vis utilization of optimal standards of care [5]. One barrier for community practice physicians has been cost; clinical trial enrollment takes time, which takes resources away from overall clinic flow, and research staff are required regardless of how robust accrual is. Understanding the types of clinical trials that readily accrue in the community setting could help improve trial selection to foster financial sustainability, since fewer trials, each of which accrue larger numbers of patients, is more efficient in the setting of having limited clinical research staff at community sites.

In addition, inadequate representation of racially diverse cancer patients has been noted to be a major problem in the applicability of most clinical trials to everyday practice. For example, clinical trials in metastatic castration-resistant prostate cancer (CRPC) were found to have 80% under-representation of African American patients [6]. In the case of geriatric patients, a study of NCI-sponsored trials found that patients over 65 made up only 32% of participants, whereas they made up 61% of patients affected by the cancers [7]. Given that community oncology practices may be located closer to patients' homes, the availability of trials in a local setting could reduce potential barriers for patients to access clinical trials. Furthermore, if community practices are located near specific ethnic enclaves, their participation in clinical trials could help alleviate the lack of racial diversity, as indicated by the NCCCP initiative [8].

City of Hope is an NCI-designated comprehensive cancer center in Duarte, California, with an extensive network of 21 community practice sites located within its vicinity in Southern California, thus allowing for delivery of specialized care near where patients reside. As part of the overall mission of City of Hope, select clinical trials have been opened to accrual at six of the community sites which service a high enough patient volume to support research recruitment. We sought to characterize and evaluate clinical trials accrual with a focus on City of Hope's community sites, and whether racial diversity was enhanced in patients accrued at community sites compared to the main cancer center campus.

2. Material and Methods

After obtaining IRB exemption for the study, we identified the individual accrual events in our clinical trials database during the calendar years 2018 and 2019 at all City of Hope sites. This dataset was extracted from our institution's secure online trial database, devoid of any personal identifiers. Inclusion criteria was prospective adult clinical trials. Study title, sponsor, location of accrual, and date of study were extracted from the dataset. We decided ahead of time to exclude trials which were felt to reflect highly tertiary patient populations, such as hematologic malignancy trials which, at City of Hope, were likely to be heavily transplant and chimeric antigen receptor T cell therapy-based, or any other trials felt to introduce bias into the analysis.

Results were tabulated for comparison between main campus and community sites and stratified by the type of trials. The Chi-square and Fisher's exact tests were used to test the differences in distribution of race, minority status, and age groups between community sites and main campus participants.

3. Results

Of the 33,558 individual accrual events identified in our analysis, 23,809 accrual events were identified to be retrospective in nature and thus excluded, along with an additional 5625 accrual events which were identified to be trials involving hematologic malignancies. Sixteen pediatric trial accrual events were also excluded, as well as 419 healthy volunteer accruals. Also excluded were two high-accruing non-therapeutic trials specifically recruiting only Hispanic women, as ethnicity was not a variable and thus biasing the minority accrual question.

Our final analysis was thus based on 3689 accrual events. Community sites in the City of Hope network accrued to 26 distinct, solid tumor clinical trials ($n = 22$ therapeutic, $n = 4$ non-therapeutic) during the years 2018–2019, compared with accrual to 93 solid tumor trials at the main campus during the same time period. A description of all therapeutic trials which accrued at least one subject at a community site is delineated in Table 1. During the same time period, an additional 57 trials were open at community sites but did not accrue patients there.

Table 1. Characteristics of therapeutic clinical trial which accrued subjects at City of Hope community practice sites from 2018–2019.

Disease	Stage of Disease	Phase of Trial	Sponsor	Community Site Accrual	Main Campus Accrual
Breast Cancer	Prevention	II	IST	6	7
Breast Cancer	Adjuvant	III, randomized	Cooperative group	2	2
Breast Cancer	Adjuvant	III, randomized	Cooperative group	3	0
Breast Cancer	Metastatic 1st line	II	IST	4	8
Breast Cancer	Metastatic, over 60, Her2+	II	IST	2	11
Breast Cancer	Survivorship	II, randomized	Cooperative group	3	20
Colorectal Cancer	Metastatic, previously treated	III, randomized	Industry	10	4
Colorectal Cancer	Metastatic RAS-mutated, previously treated	I	IST	3	18
Colorectal Cancer	Metastatic previously treated	III	Industry	5	2
Colorectal Cancer	Metastatic previously treated	Ib	Industry	1	0
Gastric/GEJ	Metastatic, previously treated	I/II	NCI	2	2
Hepatocellular carcinoma	Advanced/Metastatic 1st line	III, randomized	Industry	2	11
Kidney Cancer	Adjuvant	III, randomized	Industry	3	9
Nasopharyngeal	Primary	II/III, randomized	Cooperative group	1	4
NSCLC	Adjuvant	III, randomized	Cooperative Group	1	4
NSCLC	Adjuvant, EGFR mutant	III, randomized	Cooperative group	1	4
NSCLC	Metastatic	I/II	IST	2	3
NSCLC	Metastatic(oligo) add SBRT	II/III, randomized	Cooperative Group	1	2
NSCLC	Metastatic, first-line, EGFR mutant	IV (elderly)	Industry	1	0
Pancreas	Advanced/Metastatic	Pilot	IST	2	4
Prostate Cancer	mCRPC	II randomized	IST	1	4
Urothelial	Neoadjuvant	II	Cooperative Group	2 *	14

* Accrued at main campus, transitioned during study treatment to community site. GEJ = gastro-esophageal junction. IST = Investigator Sponsored Trials. NSCLC = non-small cell lung cancer.

Overall, 133 subjects were accrued at 6 community sites ($n = 58$ therapeutic) and 3556 at the main campus. These included randomized phase II or III trials ($n = 13$), as well as ($n = 7$) phase II trials, and ($n = 2$) phase Ib trials. Half of the trials accrued to in the community sites ($n = 13$) were cooperative group trials, four were industry, one was NCI/CTEP sponsored, and seven were investigator-initiated trials commonly called investigator-sponsored trials (IST). Trials which did not register accrual at community sites were primarily phase II (30/57; 52.6%) and phase III (21/57; 36.8%), with only five phase I trials open and not accruing (8.8%).

Most trials that registered community accruals were for breast cancers ($n = 8$), followed by gastrointestinal (6), genitourinary (3), non-small cell lung cancer (3), melanoma (1), and all solid tumors (1). Highest accruing trials in the community sites included a phase III industry-sponsored trial in metastatic refractory colorectal cancer, which accrued more patients in the community than at the main cancer center ($n = 10$ compared to $n = 4$ respectively). The other top accruing studies ($n = 6$ in community) were for breast cancer patients, one for prevention and one for first-line treatment of metastatic disease. Studies which were open in the community, but did not accrue, were distributed across tumor types; 13 gastrointestinal (22.8%), breast and lung (each 19.3%), melanoma/sarcoma and genitourinary (each 14.0%), head and neck and gynecologic (each 5.3%).

The ethnic composition of accruals in the community sites and the main campus is summarized in Table 2. Minority accrual ranged from 20.6% to 21.8% at the main campus and 15.6% to 20.0% at community sites, although there was a higher rate of accrual of African American subjects to non-therapeutic trials at community sites. Distribution of patient age was different between accrual sites (Table 3) within therapeutic and non-therapeutic studies ($p < 0.01$), as we saw a larger proportion of older patients at community sites than on main campus. Among adult subjects, 22/58 (37.9%) subjects were > 70 years old in the community, compared to 498/1828 (27.3%) patients accrued in Duarte. In contrast, 238 (13.0%) adult subjects on main campus vs. zero patients at community sites were under the age of 40.

Table 2. Accrual at sites, stratified by race.

	Therapeutic		
Race	Main Campus Therapeutic $n = 1832$	Community Site Therapeutic $n = 58$	p-Value *
	Number (%)		
African American	76 (4.1)	3 (5.2)	0.4
American Indian or Alaska native	4 (0.2)	0	
Asian	255 (13.9)	5 (8.6)	
Native Hawaiian or Pacific Islander	7 (0.4)	1 (1.7)	
Non-White Multiracial	2 (0.1)	0	
White Multiracial	12 (0.7)	0	
White	1382 (75.4)	36 (62)	
Unknown	94 (5.1)	13 (22.4)	
%minority (non-White/total)	20.6%	20.0%	1.0

Table 2. Cont.

Race	Non-Therapeutic		
	Main Campus Non-Therapeutic n = 1192	Community Site Non-Therapeutic n = 40	
	Number (%)		p-Value
African American	64 (5.3)	5 (12.5)	0.04
American Indian or Alaska native	5 (0.4)	0	
Asian	157 (13.2)	0	
Native Hawaiian or Pacific Islander	3 (0.3)	0	
Non-White Multiracial	0	0	
White Multiracial	4 (0.3)	0	
White	837 (70.2)	27 (67.5)	
Unknown	122 (10.2)	8 (20)	
%minority (non-White/total)	29.8%	32.5%	0.5

* p values calculated for distribution of known race or ethnicity, omitting unknowns from calculations.

Table 3. Age distribution of subjects accrued to clinical trials at the main campus and at community sites.

Age Group	Therapeutic Trials		Non-Therapeutic Trials	
	Main Campus	Community Sites	Main Campus	Community Sites
19–39	238 (13.0%)	0 (0.0%)	154 (13.4%)	1 (2.5%)
40–59	563 (30.8%)	21 (36.2%)	303 (26.4%)	4 (10.0%)
60–69	528 (28.9%)	15 (25.9%)	292 (25.5%)	15 (37.5%)
70+	498 (27.3%)	22 (37.9%)	398 (34.7%)	20 (50.0%)
Unknown	0 (0.0%)	0 (0.0%)	0 (0.0%)	0 (0.0%)

A complete list of trials accrued to at each site can be found in Supplemental Table S1. Notably, trials accrued to at community sites included the full spectrum of disease, from cancer prevention to adjuvant and neoadjuvant trials, as well as trials for metastatic and refractory cancer patients. Non-interventional trials which accrued at community sites included biomarker studies, both for molecular characterization as well as for predicting toxicity, and geriatric oncology trials. Studies not open in the community included supportive care trials such as a trial studying bright light to reduce frailty during androgen deprivation therapy for prostate cancer patients and studies of the perception of genomic profiling and of immunotherapy expected outcomes. Most phase I trials were not open in the community (26/32).

4. Discussions

Community sites associated with an NCI-designated cancer center may represent a unique opportunity to expand clinical trial access into underserved and under-represented populations, given the proximity of the sites to serve their respective local communities and the ability to leverage research staff and resources from the main campus. A review of more than 33,000 individual accrual events at City of Hope revealed that affiliated community sites accrued patients to a wide selection of solid tumor trials of various cancer histology, stage of disease, and therapeutic/non-therapeutic aims. Whereas it was anticipated most trials that successfully accrued patients at community sites would be later phase, cooperative group trials, there were also a relatively high accrual of investigator-sponsored phase II, and even phase Ib, trials. Similarly, it was anticipated that the most common malignancies would make up the largest percentage of accruals in the community sites, but uncommon tumor types such as hepatocellular, kidney, and pancreatic cancers also accrued at community sites.

City of Hope community practice sites are strategically located throughout five counties across Southern California (Ventura, Los Angeles, San Bernardino, Riverside, and Orange), aiming to provide cancer care to all communities, including socioeconomically disadvantaged populations and communities with cancer disparities. Our analysis did reveal a higher accrual of African American patients to non-therapeutic trials at the community sites compared to main campus but did not significantly improve diversity of trial accrual as had been hoped. Loree et al. [9] had reported African Americans and Hispanics representing 3.1% and 6.1% of trial participants respectively, and City of Hope's rate of African American representation in trial accrual was similarly low. A limitation of our analysis is that our percentages are derived from accrued subjects rather than all subjects; that is to say, the denominator are trial participants, rather than all screened patients or all eligible patients or all patients seen at the clinic, as such data was not available for analysis. Our assessment was also limited by a relatively high rate of "unknown" ethnicity among community accruals (22.4%); this can be due to incomplete datasets or patients declining to answer the question. In order to minimize missing data, standard operating procedures for research staff and centralization of clinical data management could improve consistency and data quality.

Community sites did enroll a higher rate of geriatric patients, which may reflect the difficulty elderly patients face in traveling greater distances to a comprehensive cancer center in order to obtain oncology care. Admittedly, the City of Hope experience may be unique, as geriatric oncology is a flagship program with dedicated resources. However, this finding is an encouraging signal, and warrants further study as increasing accrual of geriatric patients to cancer protocols is an important goal for the oncology community given that many cancers have substantially higher prevalence in people over the age of 65.

Additional limitation of our study involves the inherent selection process involved in extending clinical trial offerings to the community sites. Based on limited resources and anticipated accrual rates, only a select few clinical trials were extended from the main campus to the community sites, and of the 21 community sites only six higher-volume sites were selected for clinical trial participation. Trial accrual rate could have been higher for the community sites if trial offerings were identical across main campus and community sites, but such an offering would require far greater investment into trial resources at all of the community sites and may not be practical or feasible. Our analysis also could not capture the number of patients who were referred from the community sites to the main campus for enrollment into trials not offered at the community sites, thus shifting trial accrual numbers from community sites to main campus. We did notice, however, that a bladder cancer trial enrolled subjects at the main campus and then transitioned ongoing cycles of treatment to community sites due to patient travel burden (Table 1). This flexibility is an example of how academic-community collaboration can optimize both accrual and patient-centered care and could represent an efficient "just in time" model of opening the right trials in the right areas. We concur with the value of main campus regularly meeting with community sites to review currently available clinical trials [10], and we additionally propose that the community sites must be actively engaged in and collaborate with the main campus in selecting the trials offered at the community sites based on needs assessment of their unique patient population and community site clinician interests.

In contrast to published experiences, however, we found that phase I and even non-therapeutic trials did not present an insurmountable barrier to accrual in community oncology practices. In a previous survey of 51 community practices, which included both federally sponsored and private non-academic affiliated practices, half of the practices self-reported that they did not accrue to phase I trials, 53% did not accrue to investigator-initiated trials, and 33% did not enroll on correlative science trials [11]. It is likely that many investigator-initiated trials and translational "non-therapeutic" trials can meet the needs of community oncology patients, and that academic-affiliated community sites are best poised to engage patients in accrual to these types of studies.

Supplementary Materials: The following are available online at http://www.mdpi.com/2077-0383/9/6/1970/s1, Table S1: summary of phases and disease states of trials accrued to at community sites and City of Hope main campus.

Author Contributions: Conceptualization and methodology, T.D.; data curation, D.O.; validation, D.J.K., D.O., N.R., and T.D.; formal analysis, N.R. and T.D.; writing—original draft preparation, D.J.K., N.R., N.G., and N.K.; writing—review and editing, D.K., T.D.; project administration and funding acquisition, T.D. All authors have read and agreed to the published version of the manuscript.

Funding: This research was funded by an internal core grant #P30CA033572 from City of Hope, and received no external funding.

Conflicts of Interest: The authors declare no conflicts of interest.

References

1. Community Oncology Alliance. Available online: https://communityoncology.org (accessed on 28 March 2020).
2. Carpenter, W.R.; Fortune-Greeley, A.; Zullig, L.L.; Lee, S.-Y.; Weiner, B.J. Sustainability and performance of the National Cancer Institute's Community Clinical Oncology Program. *Contemp. Clin. Trials* **2011**, *33*, 46–54. [CrossRef] [PubMed]
3. Unger, J.M.; Cook, E.; Tai, E.; Bleyer, A. Role of clinical trial participation in cancer research: barriers, evidence and strategies. *Am. Soc. Clin. Oncol. Educ. Book* **2016**, *35*, 185–198. [CrossRef] [PubMed]
4. Comis, R.L.; Miller, J.D.; Aldigé, C.R.; Krebs, L.; Stoval, E. Public Attitudes Toward Participation in Cancer Clinical Trials. *J. Clin. Oncol.* **2003**, *21*, 830–835. [CrossRef] [PubMed]
5. Laliberte, L.; Fennell, M.L.; Papandonatos, G.D. The Relationship of Membership in Research Networks to Compliance with Treatment Guidelines for Early-Stage Breast Cancer. *Med. Care* **2005**, *43*, 471–479. [CrossRef] [PubMed]
6. Spratt, D.E.; Osborne, J. Disparities in Castration-Resistant Prostate Cancer Trials. *J. Clin. Oncol.* **2015**, *33*, 1101–1103. [CrossRef] [PubMed]
7. Lewis, J.H.; Kilgore, M.L.; Goldman, D.P.; Trimble, E.L.; Kaplan, R.; Montello, M.J.; Housman, M.G.; Escarce, J.J. Participation of Patients 65 Years of Age or Older in Cancer Clinical Trials. *J. Clin. Oncol.* **2003**, *21*, 1383–1389. [CrossRef] [PubMed]
8. Hirsch, B.R.; Locke, S.; Abernethy, A.P. Experience of the National Cancer Institute Community Cancer Centers Program on Community-Based Cancer Clinical Trials Activity. *J. Oncol. Pract.* **2016**, *12*, e350–e358. [CrossRef] [PubMed]
9. Loree, J.M.; Anand, S.; Dasari, A.; Unger, J.M.; Gothwal, A.; Ellis, L.M.; Varadhachary, G.; Kopetz, S.; Overman, M.J.; Raghav, K. Disparity of Race Reporting and Representation in Clinical Trials Leading to Cancer Drug Approvals from 2008 to 2018. *JAMA Oncol.* **2019**, *5*, e191870. [CrossRef] [PubMed]
10. Ludmir, E.B.; Adlakha, E.K.; Chun, S.G.; Reed, V.K.; Arzu, I.Y.; Ahmad, N.; Bloom, E.; Chronowski, G.M.; Delclos, M.E.; Mayo, L.L.; et al. Enhancing clinical trial enrollment at MD Anderson Cancer Center satellite community campuses. *Acta Oncol.* **2019**, *58*, 1135–1137. [CrossRef] [PubMed]
11. Good, M.J.; Lubejko, B.; Humphries, K.; Medders, A. Measuring Clinical Trial–Associated Workload in a Community Clinical Oncology Program. *J. Oncol. Pract.* **2013**, *9*, 211–215. [CrossRef] [PubMed]

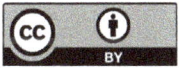

© 2020 by the authors. Licensee MDPI, Basel, Switzerland. This article is an open access article distributed under the terms and conditions of the Creative Commons Attribution (CC BY) license (http://creativecommons.org/licenses/by/4.0/).

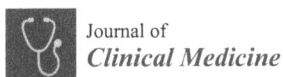

Article

Complex Oncological Decision-Making Utilizing Fast-and-Frugal Trees in a Community Setting—Role of Academic and Hybrid Modeling

Ravi Salgia [1,*], Isa Mambetsariev [1], Tingting Tan [1], Amanda Schwer [2], Daryl P. Pearlstein [3], Hazem Chehabi [2], Angel Baroz [1], Jeremy Fricke [1], Rebecca Pharaon [1], Hannah Romo [1], Thomas Waddington [4], Razmig Babikian [1], Linda Buck [1], Prakash Kulkarni [1], Mary Cianfrocca [1], Benjamin Djulbegovic [5] and Sumanta K. Pal [1]

[1] Department of Medical Oncology and Therapeutics Research, 1500 E Duarte Road, City of Hope National Medical Center, Duarte, CA 91010, USA; Imambetsariev@coh.org (I.M.); titan@coh.org (T.T.); abaroz@coh.org (A.B.); jfricke@coh.org (J.F.); rpharaon@coh.org (R.P.); hromo@coh.org (H.R.); rbabikian@coh.org (R.B.); lbuck@coh.org (L.B.); pkulkarni@coh.org (P.K.); mcianfrocca@coh.org (M.C.); spal@coh.org (S.K.P.)
[2] Newport Diagnostic Center, Newport Beach, CA 92660, USA; aschwer@newportdiagnosticcenter.com (A.S.); h.chehabi@newportdiagnosticcenter.com (H.C.)
[3] Department of Thoracic Surgery, Hoag Hospital, CA 92660, USA; darylpearlstein@gmail.com
[4] Department of Medicine, City of Hope National Medical Center, Duarte, CA 91010, USA; twaddington@coh.org
[5] Department of Hematology & Hematopoietic Cell Transplantation, City of Hope National Medical Center, Duarte, CA 91010, USA; bdjulbegovic@coh.org
* Correspondence: rsalgia@coh.org

Received: 15 May 2020; Accepted: 12 June 2020; Published: 16 June 2020

Abstract: Non-small cell lung cancer is a devastating disease and with the advent of targeted therapies and molecular testing, the decision-making process has become complex. While established guidelines and pathways offer some guidance, they are difficult to utilize in a busy community practice and are not always implemented in the community. The rationale of the study was to identify a cohort of patients with lung adenocarcinoma at a City of Hope community site (n = 11) and utilize their case studies to develop a decision-making framework utilizing fast-and-frugal tree (FFT) heuristics. Most patients had stage IV (N = 9, 81.8%) disease at the time of the first consultation. The most common symptoms at initial presentation were cough (N = 5, 45.5%), shortness of breath (N = 3, 27.2%), and weight loss (N = 3, 27.2%). The Eastern Cooperative Oncology Group (ECOG) performance status ranged from 0-1 in all patients in this study. Distribution of molecular drivers among the patients were as follows: EGFR (N = 5, 45.5%), KRAS (N = 2, 18.2%), ALK (N = 2, 18.2%), MET (N = 2, 18.2%), and RET (N = 1, 9.1%). Seven initial FFTs were developed for the various case scenarios, but ultimately the decisions were condensed into one FFT, a molecular stage IV FFT, that arrived at accurate decisions without sacrificing initial information. While these FFT decision trees may seem arbitrary to an experienced oncologist at an academic site, the simplicity of their utility is essential for community practice where patients often do not get molecular testing and are not assigned proper therapy.

Keywords: non-small cell lung cancer; actionable mutations; next-generation sequencing; fast-and-frugal trees; community practice; personalized medicine

1. Introduction

Lung cancer is a devastating disease with an overall survival rate of 16% at five years in non-small cell lung cancer (NSCLC) and 6% in small cell lung cancer (SCLC) [1]. Lung cancer incidence in 2020 is estimated at 228,820 new cases and will remain the leading cause of cancer death in the US with an estimated 135,720 deaths [2]. NSCLC accounts for approximately 85% of lung cancer cases and is a heterogeneous group of tumors comprised of adenocarcinomas, squamous cell carcinomas, and large cell carcinomas as the major subtypes [3]. These individual subtypes have different molecular characteristics, clinical features, and complex therapeutic options with unique outcomes for individual patients. More so, the advent of targeted therapy and immunotherapy have drastically shifted the therapeutic landscape of NSCLC towards precision medicine, or personalized medicine, where the individual patient is treated selectively based on their molecular characteristics [4]. Due to the rise of personalized medicine, lung cancer decision-making has grown complex, and chemotherapy, once the default treatment of choice for all patients, is no longer universally used.

This advance towards personalized medicine is primarily driven by advances in targeted therapeutic options, genomic testing, and immunotherapy that have shown improvement in patient outcomes [5–10]. EGFR therapy, once limited to first-generation tyrosine-kinase inhibitors (TKIs) such as erlotinib [11], has grown to second and third generation TKIs with osimertinib showing improvements not only in response rates and progression-free survival (PFS), but also in durable overall survival (OS) benefits as compared to chemotherapy and other TKIs [12–14]. These advances in therapeutic options for *EGFR* has further spurred greater understanding of NSCLC biology to reveal multiple distinct molecular subtypes—a widely supported theory that oncogenic "driver mutations" are responsible for NSCLC's malignant phenotype [15]. Along with *EGFR*, gene alterations in *ALK*, *ROS1*, *NTRK*, and *BRAF* have therapies that are FDA-approved and routinely tested in practice [16]. Recent long-term follow-up results from 110 ALK-positive patients who received the ALK inhibitor crizotinib, showed a median OS of 6.8 years in patients with metastatic disease [17]. Moreover, several inhibitors for MET and RET are slowly being implemented in standard clinical practice and await FDA approval [18–22]. Initial results from a phase II study of MET exon 14 inhibitor tepotinib, showed a sustained duration of response (12.4 months) and a 45% objective response rate (ORR), earning a breakthrough FDA designation [23,24]. Beyond these driver alterations, approximately 25% of lung adenocarcinomas present with KRAS alterations that occur in codons 12 or 13 [25]. No approved direct targeted therapy is available for KRAS-mutant NSCLC, but two promising inhibitors—MRTX849 and AMG 510—are currently under clinical consideration with early results reporting antitumor activity in the initial patients [26,27]. Furthermore, several studies have shown that immunotherapy is a viable treatment option for KRAS-mutant patients, with some patients showing remarkable clinical benefit from anti-PD-1/PD-L1 immunotherapy [28–30].

The availability of several targeted therapies and a variety of immunotherapies that have been approved for lung cancer has complicated oncology decision-making in clinical practice. Furthermore, advances in genomics and therapies have not been accompanied with advances in the science of medical decision-making. Clinical practice guidelines, such as the National Cancer Center Network (NCCN) and the American Society for Clinical Oncology (ASCO), are commonly used to aid in decision-making, but the recommendations are often difficult to interpret and are not easily manageable during a busy oncology clinic [31,32]. We have previously shown that a novel method of utilizing fast-and-frugal trees (FFTs) to arrive at decision-making trees can allow for physicians to make a quick but accurate decision [33]. Our previous work shows how guidelines can be converted into FFTs to allow development of individualized patient care, and the quantitative analysis of the performance characteristics of such a strategy [34,35]. The advantage of FFTs is that they are highly effective, simple decision trees composed of sequentially ordered cues (tests) and binary (yes/no) decisions formulated via a series of "if-then" statements [34]. Therefore, they can be easily applied to lung cancer decision-making where, if a genetic alteration is revealed to be actionable (e.g., EGFR exon 19 deletion), then an appropriate TKI (e.g., osimertinib) would be given [33]. While these decisions may seem arbitrary to an experienced oncologist at an academic site, the simplicity of their utility is essential for community practice where patients often do not get molecular testing and are not assigned proper therapy.

Thus, to evaluate clinical decision-making in lung cancer in the community, we have selected a cohort of community practice patients and have described their clinical complexity in detail as well as summarized the process for clinical decision-making that was employed to arrive at best the outcome for the patients. The majority of patients in this study were advanced NSCLC patients and we wanted to explore the role of personalized medicine within the community setting. We have also utilized the FFT method to develop individual simplified decision-trees that can be utilized in similar oncology cases based on patient molecular and clinical characteristics.

2. Patients and Methods

2.1. Patients

The first eleven non-small cell lung cancer patients (n = 11), evaluated at City of Hope Newport Beach community practice since its opening in January 2020, were enrolled in this analysis. De-identified patient data was obtained under the City of Hope institutional review board-approved protocol IRB 18008 with a waiver of informed consent and in accord with the Declaration of Helsinki. Data obtained from the electronic medical record included patient demographics, stage, age at diagnosis, race and ethnicity, smoking history, date of diagnosis, therapies given, histology, and outcomes. Molecular testing results were obtained from a retrospective chart review based on next-generation sequencing (NGS) tests obtained by their primary oncologist.

2.2. Fast-and-Frugal Trees

Heuristic categorization and the visualization of fast-and-frugal trees was performed according to established heuristic tree construction algorithms as previously described [36,37].

3. Results

3.1. Patients

A total of 28 patients diagnosed with cancer of the lung or bronchus were seen from January 2020 through to April 2020 at COH Newport Beach community clinic; the first 11 patients were included (Table 1). The median age at diagnosis was 70.5 years, ranging from 50–85 years. More than half of the patients were male (N = 7, 63.6%), most were white (N = 6, 54.5%), and less than half had a history of smoking (N = 5, 45.5%), with an average of 10.2 pack years. Upon initial diagnosis, all 11 patients were histologically identified with adenocarcinoma. However, one patient had a small cell lung cancer transformation status after two lines of TKI therapy (not shown on table), but also retained the original lung adenocarcinoma histology. Most patients had stage IV (N = 9, 81.8%) disease at the time of the first consultation. The most common symptoms at initial presentation were cough (N = 5, 45.5%), shortness of breath (N = 3, 27.2%), and weight loss (N = 3, 27.2%). The Eastern Cooperative Oncology Group (ECOG) performance status ranged from 0–1 in all patients in this study. Distribution of molecular drivers among the patients were as follows: *EGFR* (N = 5, 45.5%), *KRAS* (N = 2, 18.2%), *ALK* (N = 2, 18.2%), *MET* (N = 2, 18.2%), and *RET* (N = 1, 9.1%). Patients who tested positive for PD-L1 expression (N = 5, 45.5%) were considered positive if their tumor proportion score was greater than or equal to 1%.

Table 1. Patient characteristics.

Patient Characteristics	N = 11
Median Age	
Year	70.5
Range	50–85
Sex	
Male	7
Female	4
Ethnicity	
White	6
Asian	4
Hispanic/Latino	1
Smoking Status	
Never smoker	6
Former smoker	5
Average pack year	10.2
Histology	
Adenocarcinoma	11
Symptoms	
Cough	5
Sputum production	1
Shortness of breath/dyspnea	3
Weight loss	3
Chest pain	1
Other	2
Performance status	
0	4
1	7
Clinical staging	
IIIA	1
IIIB	1
IVA	6
IVB	3
Molecular driver mutation status (positive)	
EGFR	5
KRAS	2
ALK	2
MET	1
RET	1
PD-L1 Status	
Positive ≥1%	5
Negative <1%	4
Not applicable	2

Table 2. Detailed timing and order categories to address in ERAS pathways cancer surgeries.

Pre-Operative Orders Weeks Ahead Addressing:	Intra-Operative Orders Addressing:
Education visit and potential handouts	Fluid management
Assess post-op n/v risks and educate	IV/inhalational anesthetics
NSQIP surgery risk calculator	Regional anesthesia
Smoking and alcohol cessation	Deep Venus Thrombosis prophylaxis
Breathing exercise teaching	
Diet and activity guidance	**Post-Anesthesia Care Unit:**
Prehabilitation OT/PT teaching	Pain guidelines
Lab orders	Catheter guidelines
Medication education for pre-op and post-op	
Bathing instructions	**Extended Stay Orders:**
	Nursing care
Pre-Operative Orders Days or Day Before Surgery:	Medications
Patient instructions prior to surgery	DVT prophylaxis
Nasal and skin disinfection	As needed medications
Medication fills for post-op needs	
Prehabilitation OT/PT teaching	**Post-Op Orders Addressing:**
Pre-anesthesia testing	Follow-up nurse triage call
Pre-op fasting	Post-op visit scheduling
Pre-op medications	
Pre-op DVT prophylaxis	

3.2. Genomics

There were ten types of mutations identified in this cohort of patients. Eleven (100%) patients underwent NGS testing performed on tumor and/or liquid biopsies. Most patients had more than one genomic alteration reported. Figure 1 presents a heatmap of the biomarkers reported per patient, including PD-L1, TMB, and MSI status. Overall, the most frequent mutations found in this cohort were *TP53* (8/11, 66.7%), *EGFR* (5/11, 45.5%), *ALK* (2/11, 18.2%), *KRAS* (2/11, 18.2%), and *MET* (2/11, 18.2%). One patient, patient #4, is included twice in the heatmap due to NGS testing performed on two simultaneous, biologically different lung tumors (4A NGS was performed on the right lung specimen; 4B NGS was performed on the left lung specimen). The most frequent mutation types found in this cohort were substitution mutations (noted in red), deletions (noted in orange), and variant of unknown significance (VUS) mutations (noted in blue).

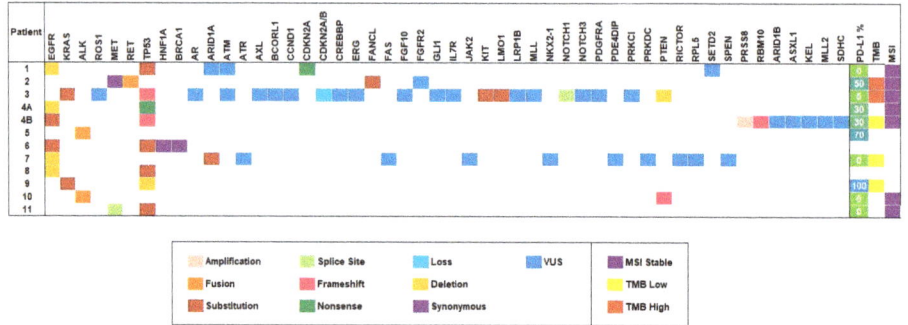

Figure 1. Mutational profile of the 11 patients as represented by heatmap. The figure displays tumor alterations reported by next-generation sequencing (NGS) testing, with the most frequent alterations on the left of the heatmap. The most frequent alteration types include substitution, deletions, and VUS mutations. The heatmap on the right reports the PD-L1, TMB, and MSI status of the cohort. Patient 4 is noted twice in the heatmap due to NGS testing performed on synchronous primary lung tumors (4A is the right lung specimen mutational profile; 4B is the left lung specimen mutational profile).

3.3. EGFR

3.3.1. Case #1

A 63-year-old Caucasian male never-smoker with a history of coughing that initially presented as throat clearing and progressed to regular frequent cough. He then developed a mild left-sided chest wall pain that improved over time, but the patient reported weight loss of about 30 pounds. He underwent a bronchoscopy that noted marked narrowing of the right middle lobe (RML) by extrinsic compression. A biopsy revealed lung adenocarcinoma of the RML, and a PET scan revealed a hypermetabolic 2.5 × 2.2 cm lesion in the left upper lobe (LUL). Molecular testing was performed on samples from both sides and showed differing results. The left-sided biopsy molecular testing showed EGFR L858R, PRSS8 amplification, RBM10 I377fs*4, and TP53 S90fs*33. The right-sided lesion showed EGFR amplification, EGFR exon 19 deletion (E746_A750del), and TP53 R306* alteration. The patient was discussed at the tumor board, and as surgery was not an option, the decision was made to treat the patient as stage IV EGFR lung cancer with a bilateral disease, and erlotinib therapy was immediately started. He was staged as a T1cN2M1a stage IVA lung adenocarcinoma. The patient had a good initial response on the right side and maintained stable disease on the left side for over 13 months. He eventually developed excess pleural effusion and liquid biopsy molecular testing revealed an EGFR T790M resistance alteration. A PleurX catheter was installed and the patient was immediately switched to osimertinib. He tolerated osimertinib well and continued on therapy for approximately 14 months until a PET/CT scan showed a mild interval increase in size of the hypermetabolic right cardiophrenic lymph node. This was considered oligoprogression, as the overall disease burden was stable and osimertinib therapy continued. A right supraclavicular, right mammary node, and a right cardiophrenic mass resection was performed and pathology showed small cell lung cancer, synaptophysin positive. Molecular testing was performed, and results showed EGFR exon 19 deletion (E746_A750del), EGFR amplification, AKT1 amplification, and TP53 R306*. EGFR TKI-small cell lung cancer transformation was suspected, and the patient immediately started carboplatin/etoposide chemotherapy alongside osimertinib. The patient tolerated combination therapy well and continues on therapy.

3.3.2. Case #2

A 66-year-old Asian female never-smoker initially presented with left shoulder pain and numbness. She underwent a chest X-ray which showed an abnormality in the lingula of the left-upper lobe.

A CT-guided biopsy was performed and revealed TTF-1 positivity, moderately differentiated pulmonary adenocarcinoma with a predominant acinar pattern. Staging CT of the chest, abdomen, and pelvis displayed a 1.5 × 2.0 × 2.2 cm left upper lobe mass. A subsequent PET/CT demonstrated F-18 fluorodeoxyglucose (FDG) activity in the left upper lobe, but also in multiple mediastinal and left hilar lymph nodes including stations 4R, 4L, 7, and 11R. These would be later confirmed for metastatic adenocarcinoma after she underwent an endobronchial ultrasound with fine needle biopsy. NGS sequencing of the station 7 lymph node revealed EGFR exon 19 deletion (E746_A750del), CDKN2A G120*, and TP53 Y163C. PD-L1 22C3 stained negative with 0% expression. The PET/CT also exhibited a 1.1 cm calcified isthmus thyroid gland nodule with an SUV of 4.9. This was also biopsied and revealed papillary carcinoma. She was referred to the endocrine surgery department but has not had surgery considering her lung cancer diagnosis. An MRI of the brain showed no metastatic disease. She was staged as a T1cN3M0 stage IIIB lung adenocarcinoma. She initiated therapy on weekly chemoradiation therapy to the left lung, hilum, and mediastinum with carboplatin and paclitaxel. She completed radiation with a few acute toxicities including chest discomfort, fatigue, and esophagitis, for which she received a 10-day course of dexamethasone. Due to her acute toxicities, she only received three weekly infusions of carboplatin and paclitaxel. She is planned to continue systemic treatment by initiating adjuvant osimertinib, and while this is not yet approved, the decision was made based on preliminary trial data and the factor that the patient could not complete chemotherapy due to toxicities.

3.3.3. Case #3

An 86-year-old male with no history of tobacco use initially presented to the emergency department with a complaint of dry cough, shortness of breath, and concern of gradual weight loss. He developed a dry cough about two months prior, without any specific or potential triggering cause. The persistent shortness of breath occurred over a few days, however, without limitations to his usual routines. Chest X-ray showed extensive consolidation and effusion on the right. Subsequent CT chest with IV contrast revealed severe right-sided pleural effusion, multiple nodular and patchy opacities in the right lung, with possible combination of atelectasis and edema. There were multiple sub-centimeter lesions throughout the lungs bilaterally, suspicious for pulmonary metastasis of more than 20 lesions. During his admission, he underwent thoracenteses that identified rare atypical cells suggestive of adenocarcinoma with lung primary (TTF-1 positive, Napsin A positive, mucicarmine cytochemistry negative). His disease progressed one month after admission. PET/CT confirmed diffuse FDG avid right pulmonary consolidation and bilateral pulmonary nodules with a max SUV of 11.6, FDG avid cervical and thoracic lymphadenopathy, and FDG avid osseous lesions. Brain MRI showed a motion-limited exam without findings to suggest intracranial metastatic disease. Single gene NGS panels showed EGFR exon 21 L858R mutation. Approximately 2.5 months after diagnosis, the patient had an initial consultation at COH community site. He was staged as a T2N3M1c stage IVB lung adenocarcinoma. He was treatment-naïve prior to consultation. Osimertinib was immediately administered after liquid biopsy confirmed EGFR exon 21 L858R and TP53 R273L. However, he experienced severe diarrhea 19 days after treatment start date. Osimertinib was held for 20 days and dosing was reduced to 40 mg daily. A few weeks following treatment re-initiation, the patient was admitted to the hospital for worsening shortness of breath associated with decreased output from his pleural catheter. Oxygen saturation ranged from 88–92% on room air. He transitioned from supplemental oxygen to high flow oxygen-enriched FiO2. Empiric antibiotics were administered for hospital-acquired pneumonia. His respiratory distress continued to deteriorate with drops in oxygen saturation, requiring continuous BIPAP treatment and nebulizer therapy. When he required BIPAP support, his family decided on comfort care. In combination with his comorbidities of atrial fibrillation, chronic respiratory failure with hypoxia, and bilateral DVT of lower extremities, the patient unfortunately passed away 23 weeks after diagnosis due to post-obstructive pneumonia and respiratory complications.

3.3.4. Case #4

A 63-year-old male never-smoker with a history of well-controlled type II diabetes without retinopathy initially presented to his ophthalmologist with blurred vision over the left eye with intermittent, mild irritation ongoing for one month. He denied any focal neurological deficits. On examination, an amelanotic choroidal lesion with subretinal fluid on the left eye was prominent and appeared malignant. CT of chest revealed a large spiculated centrally necrotic right upper lobe mass that extended to the suprahilar region measuring approximately 5.0 × 4.3 cm. There were enlarged centrally necrotic conglomerated right lower paratracheal lymph nodes, measuring up to 20 mm in maximum short axis. Subsequent CT of chest, abdomen, and pelvis demonstrated an indeterminate 1.6 cm left adrenal nodule, and an indeterminate 8 mm lucent lesion in the L4 spinous process, metastasis not excluded. The patient followed up with pulmonologist and his symptoms of mild fatigue and recent weight loss were noted. Further workup involved endobronchial ultrasound bronchoscopy of right upper lobe mass and lymph node stations. Pathology showed adenocarcinoma immunohistochemically consistent with lung primary (TTF-1 positive, Napsin A positive, CK7 positive, CK20 negative, synaptophysin negative, chromogranin negative). PET/CT confirmed the large FDG avid right upper lobe pulmonary mass extending to the right suprahilar region measuring 7.7 SUV, ground glass and consolidative opacities involving right upper lobe, FDG right level 4 and mediastinal lymph nodes, FDG avid osseous lesions involving the T1 vertebral body, right posterior iliac bone and left acetabulum, and a 14 mm FDG avid left adrenal nodule. Brain MRI showed 4 mm enhancement in the left superior frontal gyrus, concerning for metastasis. He had his first initial consultation at COH community site approximately two months after his ophthalmology visit. He was staged as a T3N2M1c stage IVB lung adenocarcinoma. Complete NGS testing demonstrated EGFR exon 19 deletion (L747_A750 delinsP). No other driver mutations were found. Osimertinib was administered six weeks after pathologic diagnosis. Patient continues on medication and osimertinib is well tolerated. A recommendation to treat brain metastasis with radiation was withdrawn due to osimertinib's CNS penetration.

3.3.5. Case #5

A 50-year-old Asian male never-smoker presented with a productive cough and clear sputum with specks of blood approximately two years ago. His primary care doctor directed him to his gastroenterologist with the belief that the cough was secondary to gastroesophageal reflux disease. A chest X-ray ordered by the gastroenterologist revealed right lower lobe consolidation. The patient underwent a CT scan of the chest, abdomen, and pelvis a month later which showed a moderate mass-like consolidation and multifocal nodular opacities in the right lower lobe, possibly obscuring an underlying mass. Additionally, there were bilateral small 0.4 cm lung nodules, a 0.7 cm AP window lymph node, a 1.3 cm subcarinal lymph node, and a 2.2 cm right infra-hilar lymph node. The patient underwent further workup in hospital. A sputum test ruled out tuberculosis and a CT-guided lung biopsy was negative for malignancy. The patient then underwent a transbronchial lung bronchoscopy which also did not reveal malignancy. However, the bronchial brushing and washing demonstrated malignant cells consistent with adenocarcinoma with weak TTF-1 positive staining. Two months later, the patient endorsed chest wall pain and shortness of breath after long periods of coughing. An MRI scan of the brain demonstrated no evidence of brain metastasis. A PET/CT scan performed revealed strong FDG uptake in mediastinal lymph nodes, small right supraclavicular lymph nodes, and hypermetabolic pulmonary nodules bilaterally. He was staged as a TXN3M1a stage IVA lung adenocarcinoma. Molecular testing was performed and showed EGFR exon 19 deletion (E746_A750del) and TP53 286K mutation. Osimertinib was administered with good tolerance. Figure 2A–C shows the representative FFTs developed from the EGFR cases above.

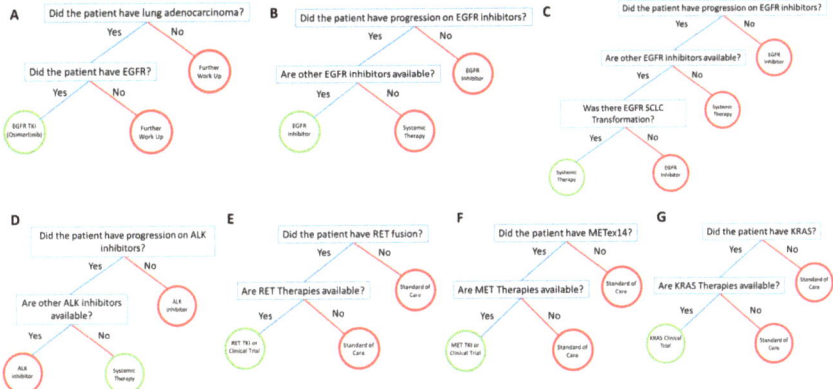

Figure 2. Fast-and-Frugal trees developed from community practice cases. (**A–C**) Representative fast-and-frugal trees for EGFR-mutated patient case scenarios. (**D**) Fast-and-frugal tree applicable to ALK mutated patient scenarios. (**E**) Fast-and-frugal tree for RET decision-making. (**F**) Fast-and-frugal tree for MET decision-making. (**G**) KRAS mutated fast-and-frugal decision-making tree.

3.4. ALK

3.4.1. Case #1

A 67-year-old Caucasian female never-smoker presented to City of Hope with an extensive history of lung cancer treated with several lines of therapy. She was staged as a T2N3M1c stage IVB lung adenocarcinoma. Initially, the patient was treated with carboplatin, taxol, and bevacizumab, but did not tolerate it well and continued pemetrexed maintenance. A few years after diagnosis, she was found to have progression and metastatic disease in the right ribs and chest wall. Molecular testing revealed an ALK-positive tumor. The patient was then started on crizotinib, ceritinib, and alectinib in sequence. Ceritinib was poorly tolerated due to significant gastrointestinal symptoms and she was switched to alectinib which she continued on for two years until the disease progressed. The patient was then started on lorlatinib and received three courses of radiation therapy due to the growing chest wall lesion. The chest wall mass measured as 2.5 to 3 cm and the patient reported pain due to the lesion. Pemetrexed was added to lorlatinib during this time. She subsequently presented to City of Hope with increased pain in the chest wall lesion with it visibly growing on the chest. Pemetrexed and lorlatinib were placed on hold as the patient had become anemic and neutropenic secondary to therapy. Due to the growing chest wall lesion, she was switched to docetaxel and ramucirumab, while also receiving 25 Gy in five fractions to the chest wall mass. The patient unfortunately developed a growing pelvic mass on the right pelvis and therapy was switched to ceritinib, as her records reported a good response to ceritinib in the past, although she did suffer from toxicity. There was improvement in the size of the chest wall lesion and the patient continues ceritinib therapy almost ten years after her initial diagnosis.

3.4.2. Case #2

An 81-year-old Asian male former smoker (12.5 pack years) presented with a history of pT3N0 poorly differentiated gastric adenocarcinoma. A robotic-converted-to-open-gastrectomy with D1+ lymphadenectomy was performed. Following the surgery, he declined adjuvant therapy and was followed on active surveillance for almost two years. During surveillance imaging, he was found to have an enlarged lower lung nodule, although he was asymptomatic for lung cancer at that time. An MRI scan of the brain demonstrated no evidence of metastatic disease within the brain. A staging PET/CT scan showed an avid mass in the posterior medial left lower lobe lung measuring up to 31 × 21 mm. The patient underwent a flexible bronchoscopy with robotic assisted left lower lobectomy and mediastinal lymph node dissection. The results revealed adenocarcinoma of lower lobe of the left lung measuring approximately 3.5 × 3 × 2.5 cm in size, with one lymph node involved. The initial immunohistochemistry performed on the specimen was positive for CK7, TTF-1, and Napsin A. Following surgical resection, the patient endorsed symptoms of productive cough with clear sputum, fatigue, poor appetite, and weight loss. Molecular testing was performed and revealed EML4-ALK fusion, PTEN R74Tfs, and SMARCA4 D696Vfs*3. He was staged as a T2aN2M0 stage IIIA lung adenocarcinoma. The patient was planned to initiate alectinib, but has not yet begun due to fear of side effects (Figure 2D). While adjuvant alectinib is not yet officially approved, the patient was deemed a poor candidate for chemotherapy due to his frailty and did not wish to have chemotherapy. Thus, based on the ALK mutation, alectinib was recommended due to the early trial results.

3.5. RET

Case #1

An 80-year-old Caucasian male with a light smoking history (<1 pack years) developed a cough, and a chest X-ray was performed that showed a persistent right upper lobe (RUL) airspace opacity consistent with pneumonia. A week later, a chest CT showed a 2.5 × 3.2 × 5 cm right upper lobe consolidation extending from the right suprahilar region to the right lung apex, and a narrowing of the right mainstem bronchus. There were also multiple right and left sub-centimeter nodules, and lesions within the superior aspect of the T4 and T9 spine. He underwent a CT-guided biopsy of the RUL which was consistent with moderate to poorly differentiated lung adenocarcinoma staining positive for TTF-1 and Napsin A and negative for p63. Partial molecular testing was negative for EGFR mutations or ALK rearrangements but stained positive for PD-L1 at 50%. Further work-up with a diagnostic PET/CT also showed an FDG-avid hepatic lesion. A brain MRI was unremarkable, with no evidence of metastatic disease. A CT-guided biopsy of the T9 lesion confirmed metastatic lung adenocarcinoma and was used for complete molecular profiling. This test revealed a RET-KIF5B fusion, TMB-high with 11 Muts/Mb, and FANCL exon 12 c.1020 + 2T > C detected. He was staged as a T3N2M1c stage IVB lung adenocarcinoma. The patient started first line systemic therapy with a combination of carboplatin, pemetrexed, and pembrolizumab and received four cycles before starting maintenance pemetrexed/pembrolizumab. He received nine maintenance cycles before developing diarrhea. A CT of the chest, abdomen, and pelvis showed rectosigmoid and proximal transverse colitis for which he was treated with prednisone, and maintenance therapy was discontinued. He remained off therapy for six months before a CT of the chest, abdomen, and pelvis showed new low-density hepatic lesions and pathologic compression fractures at T4 and T9, consistent with progressive disease. He was screened and consented for a clinical trial for the expanded access of selpercatinib (LOXO-292) for RET fusions; however, he needed to control his hypertension prior to trial initiation. After multiple adjustments of his hypertensive medications by his cardiologist, he was able to start treatment with selpercatinib (Figure 2E).

3.6. MET

Case #1

A 70-year-old female never-smoker with a past medical history of arthritis presented to an outside institution with shortness of breath and a cough. CT abdomen was performed and showed a small right pleural effusion and no evidence of an acute intra-abdominopelvic process. The patient underwent a PET/CT scan which demonstrated a medial right apical hypermetabolic pulmonary mass measuring approximately 3.1 x 2.7 cm (SUV max 12.5), with extension into the adjacent pleura, multiple additional hypermetabolic pleural-based soft tissue masses within the right hemithorax, interval mild to moderate increase in right-sided pleural effusion, and no evidence of distant metastatic disease. A CT-guided biopsy was performed on the right upper lobe mass and revealed lung adenocarcinoma. Both NGS tests demonstrated MET exon 14 splice site mutation (2888-42_2892del47) (MAF: 1.1%), TP53 G334V missense mutation (MAF: 1.5%), MSI Stable, TMB-low (9 Muts/Mb), and PD-L1 0%. She underwent an MRI of her lumbar and thoracic spine that showed a loculated pleural effusion with enhancing pleural lesions compatible with metastatic disease, lytic changes to the medial right 12th rib compatible with osseous metastatic disease, disk bulging was incidentally noted at T8, and a nonspecific 0.6 cm lesion at L1. Brain MRI at the time was negative for metastatic disease. She was staged as a T3N2M1c stage IVB lung adenocarcinoma. The patient was subsequently enrolled in a clinical trial investigating MET inhibitor capmatinib 400 BID and continued with symptomatic improvement with the first restaging scan showing response. The second interval scan showed progression with a slight increase in the right apical pleural-based mass, multiple right basilar pleural-based lesions, and a loculated right pleural effusion. The patient underwent liquid NGS testing that revealed MET exon 14 splice site (2888-42_2892del47) (MAF: 0.63% deceased from 1.1%) and TP53 G334V (MAF: 0.78% decreased from 1.5%). Progression of disease was confirmed on the third interval scan and the patient was taken off trial. She was subsequently started on carboplatin and nab-paclitaxel. Unfortunately, a restaging scan after two cycles showed interval progression of disease in the pleural-based mass, lymph nodes, and pleura. The patient presented to City of Hope for treatment options and was started on a clinical trial examining a bispecific monoclonal antibody targeting MET. She is status/post three cycles of the drug and is exhibiting stable disease thus far (Figure 2F).

3.7. KRAS

3.7.1. Case #1

A 68-year-old Caucasian female former smoker (20 pack years) presented with a cough. An initial chest CT showed a 5.4 × 5.7 cm left upper lobe lesion with numerous bilateral sub-centimeter nodules. CT-guided core needle biopsy of the left upper lobe mass revealed moderately differentiated lung adenocarcinoma. Molecular profiling of the biopsy was negative for EGFR mutations, ALK rearrangements, ROS1 rearrangements, and PD-L1. Subsequent NGS of the biopsy revealed KRAS G12A, CDKN2A/B loss, LMO1 R34H, NOTCH1 splice site 2467 + 1G > TA, and TMB-intermediate with 13 Muts/Mb. A brain MRI showed a 2 mm lesion in the right prefrontal gyrus adjacent to the central sulcus of unclear etiology. In repeat brain MRIs, this lesion had resolved and was no longer present. To finish staging, a diagnostic PET/CT showed a 6 cm mass FDG avid with an SUV of 9.6 and multiple bilateral FDG avid pulmonary nodules. She was staged as a T3NXM1a stage IVA lung adenocarcinoma. She initiated first-line systemic therapy with cisplatin and pemetrexed for three cycles with very little response. Concurrent radiation to the left upper lobe primary and mediastinum was added to regimen with no significant toxicities. With no other signs of metastatic disease, she underwent a wedge resection and one of the pulmonary nodules showed metastatic disease. Thus, the rest of the procedure was aborted. She received second-line atezolizumab without disease progression for 17 months. A new CT-guided biopsy of the right lower lobe lung was performed and was confirmed as metastatic lung adenocarcinoma. NGS molecular profiling revealed KRAS G12A, KRAS L19F, KIT A829S, PDGFRA T365N, PTEN deletion, and TMB-high with 11.4 Muts/Mb. She started third-line systemic therapy with carboplatin, paclitaxel, bevacizumab, and pembrolizumab for a total of five cycles. She is currently status/post seven cycles of maintenance bevacizumab and pembrolizumab without signs of disease progression.

3.7.2. Case #2

An 80-year-old Caucasian male never-smoker had a history of hairy cell leukemia that was treated approximately 20 years ago with chemotherapy (cladribine) for eight days and continues to follow up regularly. The patient was diagnosed with early stage lung cancer two years ago, following a biopsy of a lung nodule in the right lower lobe. He had a platinum coil as fiducial marker placed at that time. A year later, the patient underwent radiation therapy for a malignant neoplasm of the lower lobe right bronchus. Unfortunately, his disease progressed, and the patient was deemed non-operable due to medical comorbidities including diabetes mellitus, a history of coronary artery disease, and a history of hairy cell leukemia. A PET/CT scan performed ten months after radiation revealed a hypermetabolic right lower lobe pulmonary mass with central metallic fiducial marker unchanged in size and metabolic activity compared to a prior study with increased right pleural effusion. A thoracentesis performed shortly after demonstrated malignant cells seen as single cells, comprising 1–2% cellularity. Following the thoracentesis procedure, the patient reported improvement to his shortness of breath. Additionally, he reported neuropathy secondary to diabetes mellitus onset eight years ago, which is controlled, and he continues to follow up with endocrinology. He was staged as a T2NXM1a stage IVA lung adenocarcinoma. Molecular testing was performed, and results revealed BRAF V600E, NRAS G12D, KRAS G12S, PDL1 100%, meanwhile the BRAF V600E IHC was negative. The patient was subsequently initiated on pembrolizumab. One week after his first cycle, he was admitted to hospital for pneumonitis, chest pain, onset fever, transaminitis, and elevated blood pressure without previous diagnosis of HTN, thrombocytopenia, and nephrolithiasis. He was treated with IV Rocephin, oral oxycline, pain control, and given a pulmonary consultation. The patient was discharged with antibiotics. The patient continues on pembrolizumab with continued symptoms of fatigue and decreased appetite (Figure 2G).

4. Discussion

Between 2013–2017, there were 68,369 total cases of invasive cancers and 6,541 cases of lung cancer in Orange County, according to the California Cancer Registry. Age-adjusted invasive cancer incidence demonstrates that Orange County accounted for higher cancer rates compared to Los Angeles County (394.93 vs. 371.36 per 100,000 cases, respectively). Similarly, age-adjusted lung cancer incidence rate in Orange County is higher than in Los Angeles county (38.29 vs. 35.88 per 100,000 cases, respectively) [38]. Located in Orange County, Newport Beach is the newest community site in the City of Hope network. Demographic information was assessed for new patients in the first four months of operation, beginning in January 2020. Only initial new patient visits were accounted for, thereby excluding subsequent follow-up visits from the count. We identified 182 new patients, 118 (64.8%) of whom were female and 64 (35.2%) of whom were male. The median age of the patients was 63 years, ranging from 22 to 90 years. The most prevalent ethnicities were Caucasian (n = 96, 52.7%) and Asian (n = 16, 8.8%). Among the 182 patients, 28 were diagnosed with cancer in the lung or bronchus, 11 of whom were presented in this report.

Fast-and-frugal trees (FFTs) are an effective way to make binary classification decisions under time pressure conditions with only limited information [36,39]. One example to illustrate this is the decision of whether to send a patient to coronary care or a regular hospital bed if a patient reports chest pain [40]. FFTs can be used to evaluate standard guidelines and establish new decision-making heuristic strategies, allowing physicians to make fast and accurate decisions without relying on statistical training or calculation devices. An FFT is a decision tree composed of sequentially ordered cues such as diagnostic test results or clinical information and the accompanying binary decision (yes/no) of those cues [36,41–43]. The relationship between the cues can be framed as "if-then" statements; for instance, if a patient has severe chest pain, then the physician should perform tests for myocardial infraction. If the condition of the cues is met, then the decision can be made, and the FFT exited. If the condition is not met, the FFT sequentially considers other cues, until a cue's exit condition is met. The last cue of an FFT has two exits to ensure that a decision is ultimately made [36,41–44]. Formally, an FFT is defined as a decision tree that has m + 1 exits, with one exit for each of the first m-1 cues, and two exits for the last cue [36,41–44]. The FFT tool is robust, and it can be used to both evaluate established clinical pathways and guidelines, but also to develop new FFT-based decision-making trees that incorporate additional clinical data like molecular testing results. The identification of driver mutations for NSCLC has transformed patient care, such that patients who are properly screened with molecular testing have better outcomes than those who are not [45]. We wanted to develop an omics-based FFT that would outline the clinical course of action a physician should undertake when facing molecular cues.

In our analysis, we had identified individual mutational subgroups to develop fast-and-frugal trees. From the five cases of *EGFR* patients, three FFTs were developed according to their individual cases. The heuristic steps in these FFTs were similar for most patients except for one who had small cell lung cancer transformation, which has been previously associated with prolonged EGFR TKI treatment [46,47]. However, the FFT was flexible enough and the addition of one additional step resolved the issue of systemic therapy (platinum/etoposide) for the SCLC transformation. These experiences were similar for the other molecular cases including *ALK, RET, MET,* and *KRAS*. Decisions could be made with either two or three queues without sacrificing the accurate decision based on limited information. As FFTs can be used to give form and structure to patterns, our analysis introduced a pattern regarding molecular decision-making. In each case, the final decision was dependent on the first question to be asked: "Was a molecular target detected?". Without first answering that question, the oncologist cannot move on in their decision-making and should therefore consider ordering molecular testing. The subsequent question was also directly related: "Are targeted therapies available?". This question would allow physicians to consider targeted therapies for all molecular markers in our analysis. Furthermore, we found this question to be important as it applied to even novel genetic targets such as KRAS whose targeted therapies are still under clinical trials. Therefore, the final question to be asked is: "Are trials available?". The versatility of this question is that it allows an interpretation of genomic data not only based on FDA-approved therapies, but also on novel clinical trial drugs, such as KRAS inhibitor MRTX849 [26], that are still under evaluation. With these questions, we developed a comprehensive molecular decision-making FFT for stage IV lung cancer patients (Figure 3).

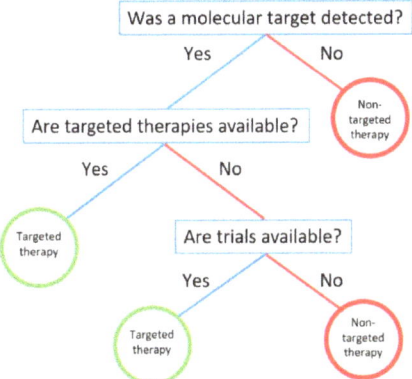

Figure 3. Comprehensive fast-and-frugal decision tree for lung cancer. A comprehensive molecular fast-and-frugal tree for stage IV lung cancer decision-making.

The advantage of a molecular FFT is that it applies to all molecular targets and while NCCN guidelines and other pathways have incorporated a few molecular targets such as EGFR, ALK, ROS1, and BRAF, they do not include MET, RET, NTRK or KRAS, for which therapies are quickly emerging and showing immense benefits to patients [48–52]. Our FFT would benefit community practice as it would incorporate those molecular targets into the decision-making strategy regardless of whether the therapy is FDA-approved or if it is in a clinical trial. The versatility of the FFT strategy shows that simple heuristics can be utilized efficiently to arrive at accurate decisions, and incorporating such FFTs into community practice can not only help with decision-making, but can also transform the decisions that oncologists make daily into a cognitive science.

4.1. EGFR

EGFR is a transmembrane protein that exists as a monomer on the surface of a cell. EGFR is a receptor tyrosine kinase, therefore it dimerizes with its specific ligand to activate the tyrosine kinase (TK) [53]. Once activated, the EGFR TK activates pathways which synthesize DNA and cause cell proliferation [54]. Thus, mutations or amplification of EGFR result in tumor growth/cancer. Predominant mutation locations include exon 19 deletions and exon 21 L858R point mutations [55]. EGFR mutations also occur more commonly in nonsmokers, women, and in people of Asian descent. A study demonstrated that EGFR mutations occurred in 42% of females compared to 14% of males and in 51% of nonsmokers compared to 10% of smokers [56]. EGFR TKIs have been heavily explored and single agent TKIs such as erlotinib, gefitinib (first generation), and afatinib (second generation) have become standard of care for EGFR mutant NSCLC patients. Osimertinib (a third generation TKI) emerged as a first-line treatment when it demonstrated improved outcomes when compared to outcomes with erlotinib and gefitinib in the FLAURA trial [57]. The FLAURA trial was conducted with 556 NSCLC patients with EGFR exon deletion or exon 21 L858R point mutation. Osimertinib showed improved PFS (18.9 vs. 10.2 months) and OS (83% vs. 71% at 18 months) when compared to standard of care treatment with gefitinib or erlotinib [58]. Dacomitinib, a second-generation single agent EGFR TKI, was approved by the FDA in 2018 as a first-line treatment for metastatic NSCLC based on the ARCHER 1050 trial [59]. The ARCHER 1050 trial compared dacomitinib to gefitinib in 452 patients with metastatic NSCLC and demonstrated a survival benefit in PFS (14.7 vs. 9.2 months) and OS (34.1 vs. 26.8 months) [60]. Several studies have demonstrated that patients who initially respond well to an EGFR TKI develop resistance, and subsequently their disease progresses [61–63]. Secondary EGFR mutations and MET amplifications are the most well-known causes of resistance [64,65]. Osimertinib selectively inhibits both EGFR-TKI-sensitizing and EGFR T790M resistance mutations, making it a valuable treatment against TKI-acquired resistance [12]. Alternative treatment options currently explored are combination therapies such as EGFR inhibitors along with bevacizumab or ramucirumab, vascular endothelial growth factor receptor inhibitors, EGFR inhibitors with chemotherapy, and EGFR inhibitors with other targeted therapy [66–68].

4.2. ALK

Initially identified in 2007, the formation of echinoderm microtubule-associated protein like-4 (EML4)-ALK fusion protein in NSCLC leads to constitutive oncogenic signaling. Patients with NSCLC harboring ALK translocations were estimated to be in approximately 6% of all NSCLC cases. Four years later, crizotinib became the first oral, ALK TKI approved by the FDA [69]. As a first-line treatment, crizotinib was shown to be safe and effective in a single arm, open-label, phase III clinical trial [70,71]. Among the patients who received prior systemic therapy, crizotinib showed an ORR of 50% and an improved quality of life compared to those on chemotherapy. PFS was improved for patients on crizotinib compared to standard of care chemotherapy by 3.9 months (10.9 vs. 7.0 months, respectively). However, the study showed that there was no difference in OS (approximately 12 months). Subsequently, other targeted therapies were developed as resistance eventually developed in advanced ALK-positive NSCLC patients. Acquired resistance mechanisms such as the amino acid substitution L1196M in the ALK gene against crizotinib have been explored [72]. Acting as a gatekeeper mutation, ALK L1196M impedes crizotinib's efficacy in ALK-positive NSCLC patients. A hypothesis of resistance involves decreased binding energy within an unstable secondary structure of the mutant ALK complex [73]. The equivalence of this mutation is the EGFR mutation T790M that confers resistance to erlotinib or gefitinib [74]. Development of second-generation ALK inhibitors including ceritinib, alectinib, and brigatinib, were sequentially approved after crizotinib in 2011. Barrows et al. outlined observational studies of sequential treatment with several ALK inhibitors [75]. Effects from consecutive treatment with ALK inhibitors may be additive in terms of survival outcomes in patients. In order to overcome ALK resistance, the discovery of new ALK inhibitors is pivotal and essential in the clinical setting.

4.3. RET

Activation of the RET gene leads to cell proliferation, migration, and differentiation, and can be found on chromosome 10q11.2 [76,77]. The proto-oncogene *RET* interacts with multiple downstream pathways including JAK/STAT, MAPK/ERK, and PI3K/AKT [78]. In 1985, the RET rearrangement was seen for the first time when lymphoma DNA was transfected in NIH-3T3 cells [79]. Mutations and rearrangements in RET are most commonly observed in papillary thyroid carcinomas and in lung cancer [80]. RET fusions lead to tumorigenesis by continuous activation via ligand-independent dimerization and autophosphorylation of the RET kinase and its downstream partners [81]. RET most frequently fuses with KIF5B in NSCLC but other fusion gene partners have been observed in CCDC6, NCOA4, and TRIM33 [82]. In NSCLC, RET rearrangement is detected in 1–2% of cases, typically adenocarcinoma histology, and without a history of smoking [83,84]. Several multi-kinase TKIs have been utilized in targeting RET rearrangements in NSCLC. In a phase II study, cabozantinib, targeting VEGFR, MET, and RET, was shown to have an ORR of 28%, a median PFS of 5.5 months, and a median OS of 9.9 months in 26 RET fusion-positive NSCLC patients [20]. A phase II study of 17 RET fusion-positive NSCLC patients previously treated with chemotherapy received vandetanib, targeting VEGFR 2 and 3, EGFR, and RET, and the trial demonstrated a 53% ORR, a median PFS of 4.7 months, and a median OS of 11.1 months [85]. A new generation of novel RET inhibitors are currently being investigated such as selpercatinib (LOXO-292) and pralsetinib (BLU-667). The phase I/II LIBRETTO-001 trial investigating selpercatinib RET-rearranged NSCLC patients with previous therapy found an ORR of 68% [86,87]. Selpercatinib was recently awarded FDA approval for adult patients with RET-positive NSCLC based on the previous trial with an ORR of 85% in treatment of naïve patients [88]. In a phase I study of pralsetinib, an ORR of 58% was demonstrated for all patients regardless of RET fusion type and was effective against intracranial metastases [89].

4.4. MET

MET proto-oncogene encodes for c-Met, a member of the receptor tyrosine kinase (RTK) family. Once activated, c-MET is involved in various signaling cascades linked to cell growth, apoptosis, motility, and invasion. Mutations in MET represent 6% of all NSCLC cases with frequent alterations including MET exon 14 skipping mutation and MET amplification [90]. Since its discovery in lung cancer and other solid tumor malignancies, research has been investigating potential targeting of MET through small molecule inhibitors or monoclonal antibodies. Initially, a phase II clinical trial enrolled recurrent NSCLC, which were randomized to receive onartuzumab with erlotinib or placebo with erlotinib [91]. In NSCLC patients with MET-mutated disease, treatment with onartuzumab plus erlotinib demonstrated improved PFS and OS, although the drug combination failed in a subsequent phase III trial [92]. A landmark study of 4,622 NSCLC patients with ALK rearrangement or MET amplification, of which 16 exhibited both alterations. The ORR was 86.7% in that subset of patients, suggesting a role of MET TKI treatment in MET-expressing tumors [93]. METROS, a phase II clinical trial, investigated the use of crizotinib—a multikinase inhibitor against ALK, ROS1, and MET—in MET or ROS1-positive pretreated, advanced NSCLC [94]. The trial confirmed anti-tumor activity with an ORR of 27%, a median PFS of 4.4 months, and an OS of 5.4 months. Another recent trial of 69 patients with MET exon 14 skipping mutated-NSCLC treated with crizotinib demonstrated encouraging data with an ORR of 32%, a median PFS of 7.3 months, and a median OS of 20.5 months [95]. Currently, there are several promising trials examining the therapeutic efficacy of other MET TKIs, such as cabozantinib (NCT03911193), cabozantinib (NCT02750215), REGN5093 (NCT04077099), tepotinib monotherapy (NCT02864992) plus osimertinib (NCT03940703), and telisotuzumab vedotin (NCT03539536). Of note, capmantinib was recently approved by the FDA for treatment of MET exon 14 skipping mutated-NSCLC due to results from the GEOMETRY mono-1 clinical trial [96].

4.5. KRAS

With an incidence rate of up to 22% in solid tumor malignancies, KRAS is one of the most prevalent oncogenic driver mutations in cancer [97]. In 1973, a murine sarcoma virus transformed mammalian genes into an oncogene in KRAS, and nearly a decade later, a human lung carcinoma cell line first showed human sequences analogous to the KRAS oncogenes in mice [98,99]. KRAS mutations in patients with advanced NSCLC are shown to have a poorer prognosis and often lack a response to standard therapies [100]. The KRAS oncoprotein triggers tumor cell growth and survival because it acts as a crucial mediator of intrasellar signaling pathways [101,102]. KRAS activating point mutations generally cause a loss of GTPase activity, and consequentially allow for the continuous activation of downstream signaling pathways such as MAPK and PI3K [103]. KRAS mutations have most recently been seen in exon 12 and 13 with the most common being G12C at 39%, G12V between 18–21%, and G12D between 17–18% [104]. In patients with lung adenocarcinoma, approximately 13% harbor a mutation of KRAS G12C [105]. KRAS mutant lung adenocarcinoma patients with concurrent inactivating mutations in the tumor suppressor genes of KEAP1 and STK11 have demonstrated lower clinical response rates treated with standard chemotherapy or immunotherapies [30,106]. KRAS G12C small molecule inhibitor, AMG-510, is the first in-human, phase I investigation in patients with advanced KRAS G12C solid tumors (NCT03600883). Taken orally, once daily, AMG-510 is a specific and irreversible inhibitor of KRAS G12C by fixing the guanosine diphosphate-bound state of the protein at an His95 groove in the P2 pocket of KRAS. Overall, the treatment was well tolerated. Twenty-two patients with results were presented and six of these patients had NSCLC. The median duration of treatment was 9.7 weeks. Two patients experienced a partial response and two had stable disease after six weeks [27,107]. Several other inhibitors including MRTX849 (NCT03785249) that target KRAS G12C and other KRAS mutation variants are currently being investigated in clinical trials.

4.6. Future Directions

The advantage of FFTs is that they are quick and accurate decisions based on limited information. This is useful in the world of oncology as unlike guidelines and pathways, FFTs do not restrict physicians to "on-pathway" and "off-pathway" decisions. FFTs incorporate physician's "instinct" and "personal expertise" to arrive at a quick decision most beneficial to the patient. While this study was limited by sample size and a relatively focused cohort to one community oncology practice, the lesson of a standardized FFT frameworks have been shown to be applicable to not only stage IV lung cancer, but also to the early stage setting in the future. This study was limited to patients from one community practice, with a majority of patients demonstrating actionable mutations which does not completely represent the comprehensive population in community practice. Evaluating a larger cohort would be needed to further understand other treatment paradigms in NSCLC. However, in the future, it will be important to standardize the utilization of these FFTs to a usable application that physicians can refer to when reviewing their cases. This application would be most beneficial to community sites, as it would be a direct translation of the academic model to the community and would guide physicians towards the accurate decision without sacrificing their expertise. At the same time, we understand that the complexity of oncology practice varies from the cancer and the stage of the disease. Therefore, it will be important in certain situations to apply not only FFT heuristics, but also to incorporate multi-layered decisions of convolutional neural networks [108] and the quick capabilities of fast-and-frugal decision trees [33,35] into a hybrid model, conditional neural network. This would allow for the model to utilize the efficiency of fast-and-frugal decision trees and the accuracy of convolutional neural networks in a unified model.

Author Contributions: Conceptualization, R.S., I.M., T.T., D.P.P., H.C., A.B., J.F., R.P., H.R., T.W., R.B., L.B., P.K., M.C., B.D., S.K.P.; Methodology, I.M., T.T., A.S., A.B., J.F., R.P., H.R., P.K., M.C., B.D., S.K.P.; Validation, R.S., I.M., T.T., J.F., R.P., H.R., T.W., L.B., M.C., S.K.P.; Investigation, R.S., I.M., T.T., A.S., D.P.P., H.C., A.B., J.F., R.P., R.B., P.K., B.D., S.K.P.; Formal Analysis, R.S., I.M., A.S., D.P.P., A.B., J.F., R.P., H.R., B.D.; Data Curation, R.S., I.M., T.T., A.S., A.B., J.F., R.P., H.R., B.D., S.K.P.; Funding acquisition, R.S.; Project administration, R.S.; Resources, R.S., T.T., H.C.; Software, I.M.; Supervision, R.S., D.P.P.; Visualization, I.M., T.T., H.C., R.P.; Writing—Original Draft Preparation; R.S., I.M.; Writing—Review and Editing, R.S., I.M., T.T., A.S., D.P.P., H.C., A.B., J.F., R.P., H.R., T.W., R.B., L.B., P.K., M.C., B.D., S.K.P. All authors have read and agreed to the published version of the manuscript.

Funding: This research received no external funding.

Acknowledgments: We would like to thank Newport Beach City of Hope staff for their skill and dedication in helping the patients. We would also like to express our deepest gratitude for the philanthropic funding by the Tenenblatt Family. The work was supported by the National Cancer Institute of the National Institutes of Health under award numbers P30CA033572, U54CA209978, R01CA247471, and R01CA218545.

Conflicts of Interest: The authors declare no conflict of interest.

References

1. Jemal, A.; Siegel, R.; Ward, E.; Murray, T.; Xu, J.; Smigal, C.; Thun, M.J. Cancer statistics, 2006. *CA Cancer J. Clin.* **2006**, *56*, 106–130. [CrossRef] [PubMed]
2. Siegel, R.L.; Miller, K.D.; Jemal, A. Cancer statistics, 2020. *CA Cancer J. Clin.* **2020**, *70*, 7–30. [CrossRef] [PubMed]
3. Salgia, R. Mutation testing for directing upfront targeted therapy and post-progression combination therapy strategies in lung adenocarcinoma. *Expert Rev. Mol. Diagn.* **2016**, *16*, 737–749. [CrossRef] [PubMed]
4. Hensing, T.; Chawla, A.; Batra, R.; Salgia, R. A Personalized Treatment for Lung Cancer: Molecular Pathways, Targeted Therapies, and Genomic Characterization. *Adv. Exp. Med. Biol.* **2014**, *799*, 85–117. [CrossRef]
5. Mok, T.S.; Wu, Y.-L.; Thongprasert, S.; Yang, J.C.-H.; Chu, D.-T.; Saijo, N.; Sunpaweravong, P.; Han, B.; Margono, B.; Ichinose, Y.; et al. Gefitinib or Carboplatin–Paclitaxel in Pulmonary Adenocarcinoma. *N. Engl. J. Med.* **2009**, *361*, 947–957. [CrossRef]
6. Planchard, D.; Besse, B.; Groen, H.J.M.; Souquet, P.-J.; Quoix, E.; Baik, C.S.; Barlesi, F.; Kim, T.M.; Mazieres, J.; Novello, S.; et al. Dabrafenib plus trametinib in patients with previously treated BRAF(V600E)-mutant metastatic non-small cell lung cancer: An open-label, phase 2 trial. *Lancet Oncol.* **2017**, *18*, 1307–1316. [CrossRef]
7. Soria, J.-C.; Wu, Y.-L.; Nakagawa, K.; Kim, S.-W.; Yang, J.-J.; Ahn, M.-J.; Wang, J.; Yang, J.C.-H.; Lu, Y.; Atagi, S.; et al. Gefitinib plus chemotherapy versus placebo plus chemotherapy in EGFR-mutation-positive non-small-cell lung cancer after progression on first-line gefitinib (IMPRESS): A phase 3 randomised trial. *Lancet Oncol.* **2015**, *16*, 990–998. [CrossRef]
8. Rosell, R.; Carcereny, E.; Gervais, R.; Vergnenègre, A.; Massuti, B.; Felip, E.; Palmero, R.; Garcia-Gomez, R.; Pallares, C.; Sanchez, J.M.; et al. Erlotinib versus standard chemotherapy as first-line treatment for European patients with advanced EGFR mutation-positive non-small-cell lung cancer (EURTAC): A multicentre, open-label, randomised phase 3 trial. *Lancet Oncol.* **2012**, *13*, 239–246. [CrossRef]
9. Sequist, L.V.; Yang, J.C.-H.; Yamamoto, N.; O'Byrne, K.; Hirsh, V.; Mok, T.S.; Geater, S.L.; Orlov, S.V.; Tsai, C.-M.; Boyer, M.; et al. Phase III Study of Afatinib or Cisplatin Plus Pemetrexed in Patients with Metastatic Lung Adenocarcinoma with EGFR Mutations. *J. Clin. Oncol.* **2013**, *31*, 3327–3334. [CrossRef]
10. Le Tourneau, C.; Delord, J.-P.; Gonçalves, A.; Gavoille, C.; Dubot, C.; Isambert, N.; Campone, M.; Tredan, O.; Massiani, M.-A.; Mauborgne, C.; et al. Molecularly targeted therapy based on tumour molecular profiling versus conventional therapy for advanced cancer (SHIVA): A multicentre, open-label, proof-of-concept, randomised, controlled phase 2 trial. *Lancet Oncol.* **2015**, *16*, 1324–1334. [CrossRef]
11. Shepherd, F.A.; Pereira, J.R.; Ciuleanu, T.; Tan, E.H.; Hirsh, V.; Thongprasert, S.; Campos, D.; Maoleekoonpiroj, S.; Smylie, M.; Martins, R.; et al. Erlotinib in Previously Treated Non–Small-Cell Lung Cancer. *N. Engl. J. Med.* **2005**, *353*, 123–132. [CrossRef]
12. Ramalingam, S.S.; Vansteenkiste, J.; Planchard, D.; Cho, B.C.; Gray, J.E.; Ohe, Y.; Zhou, C.; Reungwetwattana, T.; Cheng, Y.; Chewaskulyong, B.; et al. Overall Survival with Osimertinib in Untreated, EGFR-Mutated Advanced NSCLC. *N. Engl. J. Med.* **2020**, *382*, 41–50. [CrossRef]

13. Zhou, C.; Wu, Y.L.; Chen, G.; Feng, J.; Liu, X.-Q.; Wang, C.; Zhang, S.; Wang, J.; Zhou, S.; Ren, S.; et al. Final overall survival results from a randomised, phase III study of erlotinib versus chemotherapy as first-line treatment of EGFR mutation-positive advanced non-small-cell lung cancer (OPTIMAL, CTONG-0802). *Ann. Oncol.* **2015**, *26*, 1877–1883. [CrossRef]
14. Leighl, N.B.; Karaseva, N.; Nakagawa, K.; Cho, B.C.; Gray, J.E.; Hovey, T.; Walding, A.; Rydén, A.; Novello, S. Patient-reported outcomes from FLAURA: Osimertinib versus erlotinib or gefitinib in patients with EGFR-mutated advanced non-small-cell lung cancer. *Eur. J. Cancer* **2020**, *125*, 49–57. [CrossRef]
15. Kris, M.G.; Johnson, B.E.; Kwiatkowski, D.J.; Iafrate, A.J.; Wistuba, I.I.; Aronson, S.L.; Engelman, J.A.; Shyr, Y.; Khuri, F.R.; Rudin, C.M.; et al. Identification of driver mutations in tumor specimens from 1,000 patients with lung adenocarcinoma: The NCI's Lung Cancer Mutation Consortium (LCMC). *J. Clin. Oncol.* **2011**, *29* (Suppl. 18). [CrossRef]
16. Lindeman, N.I.; Cagle, P.T.; Aisner, D.L.; Arcila, M.E.; Beasley, M.B.; Bernicker, E.H.; Colasacco, C.; Dacic, S.; Hirsch, F.R.; Kerr, K.; et al. Updated Molecular Testing Guideline for the Selection of Lung Cancer Patients for Treatment With Targeted Tyrosine Kinase Inhibitors: Guideline From the College of American Pathologists, the International Association for the Study of Lung Cancer, and the Association for Molecular Pathology. *J. Thorac. Oncol.* **2018**, *13*, 323–358.
17. Pacheco, J.M.; Gao, D.; Smith, D.; Purcell, T.; Hancock, M.; Bunn, P.; Robin, T.; Liu, A.; Karam, S.; Gaspar, L.; et al. Natural History and Factors Associated with Overall Survival in Stage IV ALK-Rearranged Non–Small Cell Lung Cancer. *J. Thorac. Oncol.* **2019**, *14*, 691–700. [CrossRef] [PubMed]
18. Ramalingam, S.S.; Yang, J.C.-H.; Lee, C.K.; Kurata, T.; Kim, D.-W.; John, T.; Nogami, N.; Ohe, Y.; Mann, H.; Rukazenkov, Y.; et al. Osimertinib As First-Line Treatment of EGFR Mutation–Positive Advanced Non–Small-Cell Lung Cancer. *J. Clin. Oncol.* **2018**, *36*, 841–849. [CrossRef] [PubMed]
19. Shaw, A.T.; Felip, E.; Bauer, T.M.; Besse, B.; Navarro, A.; Postel-Vinay, S.; Gainor, J.; Johnson, M.; Dietrich, J.; James, L.P.; et al. Lorlatinib in non-small-cell lung cancer with ALK or ROS1 rearrangement: An international, multicentre, open-label, single-arm first-in-man phase 1 trial. *Lancet Oncol.* **2017**, *18*, 1590–1599. [CrossRef]
20. Drilon, A.; Rekhtman, N.; Arcila, M.; Wang, L.; Ni, A.; Albano, M.; Van Voorthuysen, M.; Somwar, R.; Smith, R.S.; Montecalvo, J.; et al. Cabozantinib in patients with advanced RET-rearranged non-small-cell lung cancer: An open-label, single-centre, phase 2, single-arm trial. *Lancet Oncol.* **2016**, *17*, 1653–1660. [CrossRef]
21. Hyman, D.M.; Puzanov, I.; Subbiah, V.; Faris, J.E.; Chau, I.; Blay, J.-Y.; Wolf, J.; Raje, N.S.; Diamond, E.L.; Hollebecque, A.; et al. Vemurafenib in Multiple Nonmelanoma Cancers with BRAF V600 Mutations. *N. Engl. J. Med.* **2015**, *373*, 726–736. [CrossRef]
22. Chuang, J.C.; Stehr, H.; Liang, Y.; Das, M.; Huang, J.; Diehn, M.; Wakelee, H.A.; Neal, J.W. ERBB2-Mutated Metastatic Non-Small Cell Lung Cancer: Response and Resistance to Targeted Therapies. *J. Thorac. Oncol.* **2017**, *12*, 833–842. [CrossRef]
23. Paik, P.K.; Veillon, R.; Cortot, A.B.; Felip, E.; Sakai, H.; Mazieres, J.; Griesinger, F.; Horn, L.; Senellart, H.; Van Meerbeeck, J.P.; et al. Phase II study of tepotinib in NSCLC patients with METex14 mutations. *J. Clin. Oncol.* **2019**, *37*, 9005. [CrossRef]
24. Adjei, A.A.; Mauer, A.; Bruzek, L.; Marks, R.S.; Hillman, S.; Geyer, S.; Hanson, L.J.; Wright, J.J.; Erlichman, C.; Kaufmann, S.H.; et al. Phase II Study of the Farnesyl Transferase Inhibitor R115777 in Patients With Advanced Non–Small-Cell Lung Cancer. *J. Clin. Oncol.* **2003**, *21*, 1760–1766. [CrossRef]
25. Kris, M.G.; Johnson, B.E.; Berry, L.D.; Kwiatkowski, D.J.; Iafrate, A.J.; Wistuba, I.I.; Varella-Garcia, M.; Franklin, W.A.; Aronson, S.L.; Su, P.-F.; et al. Using multiplexed assays of oncogenic drivers in lung cancers to select targeted drugs. *JAMA* **2014**, *311*, 1998–2006. [CrossRef]
26. Hallin, J.; Engstrom, L.D.; Hargis, L.; Calinisan, A.; Aranda, R.; Briere, D.M.; Sudhakar, N.; Bowcut, V.; Baer, B.R.; Ballard, J.A.; et al. The KRASG12C Inhibitor MRTX849 Provides Insight toward Therapeutic Susceptibility of KRAS-Mutant Cancers in Mouse Models and Patients. *Cancer Discov.* **2020**, *10*, 54–71. [CrossRef]
27. Canon, J.; Rex, K.; Saiki, A.Y.; Mohr, C.; Cooke, K.; Bagal, D.; Gaida, K.; Holt, T.; Knutson, C.G.; Koppada, N.; et al. The clinical KRAS(G12C) inhibitor AMG 510 drives anti-tumour immunity. *Nature* **2019**, *575*, 217–223. [CrossRef]
28. Liu, C.; Zheng, S.; Jin, R.; Wang, X.; Wang, F.; Zang, R.; Xu, H.; Lu, Z.; Huang, J.; Lei, Y.; et al. The superior efficacy of anti-PD-1/PD-L1 immunotherapy in KRAS-mutant non-small cell lung cancer that correlates with an inflammatory phenotype and increased immunogenicity. *Cancer Lett.* **2020**, *470*, 95–105. [CrossRef]

29. Amanam, I.; Mambetsariev, I.; Gupta, R.; Achuthan, S.; Wang, Y.; Pharaon, R.; Massarelli, E.; Koczywas, M.; Reckamp, K.; Salgia, R. Role of immunotherapy and co-mutations on KRAS-mutant non-small cell lung cancer survival. *J Thorac Dis.* **2020**. In Press.
30. Jeanson, A.; Tomasini, P.; Souquet-Bressand, M.; Brandone, N.; Boucekine, M.; Grangeon, M.; Chaleat, S.; Khobta, N.; Milia, J.; Mhanna, L.; et al. Efficacy of Immune Checkpoint Inhibitors in KRAS-Mutant Non-Small Cell Lung Cancer (NSCLC). *J. Thorac. Oncol.* **2019**, *14*, 1095–1101. [CrossRef]
31. Hanna, N.H.; Temin, S.; Masters, G. Therapy for Stage IV Non-Small-Cell Lung Cancer without Driver Alterations: ASCO and OH (CCO) Joint Guideline Update. *J. Oncol. Pract.* **2020**, *38*, 1608–1632. [CrossRef]
32. National Comprehensive Cancer Network. NCCN Clinical Practice Guidelines in Oncology. 2019. Available online: https://www.nccn.org/professionals/physician_gls/default.aspx (accessed on 8 May 2020).
33. Mambetsariev, I.; Pharaon, R.; Nam, A.; Knopf, K.; Djulbegovic, B.; Villaflor, V.M.; Vokes, E.E.; Salgia, R. Heuristic value-based framework for lung cancer decision-making. *Oncotarget* **2018**, *9*, 29877–29891. [CrossRef] [PubMed]
34. Hozo, I.; Djulbegovic, B.; Luan, S.; Tsalatsanis, A.; Gigerenzer, G. Towards theory integration: Threshold model as a link between signal detection theory, fast-and-frugal trees and evidence accumulation theory. *J. Eval. Clin. Pract.* **2017**, *23*, 49–65. [CrossRef] [PubMed]
35. Djulbegovic, B.; Hozo, I.; Dale, W. Transforming clinical practice guidelines and clinical pathways into fast-and-frugal decision trees to improve clinical care strategies. *J. Eval. Clin. Pract.* **2018**, *24*, 1247–1254. [CrossRef]
36. Martignon, L.; Katsikopoulos, K.V.; Woike, J.K. Categorization with limited resources: A family of simple heuristics. *J. Math. Psychol.* **2008**, *52*, 352–361. [CrossRef]
37. Woike, J.K.; Hoffrage, U.; Hertwig, R. Estimating Quantities: Comparing Simple Heuristics and Machine Learning Algorithms. In *Lecture Notes in Computer Science, Proceedings of the Artificial Neural Networks and Machine Learning—ICANN 2012, Lausanne, Switzerland, 11–14 September 2012*; Villa, A.E.P., Duch, W., Érdi, P., Masulli, F., Palm, G., Eds.; Springer: Berlin/Heidelberg, Germany; p. 7553.
38. Registry, C.C. Age-Adjusted Cancer Mortality Rates in California. Cancer Incidence and Mortality Data by Geographic Region. Cancer-Rates.Info Is a Contractual Web Service Hosted by the Kentucky Cancer Registry at the Markey Cancer Center at the University of Kentucky (http://www.kcr.uky.edu). Data Are Provided by Participating Population-Based Central Cancer Registries. Inquiries or Questions Related to Data Content Should Be Directed to California Cancer Registry. Available online: http://cancer-rates.info/ca (accessed on 9 May 2020).
39. Martignon, L.; Vitouch, O.; Takezawa, M.; Forster, R. Naive and Yet Enlightened: From Natural Frequencies to Fast and Frugal Decision Trees. In *Thinking: Psychological Perspectives on Reasoning, Judgment and Decision Making*; Hardman, D., Macchi, L., Eds.; Wiley Online Library: Hoboken, NJ, USA, 2003.
40. Green, L.; Mehr, D.R. What alters physicians' decisions to admit to the coronary care unit? *J. Fam. Pract.* **1997**, *45*, 219–226.
41. Woike, J.K.; Hoffrage, U.; Martignon, L. Integrating and testing natural frequencies, naïve Bayes, and fast-and-frugal trees. *Decision* **2017**, *4*, 234–260. [CrossRef]
42. Phillips, N.; Neth, H.; Woike, J.K.; Gaissmaier, W. FFTrees: A toolbox to create, visualize, and evaluate fast-and-frugal decision trees. *Judgm. Decis. Mak.* **2017**, *12*, 344–368.
43. Luan, S.; Schooler, L.J.; Gigerenzer, G. A signal-detection analysis of fast-and-frugal trees. *Psychol. Rev.* **2011**, *118*, 316–338. [CrossRef]
44. Gigerenzer, G.E.; Hertwig, R.E.; Pachur, T.E. *Heuristics: The Foundations of Adaptive Behavior*; Oxford University Press: Oxford, UK; New York, NY, USA, 2011; Volume xxv, p. 844.
45. Moscow, J.A.; Fojo, T.; Schilsky, R.L. The evidence framework for precision cancer medicine. *Nat. Rev. Clin. Oncol.* **2018**, *15*, 183–192. [CrossRef]
46. Oser, M.G.; Niederst, M.J.; Sequist, L.V.; Engelman, J.A. Transformation from non-small-cell lung cancer to small-cell lung cancer: Molecular drivers and cells of origin. *Lancet Oncol.* **2015**, *16*, e165–e172. [CrossRef]
47. Marcoux, N.; Gettinger, S.N.; O'Kane, G.; Arbour, K.C.; Neal, J.W.; Husain, H.; Evans, T.L.; Brahmer, J.R.; Muzikansky, A.; Bonomi, P.D.; et al. EGFR-Mutant Adenocarcinomas That Transform to Small-Cell Lung Cancer and Other Neuroendocrine Carcinomas: Clinical Outcomes. *J. Clin. Oncol.* **2019**, *37*, 278–285. [CrossRef] [PubMed]

48. National Comprehensive Cancer Network. NCCN Clinical Practice Guidelines in Oncology (NCCN Guidelines) for Non-Small Cell Lung Caner. 2019. Available online: https://www.nccn.org/professionals/physician_gls/default.aspx (accessed on 8 May 2020).
49. Salgia, R. MET in Lung Cancer: Biomarker Selection Based on Scientific Rationale. *Mol. Cancer Ther.* **2017**, *16*, 555–565. [CrossRef] [PubMed]
50. Ackermann, C.J.; Stock, G.; Tay, R.; Dawod, M.; Gomes, F.; Califano, R. Targeted Therapy For RET-Rearranged Non-Small Cell Lung Cancer: Clinical Development And Future Directions. *OncoTargets Ther.* **2019**, *12*, 7857–7864. [CrossRef]
51. Cocco, E.; Scaltriti, M.; Drilon, A. NTRK fusion-positive cancers and TRK inhibitor therapy. *Nat. Rev. Clin. Oncol.* **2018**, *15*, 731–747. [CrossRef]
52. Bar-Sagi, D.; Knelson, E.H.; Sequist, L.V. A bright future for KRAS inhibitors. *Nat. Cancer* **2020**, *1*, 25–27. [CrossRef]
53. Zhang, H.; Berezov, A.; Wang, Q.; Zhang, G.; Drebin, J.; Murali, R.; Greene, M.I. ErbB receptors: From oncogenes to targeted cancer therapies. *J. Clin. Investig.* **2007**, *117*, 2051–2058. [CrossRef]
54. Shtivelman, E.; Hensing, T.; Simon, G.R.; Dennis, P.A.; Otterson, G.A.; Bueno, R.; Salgia, R. Molecular pathways and therapeutic targets in lung cancer. *Oncotarget* **2014**, *5*, 1392–1433. [CrossRef] [PubMed]
55. Da Cunha Santos, G.; Shepherd, F.A.; Tsao, M.S. EGFR mutations and lung cancer. *Annu. Rev. Pathol.* **2011**, *6*, 49–69. [CrossRef]
56. Sakurada, A.; Shepherd, F.A.; Tsao, M.-S. Epidermal growth factor receptor tyrosine kinase inhibitors in lung cancer: Impact of primary or secondary mutations. *Clin. Lung Cancer* **2006**, *7* (Suppl. 4), S138–S144. [CrossRef]
57. FDA. FDA Approves Osimertinib for First-Line Treatment of Metastatic NSCLC with Most Common EGFR Mutations. 2018. Available online: https://www.fda.gov/drugs/resources-information-approved-drugs/fda-approves-osimertinib-first-line-treatment-metastatic-nsclc-most-common-egfr-mutations (accessed on 8 May 2020).
58. Soria, J.-C.; Ohe, Y.; Vansteenkiste, J.; Reungwetwattana, T.; Chewaskulyong, B.; Lee, K.H.; Dechaphunkul, A.; Imamura, F.; Nogami, N.; Kurata, T.; et al. Osimertinib in Untreated EGFR-Mutated Advanced Non–Small-Cell Lung Cancer. *N. Engl. J. Med.* **2018**, *378*, 113–125. [CrossRef] [PubMed]
59. FDA. FDA Approves Dacomitinib for Metastatic Non-Small Cell Lung Cancer. 2018. Available online: https://www.fda.gov/drugs/drug-approvals-and-databases/fda-approves-dacomitinib-metastatic-non-small-cell-lung-cancer-0 (accessed on 8 May 2020).
60. Wu, Y.-L.; Cheng, Y.; Zhou, X.; Lee, K.H.; Nakagawa, K.; Niho, S.; Tsuji, F.; Linke, R.; Rosell, R.; Corral, J.; et al. Dacomitinib versus gefitinib as first-line treatment for patients with EGFR-mutation-positive non-small-cell lung cancer (ARCHER 1050): A randomised, open-label, phase 3 trial. *Lancet Oncol.* **2017**, *18*, 1454–1466. [CrossRef]
61. Kosaka, T.; Yatabe, Y.; Endoh, H.; Yoshida, K.; Hida, T.; Tsuboi, M.; Tada, H.; Kuwano, H.; Mitsudomi, T. Analysis of Epidermal Growth Factor Receptor Gene Mutation in Patients with Non-Small Cell Lung Cancer and Acquired Resistance to Gefitinib. *Clin. Cancer Res.* **2006**, *12*, 5764–5769. [CrossRef]
62. Balak, M.N.; Gong, Y.; Riely, G.J.; Somwar, R.; Li, A.R.; Zakowski, M.F.; Chiang, A.; Yang, G.; Ouerfelli, O.; Kris, M.G.; et al. Novel D761Y and Common Secondary T790M Mutations in Epidermal Growth Factor Receptor-Mutant Lung Adenocarcinomas with Acquired Resistance to Kinase Inhibitors. *Clin. Cancer Res.* **2006**, *12*, 6494–6501. [CrossRef] [PubMed]
63. Kobayashi, S.; Boggon, T.J.; Dayaram, T.; Jänne, P.A.; Kocher, O.; Meyerson, M.; Johnson, B.E.; Eck, M.J.; Tenen, D.G.; Halmos, B. EGFR mutation and resistance of non-small-cell lung cancer to gefitinib. *N. Engl. J. Med.* **2005**, *352*, 786–792. [CrossRef] [PubMed]
64. Su, K.-Y.; Chen, H.-Y.; Li, K.-C.; Kuo, M.-L.; Yang, J.C.-H.; Chan, W.-K.; Ho, B.-C.; Chang, G.-C.; Shih, J.-Y.; Yu, S.-L.; et al. Pretreatment Epidermal Growth Factor Receptor (EGFR) T790M Mutation Predicts Shorter EGFR Tyrosine Kinase Inhibitor Response Duration in Patients With Non–Small-Cell Lung Cancer. *J. Clin. Oncol.* **2012**, *30*, 433–440. [CrossRef]
65. Yu, H.; Arcila, M.E.; Hellmann, M.D.; Kris, M.G.; Ladanyi, M.; Riely, G.J. Poor response to erlotinib in patients with tumors containing baseline EGFR T790M mutations found by routine clinical molecular testing. *Ann. Oncol.* **2014**, *25*, 423–428. [CrossRef]

66. Saito, H.; Fukuhara, T.; Furuya, N.; Watanabe, K.; Sugawara, S.; Iwasawa, S.; Tsunezuka, Y.; Yamaguchi, O.; Okada, M.; Yoshimori, K.; et al. Erlotinib plus bevacizumab versus erlotinib alone in patients with EGFR-positive advanced non-squamous non-small-cell lung cancer (NEJ026): Interim analysis of an open-label, randomised, multicentre, phase 3 trial. *Lancet Oncol.* **2019**, *20*, 625–635. [CrossRef]
67. Zhao, Y.; Liu, J.; Cai, X.; Pan, Z.; Liu, J.; Yin, W.; Chen, H.; Xie, Z.; Liang, H.; Wang, W.; et al. Efficacy and safety of first line treatments for patients with advanced epidermal growth factor receptor mutated, non-small cell lung cancer: Systematic review and network meta-analysis. *BMJ* **2019**, *367*, l5460. [CrossRef]
68. Nakagawa, K.; Garon, E.B.; Seto, T.; Nishio, M.; Aix, S.P.; Paz-Ares, L.; Chiu, C.-H.; Park, K.; Novello, S.; Nadal, E.; et al. Ramucirumab plus erlotinib in patients with untreated, EGFR-mutated, advanced non-small-cell lung cancer (RELAY): A randomised, double-blind, placebo-controlled, phase 3 trial. *Lancet Oncol.* **2019**, *20*, 1655–1669. [CrossRef]
69. Soda, M.; Choi, Y.L.; Enomoto, M.; Takada, S.; Yamashita, Y.; Ishikawa, S.; Fujiwara, S.-I.; Watanabe, H.; Kurashina, K.; Hatanaka, H.; et al. Identification of the transforming EML4–ALK fusion gene in non-small-cell lung cancer. *Nature* **2007**, *448*, 561–566. [CrossRef] [PubMed]
70. Solomon, B.J.; Kim, N.-W.; Mekhail, T.; Paolini, J.; Usari, T.; Reisman, A.; Wilner, K.D.; Tursi, J.; Mok, T.S.; Wu, Y.-L.; et al. First-Line Crizotinib versus Chemotherapy in ALK-Positive Lung Cancer. *N. Engl. J. Med.* **2014**, *371*, 2167–2177. [CrossRef] [PubMed]
71. Lee, J.-K.; Park, H.S.; Kim, D.-W.; Kulig, K.; Kim, T.M.; Lee, S.-H.; Jeon, Y.; Chung, D.H.; Heo, D.S.; Kim, W.-H.; et al. Comparative analyses of overall survival in patients with anaplastic lymphoma kinase-positive and matched wild-type advanced nonsmall cell lung cancer. *Cancer* **2012**, *118*, 3579–3586. [CrossRef]
72. Katayama, R.; Khan, T.M.; Benes, C.; Lifshits, E.; Ebi, H.; Rivera, V.M.; Shakespeare, W.C.; Iafrate, A.J.; Engelman, J.A.; Shaw, A.T. Therapeutic strategies to overcome crizotinib resistance in non-small cell lung cancers harboring the fusion oncogene EML4-ALK. *Proc. Natl. Acad. Sci. USA* **2011**, *108*, 7535–7540. [CrossRef] [PubMed]
73. Kay, M.; Dehghanian, F. Exploring the crizotinib resistance mechanism of NSCLC with the L1196M mutation using molecular dynamics simulation. *J. Mol. Model.* **2017**, *23*, 323. [CrossRef] [PubMed]
74. Pao, W.; Miller, V.A.; Politi, K.A.; Riely, G.J.; Somwar, R.; Zakowski, M.F.; Kris, M.G.; Varmus, H. Acquired Resistance of Lung Adenocarcinomas to Gefitinib or Erlotinib Is Associated with a Second Mutation in the EGFR Kinase Domain. *PLoS Med.* **2005**, *2*, e73. [CrossRef]
75. Barrows, S.; Wright, K.; Copley-Merriman, C.; Kaye, J.A.; Chioda, M.; Wiltshire, R.; Torgersen, K.M.; Masters, E.T. Systematic review of sequencing of ALK inhibitors in ALK-positive non-small-cell lung cancer. *Lung Cancer (Auckl.)* **2019**, *10*, 11–20. [CrossRef]
76. Wang, R.; Hu, H.; Pan, Y.; Li, Y.; Ye, T.; Li, C.; Luo, X.; Wang, L.; Li, H.; Zhang, Y.; et al. RET Fusions Define a Unique Molecular and Clinicopathologic Subtype of Non–Small-Cell Lung Cancer. *J. Clin. Oncol.* **2012**, *30*, 4352–4359. [CrossRef]
77. Ishizaka, Y.; Itoh, F.; Tahira, T.; Ikeda, I.; Sugimura, T.; Tucker, J.; Fertitta, A.; Carrano, A.V.; Nagao, M. Human ret proto-oncogene mapped to chromosome 10q11.2. *Oncogene* **1989**, *4*, 1519–1521.
78. Phay, J.E.; Shah, M.H. Targeting RET Receptor Tyrosine Kinase Activation in Cancer. *Clin. Cancer Res.* **2010**, *16*, 5936–5941. [CrossRef]
79. Takahashi, M.; Ritz, J.; Cooper, G.M. Activation of a novel human transforming gene, ret, by DNA rearrangement. *Cell* **1985**, *42*, 581–588. [CrossRef]
80. Drilon, A.; Wang, L.; Hasanovic, A.; Suehara, Y.; Lipson, R.; Stephens, P.; Ross, J.; Miller, V.; Ginsberg, M.; Zakowski, M.F.; et al. Response to Cabozantinib in patients with RET fusion-positive lung adenocarcinomas. *Cancer Discov.* **2013**, *3*, 630–635. [CrossRef] [PubMed]
81. Drilon, A.; Hu, Z.I.; Lai, G.G.Y.; Tan, D.S.W. Targeting RET-driven cancers: Lessons from evolving preclinical and clinical landscapes. *Nat. Rev. Clin. Oncol.* **2018**, *15*, 151–167. [CrossRef] [PubMed]
82. Gautschi, O.; Milia, J.; Filleron, T.; Wolf, J.; Carbone, D.P.; Owen, D.H.; Camidge, R.; Narayanan, V.; Doebele, R.C.; Besse, B.; et al. Targeting RET in Patients With RET-Rearranged Lung Cancers: Results From the Global, Multicenter RET Registry. *J. Clin. Oncol.* **2017**, *35*, 1403–1410. [CrossRef] [PubMed]
83. Takeuchi, K.; Soda, M.; Togashi, Y.; Suzuki, R.; Sakata, S.; Hatano, S.; Asaka, R.; Hamanaka, W.; Ninomiya, H.; Uehara, H.; et al. RET, ROS1 and ALK fusions in lung cancer. *Nat. Med.* **2012**, *18*, 378–381. [CrossRef]
84. Gainor, J.; Shaw, A.T. Novel Targets in Non-Small Cell Lung Cancer: ROS1 and RET Fusions. *Oncologist* **2013**, *18*, 865–875. [CrossRef]

85. Yoh, K.; Seto, T.; Satouchi, M.; Nishio, M.; Yamamoto, N.; Murakami, H.; Nogami, N.; Matsumoto, S.; Kohno, T.; Tsuta, K.; et al. Vandetanib in patients with previously treated RET-rearranged advanced non-small-cell lung cancer (LURET): An open-label, multicentre phase 2 trial. *Lancet Respir. Med.* **2017**, *5*, 42–50. [CrossRef]
86. Drilon, A.; Subbiah, V.; Oxnard, G.R.; Bauer, T.M.; Velcheti, V.; Lakhani, N.J.; Besse, B.; Park, K.; Patel, J.D.; Cabanillas, M.E.; et al. A phase 1 study of LOXO-292, a potent and highly selective RET inhibitor, in patients with RET-altered cancers. *J. Clin. Oncol.* **2018**, *36*, 102. [CrossRef]
87. Oxnard, G.; Subbiah, V.; Park, K.; Bauer, T.; Wirth, L.; Velcheti, V.; Shah, M.; Besse, B.; Boni, V.; Reckamp, K.; et al. OA12.07 Clinical Activity of LOXO-292, a Highly Selective RET Inhibitor, in Patients with RET Fusion+ Non-Small Cell Lung Cancer. *J. Thorac. Oncol.* **2018**, *13*, S349–S350. [CrossRef]
88. FDA. FDA Approves First Therapy for Patients with Lung and Thyroid Cancers with a Certain Genetic Mutation or Fusion. 2020. Available online: https://www.fda.gov/news-events/press-announcements/fda-approves-first-therapy-patients-lung-and-thyroid-cancers-certain-genetic-mutation-or-fusion (accessed on 8 May 2020).
89. Gainor, J.F.; Lee, D.H.; Curigliano, G.; Doebele, R.C.; Kim, D.-W.; Baik, C.S.; Tan, D.S.-W.; Lopes, G.; Gadgeel, S.M.; Cassier, P.A.; et al. Clinical activity and tolerability of BLU-667, a highly potent and selective RET inhibitor, in patients (pts) with advanced RET-fusion+ non-small cell lung cancer (NSCLC). *J. Clin. Oncol.* **2019**, *37*, 9008. [CrossRef]
90. Cancer Genome Atlas Research Network. Comprehensive molecular profiling of lung adenocarcinoma. *Nature* **2014**, *511*, 543–550. [CrossRef] [PubMed]
91. Spigel, D.R.; Ervin, T.J.; Ramlau, R.; Daniel, D.B.; Goldschmidt, J.H.; Blumenschein, G.R.; Krzakowski, M.; Robinet, G.; Godbert, B.; Barlesi, F.; et al. Randomized Phase II Trial of Onartuzumab in Combination with Erlotinib in Patients with Advanced Non–Small-Cell Lung Cancer. *J. Clin. Oncol.* **2013**, *31*, 4105–4114. [CrossRef]
92. Spigel, D.R.; Edelman, M.J.; O'Byrne, K.; Paz-Ares, L.; Mocci, S.; Phan, S.; Shames, D.S.; Smith, D.; Yu, W.; Paton, V.E.; et al. Results From the Phase III Randomized Trial of Onartuzumab Plus Erlotinib Versus Erlotinib in Previously Treated Stage IIIB or IV Non–Small-Cell Lung Cancer: METLung. *J. Clin. Oncol.* **2017**, *35*, 412–420. [CrossRef] [PubMed]
93. Chen, R.-L.; Zhao, J.; Zhang, X.-C.; Lou, N.-N.; Chen, H.-J.; Yang, X.; Su, J.; Xie, Z.; Zhou, Q.; Tu, H.-Y.; et al. Crizotinib in advanced non-small-cell lung cancer with concomitant ALK rearrangement and c-Met overexpression. *BMC Cancer* **2018**, *18*, 1171. [CrossRef]
94. Landi, L.; Chiari, R.; Tiseo, M.; D'Incà, F.; Dazzi, C.; Chella, A.; Delmonte, A.; Bonanno, L.; Giannarelli, D.; Cortinovis, D.L.; et al. Crizotinib in MET-Deregulated or ROS1-Rearranged Pretreated Non–Small Cell Lung Cancer (METROS): A Phase II, Prospective, Multicenter, Two-Arms Trial. *Clin. Cancer Res.* **2019**, *25*, 7312–7319. [CrossRef] [PubMed]
95. Drilon, A.; Clark, J.W.; Weiss, J.; Ou, S.-H.I.; Camidge, D.R.; Solomon, B.J.; Otterson, G.A.; Villaruz, L.C.; Riely, G.J.; Heist, R.S.; et al. Antitumor activity of crizotinib in lung cancers harboring a MET exon 14 alteration. *Nat. Med.* **2020**, *26*, 47–51. [CrossRef] [PubMed]
96. Wolf, J.; Seto, T.; Han, J.-Y.; Reguart, N.; Garon, E.B.; Groen, H.J.; Tan, D.S.-W.; Hida, T.; De Jonge, M.J.; Orlov, S.V.; et al. Capmatinib (INC280) in METΔex14-mutated advanced non-small cell lung cancer (NSCLC): Efficacy data from the phase II GEOMETRY mono-1 study. *J. Clin. Oncol.* **2019**, *37*, 9004. [CrossRef]
97. Prior, I.; Lewis, K.; Mattos, C. A comprehensive survey of Ras mutations in cancer. *Cancer Res.* **2012**, *72*, 2457–2467. [CrossRef]
98. Scolnick, E.M.; Rands, E.; Williams, D.; Parks, W.P. Studies on the Nucleic Acid Sequences of Kirsten Sarcoma Virus: A Model for Formation of a Mammalian RNA-Containing Sarcoma Virus. *J. Virol.* **1973**, *12*, 458–463. [CrossRef] [PubMed]
99. Der, C.J.; Krontiris, T.G.; Cooper, G.M. Transforming genes of human bladder and lung carcinoma cell lines are homologous to the ras genes of Harvey and Kirsten sarcoma viruses. *Proc. Natl. Acad. Sci. USA* **1982**, *79*, 3637–3640. [CrossRef]
100. Johnson, M.L.; Sima, C.S.; Chaft, J.E.; Paik, P.K.; Pao, W.; Kris, M.G.; Ladanyi, M.; Riely, G.J. Association of KRAS and EGFR mutations with survival in patients with advanced lung adenocarcinomas. *Cancer* **2013**, *119*, 356–362. [CrossRef]
101. Barbacid, M. Ras genes. *Annu. Rev. Biochem.* **1987**, *56*, 779–827. [CrossRef] [PubMed]

102. Simanshu, D.K.; Nissley, D.V.; McCormick, F. RAS Proteins and Their Regulators in Human Disease. *Cell* **2017**, *170*, 17–33. [CrossRef] [PubMed]
103. Campbell, S.L.; Khosravi-Far, R.; Rossman, K.L.; Clark, G.J.; Der, C.J. Increasing complexity of Ras signaling. *Oncogene* **1998**, *17*, 1395–1413. [CrossRef] [PubMed]
104. Dogan, S.; Shen, R.; Ang, D.C.; Johnson, M.L.; D'Angelo, S.P.; Paik, P.K.; Brzostowski, E.B.; Riely, G.J.; Kris, M.G.; Zakowski, M.F.; et al. Molecular epidemiology of EGFR and KRAS mutations in 3,026 lung adenocarcinomas: Higher susceptibility of women to smoking-related KRAS-mutant cancers. *Clin. Cancer Res.* **2012**, *18*, 6169–6177. [CrossRef] [PubMed]
105. AACR Project GENIE Consortium. AACR Project GENIE: Powering Precision Medicine through an International Consortium. *Cancer Discov.* **2017**, *7*, 818–831. [CrossRef]
106. Skoulidis, F.; Goldberg, M.E.; Greenawalt, D.M.; Hellmann, M.D.; Awad, M.M.; Gainor, J.F.; Schrock, A.B.; Hartmaier, R.J.; Trabucco, S.E.; Gay, L.; et al. STK11/LKB1 Mutations and PD-1 Inhibitor Resistance in KRAS-Mutant Lung Adenocarcinoma. *Cancer Discov.* **2018**, *8*, 822–835. [CrossRef]
107. Fakih, M.; O'Neil, B.; Price, T.J.; Falchook, G.S.; Desai, J.; Kuo, J.; Govindan, R.; Rasmussen, E.; Morrow, P.K.H.; Ngang, J.; et al. Phase 1 study evaluating the safety, tolerability, pharmacokinetics (PK), and efficacy of AMG 510, a novel small molecule KRASG12C inhibitor, in advanced solid tumors. *J. Clin. Oncol.* **2019**, *37*, 3003. [CrossRef]
108. Wang, J.X.; Sullivan, D.K.; Wells, A.J.; Wells, A.C.; Chen, J.H. Neural Networks for Clinical Order Decision Support. *AMIA Jt. Summits Transl. Sci. Proc.* **2019**, *2019*, 315–324.

© 2020 by the authors. Licensee MDPI, Basel, Switzerland. This article is an open access article distributed under the terms and conditions of the Creative Commons Attribution (CC BY) license (http://creativecommons.org/licenses/by/4.0/).

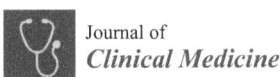

Article

Implementing Lung Cancer Screening and Prevention in Academic Centers, Affiliated Network Offices and Collaborating Care Sites

Cary A. Presant [1,2,*], Ravi Salgia [1,2], Prakash Kulkarni [1,2], Brian L. Tiep [1,2], Shamel Sanani [1,2], Benjamin Leach [1,2], Kimlin Ashing [1,2], Jossie Sandoval [1,2], Mina S. Sedrak [1,2], Shana Landau [1,2], Sophia Yeung [1,2], Dan Raz [1,2] and Shanmugga Subbiah [1,2]

1. City of Hope Medical Center, Duarte, CA 91010, USA; rsalgia@coh.org (R.S.); pkulkarni@coh.org (P.K.); btiep@coh.org (B.L.T.); ssanani@coh.org (S.S.); bleach@coh.org (B.L.); kashing@coh.org (K.A.); asandoval@coh.org (J.S.); msedrak@coh.org (M.S.S.); slandau@coh.org (S.L.); syeung@coh.org (S.Y.); draz@coh.org (D.R.); ssubbiah@coh.org (S.S.)
2. City of Hope Medical Center, West Covina, CA 91790, USA
* Correspondence: cpresant@coh.org

Received: 18 April 2020; Accepted: 9 June 2020; Published: 11 June 2020

Abstract: Lung cancer is one of the deadliest and yet largely preventable neoplasms. Smoking cessation and lung cancer screening are effective yet underutilized lung cancer interventions. City of Hope Medical Center, a National Cancer Institute (NCI)- designated comprehensive cancer center, has 27 community cancer centers and has prioritized tobacco control and lung cancer screening throughout its network. Despite challenges, we are implementing and monitoring the City of Hope Tobacco Control Initiative including (1) a Planning and Implementation Committee; (2) integration of IT, e.g., medical records and clinician notification/prompts to facilitate screening, cessation referral, and digital health, e.g., telehealth and social media; (3) clinician training and endorsing national guidelines; (4) providing clinical champions at all sites for site leadership; (5) Coverage and Payment reform and aids to facilitate patient access and reduce cost barriers; (6) increasing tobacco exposure screening for all patients; (7) smoking cessation intervention and evaluation—patient-centered recommendations for smoking cessation for all current and recent quitters along with including QuitLine referral for current smokers and smoking care-givers; and (8) establishing a Tobacco Registry for advancing science and discoveries including team science for basic, translation and clinical studies. These strategies are intended to inform screening, prevention and treatment research and patient-centered care.

Keywords: cancer center; lung cancer; lung cancer screening; low-dose CT scans; cancer prevention; smoking cessation; tobacco control; national guidelines for screening and prevention; pharmaceutical aids to smoking cessation

1. Introduction

Lung cancer is the leading cause of cancer-related deaths. However, lung cancer is one of the most preventable human malignancies. A screening program is able to detect lung cancer at an earlier and more successfully treatable stage, and thus improves survival. In order to control lung cancer incidence, morbidity and mortality, it is important for a health care delivery system to provide and monitor screening and prevention programs including tobacco cessation. In this report, we will review the experience of the City of Hope Medical Center at its academic campus in Duarte, CA, as well as its 27 community practice sites throughout much of Southern California. This is an observational descriptive study, and broader results of our experience are under study and will be published separately.

1.1. City of Hope's Experience in Lung Cancer Screening and Prevention

City of Hope is an NCI-designated comprehensive cancer center and a member of the National Comprehensive Cancer Network (NCCN) network. City of Hope utilizes the NCCN guidelines for lung cancer screening and prevention. In addition, all clinical sites (the academic center in Duarte and all 27 community centers) follow the NCCN lung cancer care and screening guidelines and comply with Via Oncology Pathways (as modified by City of Hope) for evaluation, anti-tumor treatment and surveillance after treatments. A map of these sites indicates the broad coverage of communities in the greater Los Angeles area (Figure 1). Compliance with these pathways is monitored for every physician and advanced practice practitioner (APP). Pathway compliance is very strongly encouraged. We follow the NCCN guidelines on smoking cessation, since smoking cessation is conceptually an integral component of cancer care.

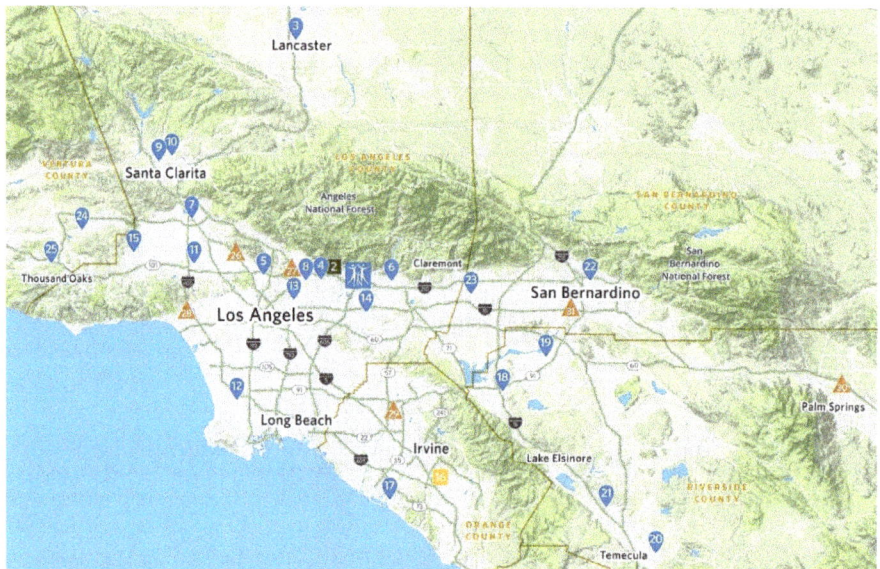

Figure 1. Map of City of Hope Locations in Southern California. Blue Square, Duarte National Medical Center Academic Site; Blue Teardrops, Community Cancer Center Practice Sites; Orange Triangles, City of Hope Oncologist-Staffed Community Hospitals; Yellow Square, Orange County Campus (under construction). Map designed at City of Hope Medical Center.

Lung cancer team leadership at City of Hope is provided by Dr. Ravi Salgia, Dr. Dan Raz and Dr. Erminia Massarelli. Under their direction as champions, the lung cancer disease team promotes lung cancer screening and prevention in Duarte and in all network community centers. The relationships between these components of the program are pictured in Figure 2. This model following the team leadership with advice of the Department of Population Science allows interactive design of the initiative and modifications, and implementation in Duarte and community sites and a synergistic effect implementing screening and prevention.

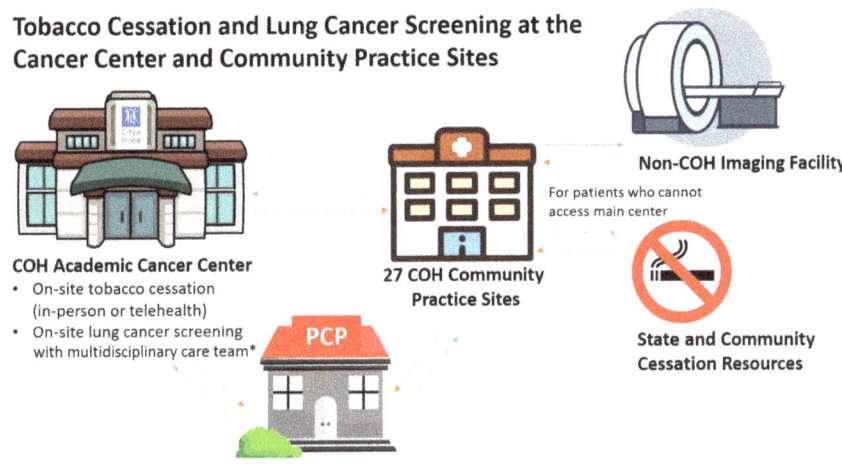

Figure 2. Lung Cancer Prevention and Screening Model. The City of Hope Lung Cancer Tobacco Control and Cancer Screening Initiative Is Implemented in the above Model. Model was designed by City of Hope Medical Center.

1.2. Academic Center Experience

At the academic center, City of Hope conducts preclinical laboratory investigations into genetic factors associated with lung cancer. This research helps to define which patients are at risk for developing lung cancer. Genomic alterations are identified which may help in screening and development of drugs targeted for cancer prevention. Population science research further aids in cancer control activities. Clinical trials, developed from these research activities, are initiated at the academic campus in Duarte as well as at one or more of our 27 affiliated network community cancer centers.

At the academic center, cancer program members (67 physicians, 67 APPs, 12 research faculty, 14 graduate students and fellows and 10 additional data analysts, and clinical trial coordinators) and specifically the lung cancer team conduct weekly disease team-based meetings/tumor boards/research seminars and invite participation of physicians at the network community cancer center offices. At the academic center, screening with low-dose CT (LDCT), smoking cessation, and patient education are provided.

At the academic center, 8623 total new patients including 3255 new cancer patients are seen annually (data from 2019), with 252 new lung cancer patients evaluated per year. Racial/ethnic diversity exists, with 61.4% Caucasian, 19.9% Hispanic, 14.7% Asian/Pacific Islander, and 3.9% African-American patients. Overall, 4.2% of all patients at the academic center self-report as current smokers, 27.8% are former smokers, and 61% of patients are never smokers. Medicare is the payer in 37.9%, Medicare Advantage in 1.7%, Medicaid in 9.3%, PPO or commercial in 29.1%, HMO or managed care in 17.9%, and other payers in 3.4% of patients. This patient population is different compared to the 27 community centers, which has implications for screening and tobacco control. Actual practices in tobacco control vary by treatment site. At the academic center, there is a formal smoking cessation program, while there are no formal smoking cessation resources at network community offices. At all sites, patients are referred to the California Smokers Helpline 800 No Butts program (800-No-Butts) or to the California QuitLine operated out of the University of California San Diego (800 Quit Now).

At the academic center, LDCT screenings were ordered in 434 patients over a 4 year period, and 424 (98%) completed the procedure. We universally use the Lung-RADS system of evaluation of LDCT scans [1]. Of those patients undergoing LDCT, Lung-RADS results showed suspicious lung cancer category 4A results in 3.3% and highly suspicious category 4B results in 1.7%. Of the six patients who had biopsies performed at the academic center, four (67%) had stage 1 lung cancer diagnosed, and two (33%) had stage 4 lung cancer. Other patients were referred back to their primary care physicians for diagnostic biopsies. Long-term follow up of patients diagnosed through our LDCT screening program will determine reductions in risk of death and will be reported in the future. Any cost savings associated with earlier diagnosis depend on the health system, and different health payers are involved with our patients (see above).

One of the issues in lung cancer screening is the excessive use of scans. At City of Hope, Shared Decision-Making Consults and Lung-RADS are some of our tools to address the issue of reducing excessive imaging, false positives, excessive harm as a result of the additional testing, patient anxiety, and cost. During the Shared Decision-Making Consults, ordering clinicians use checklist and visual tools to discuss the risk and benefits with the patients, address patients' concerns, and assist patients to determine whether the lung cancer screening is suitable. The clinician also educates patients on what is low-dose CT, and advises postponing the screening if they have had a chest/PET-CT in the past 12 months. In the Duarte cancer center LCS program, we also coordinate with the attending clinicians to prevent excessive imaging. Lung-RADS is a widely accepted and logical nodule reporting and management tool used by the radiologists to minimize false-positive findings, excessive imaging, and unnecessary procedures. As part of our lung cancer screening initiative, we are developing educational tools and informational aids to help patients understand these issues before screening.

1.3. Community Centers Experience

Our community cancer centers are staffed with 43 medical oncologists, 40 radiation oncologists, 7 APPs and a clinical trials coordinator. In order to improve lung cancer control, physicians and APPs at the 27 network community cancer centers advise screening and prevention at local tumor boards and medical lectures, and depend on collaborating/referring community primary care physicians, pulmonologists, radiologists and hospitals for lung cancer control. Primary care physicians who are the referring doctors of patients to City of Hope, as well as City of Hope providers themselves (to varying degrees), make assessments of lung cancer risk, order LDCT screening exams, advise or provide smoking cessation to current smokers or recently quit patients, refer patients to other local smoking cessation programs if available, prescribe smoking cessation medications, and provide behavior intervention and counseling with follow-up visits to assess compliance.

In only one-half of the network community practices do the oncologists prescribe medications to assist in smoking cessation, while the other half simply refer the patients back to their primary care physicians with recommendations. In a current survey of community practice sites, almost all of the network community center physicians discuss screening and prevention at tumor boards or hospital meetings where primary physicians and pulmonologists are in attendance, but a few still do not, even today.

At the 27 community centers, 22,000 new patients are seen annually (data from 2019). In total, 19,201 patients are seen by medical oncology/hematology specialists. The incidence of current smokers is 7.2%. Of the patients, 49.4% are Caucasian, 20.3% are Hispanic, 4.5% are African-American, and 6% are Asian/Pacific Islander. Among our patients, 43.7% are insured by government programs, 22.9% are PPO/commercially insured, and 22.7% are insured by HMOs or IPA medical groups.

1.4. Institutional Vision

Even in an integrated oncology network, there remain challenges with opportunities for improvement. In our vision, there is a focus on team medicine. The academic center uses its knowledge, skills and experience to set standards and create pathways so as to encourage its network community centers to implement the science and evidence base (Table 1). The community center encourages the local collaborating physicians, medical groups, IPAs, and hospitals to utilize their resources to implement the screening and prevention activities as well as providing smoking cessation advice and medications and/or nicotine replacement treatments for some patients. Naturally, these necessitate that the primary care physician, pulmonologist and/or oncologist order the interventions necessary to reduce the risks of lung cancer. The component activities or interventions seen in Table 1 are most appropriately (indicated by +++) taking place at the academic center or network community cancer center.

Table 1. Sites for Lung Cancer Screening and Prevention.

Program	Academic Center	Affiliated Network Community Clinical Center	Collaborating Physicians and Hospitals
Screening Research	+++	+	−
Screening Implementation	+	++	+++
Prevention Research	+++	+	−
Prevention Implementation	+	++	+++
Provider Education	+++	+++	+
Patient Education	+++	+++	+++

To address these, we have developed the City of Hope Tobacco Control Initiative. Elements of the initiative were begun in 2013. As the program elements matured and new information informed needed improvements and coordination, the initiative was revised. The current initiative was formulated in January 2020. It includes (1) a Planning and Implementation Committee; (2) integration of IT including medical records and clinician notification/prompts to facilitate screening, cessation referral; (3) physician and clinician training and supervision that endorses national guidelines and refer and encourage lung cancer screening and smoking cessation interventions; (4) providing a clinical champion at the community sites, and at the academic center for program leadership; (5) Coverage and Payment reform and aide to facilitate patient access and utilization and reduce cost barriers; (6) implementing systemic tobacco exposure screen for new and existing patients; (7) smoking cessation intervention and evaluation—patient-centered recommendation for smoking cessation for all current and recent quitters along with QuitLine referral for all current smokers and the smoking care-givers; and (8) establishing a Tobacco Registry for advancing science and discoveries including team science for basic, translation and clinical studies.

The implementation of the initiative is in progress at Duarte and in community sites, as led by the lung cancer disease team, clinical departments, and the network, regional and individual site leaders, and community center lung cancer champions. Evaluation methods include a review of electronic health records for LDCT screening orders in patients with higher risk based on smoking history and other clinical and epidemiologic factors, referral for smoking cessation, continuing visits for monitoring cessation efforts, and frequency of prescribing anti-smoking medications and/or nicotine replacement therapy medications. Compliance measures are thus multifactorial. At present, we have demonstrated that all 27 community cancer centers can operate together, in a coordinated well-integrated effort with the academic site.

2. Focus on Lung Cancer Screening

The Science

Unfortunately, LDCT is a lung cancer screening method which is underused [2]. The frequency of performing lung cancer screening in patients who are eligible for screening by nationally accepted criteria is 3.9% as of 2015 [2]. However, this may be improving, since a recent study suggests that in a survey of 10 states in 2017, 12.7% of people 55–80 years old were eligible for screening by national criteria, and 12.5% actually had received screening [3]. There was a variation by state ranging from 9.7% to 16%.

As summarized in NCCN guidelines [4], patients who are generally eligible for LDCT screening are those at high risk, defined as 55 to 77 years old, have a 30 or more pack year history of smoking, and are active smokers or have stopped smoking within the last 15 years. Although not defined in the screening trials as high risk, other patients who are also at higher risk are those who are age 50 years or over, with a 20 or more pack year smoking history, and have other risk factors. These risk factors can include prior lung or head and neck cancer, a family history of lung cancer, prior chest radiotherapy, asbestos or radon exposure, presence of HIV or COPD or pulmonary fibrosis, or significant second-hand smoke exposure.

Criteria for evaluation are also nationally standardized as outlined in the NCCN guidelines [4]. They cover not only which findings require immediate biopsy or excision, but also which require close follow up versus those who require a repeat LDCT in 1 year.

LDCT has been shown to detect earlier state lung cancer. In fact, 63% of lung cancers which were found by LDCT were stage IA or IB [5]. Further, this earlier detection has been associated with reduced lung cancer deaths by 20% worldwide [6].

It is important to identify patient symptoms which might be associated with lung cancer. Persistent cough, hemoptysis, shortness of breath, chest pain, weight loss, and/or wheezing may be symptoms of lung cancer. Someone who has any of these symptoms should not get a low-dose CT scan, but they should get a diagnostic CT scan with and without contrast. Payment for diagnostic CT in the presence of symptoms is covered by insurance even in managed care plans. Requests for prior authorization should include diagnostic codes for the specific symptoms. For patients with prior lung cancer, annual diagnostic CT chest scans are indicated, with details included in NCCN guidelines. Clinicians both at Duarte and in community sites are committed to compliance with those guidelines.

If the LDCT is negative, patients should be counseled regarding prevention. This is addressed in the following section. Since the prevalence of LDCT screening is low among patients who meet requirements to receive it, there remains considerable need for medical leadership in local communities to encourage more widespread use.

3. Smoking Prevention

The Science

The most prevalent causative factor for lung cancer is smoking—an estimated 85–90% of patients [7]. Thus, smoking cessation is crucial. Smoking cessation programs include a recommendation from a physician to a patient to stop smoking, followed by referral to a smoking cessation program. In order to prevent withdrawal symptoms and facilitate cessation, the physician can prescribe pharmaceuticals such as varenicline, nicotine replacement therapy (NRT), or buproprion with or without NRT [8]. The success of cessation in achieving complete abstinence is poor with a 1 year abstinence rate of 20% using buproprion with NRT, and a 24 week abstinence rate of 26% with varenicline [8]. Behavioral interventions have been shown to improve odds of success over medications alone.

Therefore, follow up is most necessary to continue to promote cessation on the individual patient level. Referral to smoking cessation is best performed by the primary care physician or APP, since their relationships with the patient are generally closer than relationships with the oncologists. However, cessation is also often prescribed and facilitated by an oncologist as part of standard cancer care. Further, the oncologist has a role in promoting smoking control at the collaborating hospital or medical staff meetings. The immediate and long-term benefits of smoking cessation include not only better survival, but also critical positive impact on cancer care, improved success of treatment, reduced recurrence of the primary cancer, less frequent development of new cancers, and less progression of comorbid conditions.

If smoking cessation is achieved, lung cancer incidence rate is reduced by 83% in totally abstinent non-smokers, and by 55% in partially abstinent smokers [9]. Recidivism rate, with patients again starting to smoke, are unfortunately high. Continued motivational support for the patient is necessary. Many hospitals including the City of Hope academic center in Duarte have smoking cessation support programs. Alternative programs are provided by such organizations as the American Cancer Society California Division and state of California via phone or internet-based support program called 1-800-No-Butts.

There is high and growing use of E-cigarettes for either nicotine replacement or combustible smoking cessation. The exact impact of E-cigarettes in transitioning from combustible smoking to non-smoking remains controversial. Recent studies cast doubt on the true efficacy of substituting vaping for combustible cigarette smoking. For many individuals who turn to vaping, dual use is common. This leads to an additive effect of toxicities from smoking and vaping, which is counter to the overall goal of tobacco cessation.

City of Hope has helped to develop and adheres to NCCN guidelines on smoking cessation. We do not recommend E-cigarettes or vaping as a smoking cessation or smoking replacement tool either for single use or in combination with FDA-approved smoking cessation medication. If a patient has quit smoking using E-cigarettes, we support continuation of non-smoking status, encourage transition to approved smoking cessation medications, encourage behavior support, and provide support to reduce the risk of lapses or relapses. Of special concerns are the dual use of tobacco and E-cigarettes and E-cigarettes in children where lifetime addiction to nicotine products are of particular concern.

In addition to smoking cessation, other interventions are known to be effective in reducing lung cancer rates and are advised by the National Institutes of Health [10,11]. Patients should avoid second-hand smoke, avoid excessive radiologic scans, reduce exposure to radon (present in 1 of every 15 homes), not be exposed to asbestos (and also chromium, nickel, beryllium, cadmium, tar, uranium, coal products and diesel fuel), and avoid beta carotene use in smokers.

Other interventions to reduce lung cancer risk which have evidence to support them but not yet accepted in national guidelines include eating a Mediterranean-style diet with increased fruits and vegetables, possibly leading to a 33–50% reduction in lung cancer [12]; increasing exercise, with possibly a 25% reduction [13]; or using green tea, with possibly a 22% reduction [14].

A number of nutritional interventions have been recommended without clear evidence of possible improvement. These interventions include red wine, flax seed, garlic, ginger, selenium, turmeric and vitamin D.

4. Translating Screening and Prevention from the Academic Center

It is difficult to successfully promote lung cancer screening and prevention at the local community since insurance often does not adequately reimburse for these programs or for pharmaceuticals. The evidence base is clear that screening and prevention should be strongly encouraged. Our survey of primary care physicians in our catchment area of greater Los Angeles indicated that these physicians were aware of LDCT screening guidelines—only 12% of primary care physicians in the community (not at academic centers) had referred patients for lung cancer screening in the past year [15]. This indicates a need for community leadership by City of Hope oncologists at local hospital meetings and tumor boards to promote appropriate LDCT screening.

There are many factors that help to promote these programs (Table 2). Guidelines exist for screening and prevention, but they must be more widely accepted by physicians, medical groups, IPAs, HMOs, and hospitals. This must be based on a collaborative relationship, which must be fostered by network community cancer centers and collaborating local physicians and APPs. Promotion can be most effective at tumor boards, at continuing medical education presentations, and even in lunchrooms. Hospitals often need to differentiate themselves from competing institutions, and controlling lung cancer can be an important factor. Having champions in the hospital and on the medical staff can help, and often philanthropy can foster a successful program of smoking cessation. Coordination with voluntary health care organizations can provide educational and patient-support resources not otherwise available in the community.

Table 2. Factors in Translating Screening and Prevention Science from Academic Centers to Affiliated Network Community Centers and Collaborating Community Sites.

Factors Promoting Translation	Factors Limiting Translation
Establishing or accepting clear guidelines for screening and prevention	Insurers and IPAs desire reduced spending
Atmosphere of Collaboration and Congeniality	Contracts with physicians to reduce spending
Education at tumor boards and presentations	Limited resources at hospitals
Establishing screening and prevention programs at hospitals	Constricted time to focus on screening and prevention
Coordinating with voluntary health care organizations	Lack of payment for services or medications
American Cancer Society	Compliance surveys not focused on screening and prevention
American Lung Association	Lack of coordination
Cancer Support Community	High cost to patients
	Need to distinguish between screening for lung cancer versus diagnostic services to evaluate symptoms

However, many obstacles exist in successfully controlling lung cancer. Pressure to reduce health care spending is part of the national debate, and motivates lower authorization of screening and prevention efforts at the insurer, IPA, HMO, alternative payment model (APM) and medical group administrative level. Contracts between those organizations and individual physicians and APPs may limit ability to refer for screening and prevention interventions. Even with approval for LDCT screening or smoking cessation, many hospitals do not have resources available. Since it takes time to evaluate lung cancer risk, and order tests and preventive interventions, there is often a lack of reimbursement for those individual patient visits.

Importantly, compliance surveys on which contracts and payments are based only infrequently assess lung cancer screening and prevention activities. There is poor coordination of patient care in the area of lung cancer screening and prevention. Even when a health plan approves screening or smoking cessation, copayments by patients may still be high for those interventions as well as for medications to suppress withdrawal symptoms.

Just to reemphasize, physicians and APPs should always distinguish between screening LDCT, versus the need for diagnostic chest CT. A diagnostic CT is appropriate and indicated if patients have any symptoms that could be associated with lung cancer. Ordering the appropriate test is most important.

Another opportunity for enhancing local community hospital implementation of lung cancer screening is the evolution of algorithms for interpreting LDCT scans. As software and analytics improves, we expect to see new criteria for identifying lung nodules likely to be neoplastic. Although sometimes difficult for a local community radiologist to remain current in updates, the City of Hope Department of Radiology can provide educational updates for local community hospital radiologists to be immediately aware of the new algorithms necessary for earliest diagnosis of lung cancers more amenable to curative interventions.

5. Recommendations for Translating Screening and Prevention into Local Medical Communities

Although there are obstacles for lung cancer control, advances in the science of lung cancer screening, prevention and treatment can favorably impact cancer care. The success of the City of Hope programs across the entire enterprise of academic center and 27 affiliated network community sites has led us to be able to recommend steps that other institutions can take to improve lung cancer care (Table 3). We recommend adoption of the NCCN guidelines for lung cancer LDCT screening and prevention by physicians, health plans, medical groups, physicians, IPAs, HMOs, APMs and hospitals. To provide leadership, a clinical champion at the community site and also a champion at the academic center are important. The electronic medical record systems used should be updated to separately identify LDCT screening, prevention counseling and smoking cessation referrals and to enable lung cancer risk assessments. Compliance with guidelines should be measured, with reports back to physicians of their success rate or impact. High compliance should be promoted and rewarded. Additionally, the electronic health record can be better programmed to prompt or "nudge" health care providers to implement appropriate cancer screening [16]. Nudge interventions, such as automated alerts directed to the medical team to discuss breast cancer and colorectal cancer screening with patients, showed a dramatic increase in the number of ordered screening tests [17], but it did not affect how likely the patient was to actually complete the test within a year. Once cancer screening is ordered, the patient still has to take the right steps to complete it, such as scheduling an appointment and then going to the appointment. Hence, interventions should test methods to nudge both providers and patients to complete lung cancer screening, while also attempting to eliminate or mitigate some of the hurdles to these tests.

Table 3. Recommendations for Improving Integration of Lung Cancer Screening and Prevention in Clinical Networks.

Recommendation	Responsibility of the Academic Center	Responsibility of Community Network Sites
Establish guidelines for ling cancer screening and prevention	+	
Identify clinical champions at the academic center and community site	+	+
Enhance electronic medical records to include screening LDCT and prevention counseling	+	+
Measure and reward compliance with guidelines	+	+
Promote screening with LDCT	+	+
Promote smoking cessation	+	+
Establish payment coverage for screening/prevention services	+	
Screening tests	+	
Prevention visits	+	
Counseling	+	
Smoking cessation program	+	
Smoking cessation drugs	+	
Fund prevention trials and fund medication trials for smoking cessation	+	

Medical community and public promotion of lung cancer screening and prevention should be implemented. This will only be successful if each of the elements of screening and prevention are covered by insurance with reasonable copayments by patients.

As science improves, there continues to be a need for clinical trials of the possibly beneficial improvements. These trials should be funded by government programs and/or voluntary health care agencies. As leaders in our communities, we should support these trials.

6. Limitations of This Study

This study is at present observational and descriptive, and results will be determined prospectively with additional implementation of the initiative. The short follow up at present precludes detailed reporting of results on cessation success, reductions in lung cancer mortality, and cost savings. Results will be analyzed and published in future communications. Comparisons of lung cancer staging results with LDCT compared to staging resulting from diagnosis when symptoms were present will be evaluated when more patients have been diagnosed at Duarte and in the community network.

7. Conclusions

Lung cancer continues to be a challenge to patients, providers, and health care systems despite dramatic improvements in treatment. We can use successful screening and prevention programs to reduce these life-threatening diagnoses and give patients more hope for the future. Smoking cessation in particular must become an integral component of cancer care and prevention. Reporting on the experience at City of Hope, the recommendations of the translational medical system of City of Hope, and the City of Hope Tobacco Control Initiative is designed to promote broader lung cancer screening and prevention efforts at other institutions and in other communities. We hope our experience will help contribute to improved patient outcomes and increase tobacco control.

Author Contributions: Conceptualization, C.A.P., S.S. (Shamel Sanani), B.L., K.A., B.L.T., R.S., P.K., J.S., M.S.S., S.L., and S.S. (Shanmugga Subbiah); Methodology, C.A.P., S.S. (Shamel Sanani), B.L., K.A., B.L.T., R.S., P.K., J.S., M.S.S., S.L., S.Y., D.R., and S.S. (Shanmugga Subbiah); Investigation, C.A.P., S.S. (Shamel Sanani), B.L., K.A., B.L.T., R.S., P.K., J.S., M.S.S., S.L., D.R., and S.S. (Shanmugga Subbiah); Data Evaluation, C.A.P., S.S. (Shamel Sanani), B.L., K.A., B.L.T., R.S., P.K., and S.S. (Shanmugga Subbiah); Writing—Initial Draft, C.A.P.; Writing—Review and Editing, C.A.P., S.S. (Shamel Sanani), B.L., K.A., B.L.T., R.S., P.K., J.S., M.S.S., S.L., S.Y., D.R., and S.S. (Shanmugga Subbiah); Supervision, C.A.P. and R.S.; Project Administration, C.A.P., B.T., R.S., P.K., and S.S. (Shanmugga Subbiah). All authors have read and agreed to the published version of the manuscript.

Funding: This work was funded in part by NIH Grant P30 CA033572

Conflicts of Interest: The authors declare no conflicts of interest.

List of Abbreviations

APM—alternative payment model organization; APP—advanced practice provider; COH—City of Hope; COPD—chronic obstructive pulmonary disease; HMO—health maintenance organization; IPA—independent practice association; IT—information technology; LDCT—low-dose computed chest tomography; L-RADS—lung imaging reporting and data system; NCI—National Cancer Institute; NCCN—National Comprehensive Cancer Network; NRT—nicotine replacement therapy; PPO—preferred provider organization; Via—Via Oncology Clinical Pathways, now also known as ClinicalPath (Elsevier)

References

1. Pinsky, P.F.; Gierada, D.S.; Black, W.; Munden, R.; Nath, H.; Aberle, D.; Kazerooni, E. Performance of Lung-RADS in the national screening trial—A retrospective assessment. *Ann. Int. Med.* **2015**, *162*, 485–491. [CrossRef] [PubMed]
2. Jemal, A.; Fedewa, S.A. Lung cancer screening with low dose computed tomography in the United States—2010 to 2015. *JAMA Oncol.* **2017**, *3*, 1278–1281. [CrossRef] [PubMed]
3. Richards, T.B.; Ashwini, S.; Thomas, C.C.; VanFrank, B.; Henley, J.; Gallaway, M.S. Screening for lung cancer—10 states 2017. *Morb. Mortal. Wkly.* **2020**, *69*, 201–206. [CrossRef]
4. NCCN. Available online: org/professionals/physician_gls/pdf/lung_screening.pdf (accessed on 27 February 2020).
5. Aberle, D.R.; Adams, A.M.; Berg, C.D. Reduced lung cancer mortality with low dose computed tomographic screening. *N. Engl. J. Med.* **2011**, *365*, 395–409.
6. Pinsky, P.F. Lung cancer screening with lose dose CT: A world wide view. *Transl. Lung Cancer Res.* **2018**, *7*, 234–242. [CrossRef] [PubMed]
7. Samet, J.M.; Avila-Tang, E.; Boffetta, P. Lung cancer in never smokers: Clinical epidemiology and environmental risk factors. *Clin. Cancer Res.* **2009**, *15*, 5625–5645. [CrossRef]
8. Shields, P.G.; Herbst, R.S.; Arenberg, D.; Benowitz, N.L.; Bierut, L.; Luckart, J.B.; Hitsman, B.; Lang, M.; Park, E.R.; Selzle, J.; et al. Smoking Cessation, Version 1.2016, NCCN Clinical Practice Guidelines in Oncology. *J. Natl. Compr. Cancer Netw.* **2016**, *4*, 1430–1468. [CrossRef] [PubMed]
9. Godtfredsen, N.S.; Prescott, E.; Oder, M. Effect of smoking reduction on lung cancer risk. *JAMA* **2005**, *294*, 1505–1510. [CrossRef]

10. PDQ Advisory Committee. Lung Cancer Prevention (PDQ). Available online: https://www.ncbi.nlm.nih.gov/books/NBK66063/ (accessed on 22 May 2020).
11. Beveridge, R.; Pintos, J.; Parent, M.-E.; Asselin, J.; Siemiatycki, J. Lung cancer risk associated with occupational exposure to nickel, chromium VI, and cadmium in two population based case control studies in Montreal. *Ann. Int. Med.* **2010**, *53*, 476–485. [CrossRef]
12. Gnagnarella, P.; Maisonnueve, P.; Belloni, M.; Rampinelli, C.; Bertolotti, R.; Spaggiari, L.; Veronesi, G. Red meat, Mediterranean diet and lung cancer risk among heavy smokers in the COSMOS screening study. *Ann. Oncol.* **2013**, *24*, 2606–2611. [CrossRef] [PubMed]
13. Thune, I.; Lund, E. The influence of physical activity on lung cancer risk: A prospective study of 81,516 men and women. *Int. J. Cancer* **1997**, *70*, 57–62. [CrossRef]
14. Tang, N.; Wu, Y.; Zhou, B.; Wang, B.; Yu, R. Green tea, black tea consumption and risk of lung cancer: A meta-analysis. *Lung Cancer* **2009**, *65*, 274–283. [CrossRef]
15. Raz, D.J.; Wu, G.X.; Consunji, M.; Nelson, R.; Sun, C.; Erhunmwunsee, L.; Ferrell, B.; Sun, V.; Kim, J.Y. Perceptions and utilization of lung cancer screening among primary care physicians. *J. Thorac. Oncol.* **2016**, *11*, 1856–1862. [CrossRef] [PubMed]
16. Patel, M.S.; Volpo, K.G.; Asch, D.A. Nudge units to improve the delivery of health care. *N. Engl. J. Med.* **2018**, *378*, 214–216. [CrossRef] [PubMed]
17. Hsiang, E.Y.; Mehta, S.J.; Small, D.S.; Rareshide, C.A.; Snider, C.K.; Day, S.C.; Patel, M.S. Association of an Active Choice Intervention in the electronic health record directed to medical assistants with clinician ordering and patient completion of breast and colorectal cancer screening tests. *JAMA Netw. Open* **2019**, *2*, e1915619. [CrossRef] [PubMed]

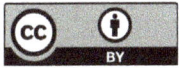

© 2020 by the authors. Licensee MDPI, Basel, Switzerland. This article is an open access article distributed under the terms and conditions of the Creative Commons Attribution (CC BY) license (http://creativecommons.org/licenses/by/4.0/).

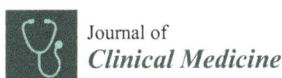

Article

Advancing the Science and Management of Renal Cell Carcinoma: Bridging the Divide between Academic and Community Practices

Nicholas J. Salgia [1], Errol J. Philip [2], Mohammadbagher Ziari [3], Kelly Yap [4] and Sumanta Kumar Pal [1,*]

1. Department of Medical Oncology & Experimental Therapeutics, City of Hope Comprehensive Cancer Center, Duarte, CA 91107, USA; nsalgia@coh.org
2. University of California San Francisco School of Medicine, San Francisco, CA 94143, USA; errol.philip@ucsf.edu
3. Department of Medical Oncology & Experimental Therapeutics, City of Hope Comprehensive Cancer Center, Corona, CA 92879, USA; mziari@coh.org
4. Department of Medical Oncology & Experimental Therapeutics, City of Hope Comprehensive Cancer Center, South Pasadena, CA 91030, USA; keyap@coh.org
* Correspondence: spal@coh.org; Tel.: +1-(626)-256-4673; Fax: +1-(626)-301-8233

Received: 29 April 2020; Accepted: 14 May 2020; Published: 17 May 2020

Abstract: The treatment of metastatic renal cell carcinoma (mRCC) has rapidly evolved; however, the progress made in the field is heavily contingent upon timely and efficient accrual to clinical trials. While a substantial proportion of accrual occurs at tertiary care centers, community sites are playing an increasing role in patient recruitment. In this article, we discuss strategies to optimize collaborations between academic and community sites to facilitate clinical research. Further, as the role of biomarker discovery has become increasingly important in tailoring therapy, we will discuss opportunities to bridge diverse accrual sites for the purpose of translational research.

Keywords: renal cell carcinoma; team medicine; translational research; community practice; clinical trials

1. Introduction

Two decades ago, the outlook for patients with metastatic renal cell carcinoma (mRCC) was bleak. Treatments such as interferon-α (IFN-α) and interleukin-2 (IL-2) yielded a median survival of approximately one year [1]. The landscape changed tremendously with the introduction of targeted therapies from 2005 onwards, and, once again, with the introduction of checkpoint blockade a decade later [2–5]. In 2020, the current standard for front-line treatment of mRCC remains either dual checkpoint inhibition or a combination of targeted therapy with checkpoint blockade [6–8]. Survival estimates have essentially tripled what was anticipated in the cytokine era.

The rapid developments in mRCC therapy have been made possible by the timely and efficient completion of both early and late phase clinical trials. In addition, the discovery of novel therapies has been fostered by translational research efforts—the intersect of the bench and bedside. This is especially true in RCC, which has directly benefitted from research discoveries that have led to both the 2018 and 2019 Nobel Prizes in Physiology or Medicine. While tertiary centers (e.g., cancer centers and academic hospitals) serve as a common ground for early phase clinical trials and translational work, there is no doubt that their efforts can be bolstered through the participation of community oncology practices. Further, late-phase clinical trials, which often require less stringent data collection and less intensive evaluation schedules, can perhaps be done equally well at community and academic sites.

Whereas the prognosis of mRCC has improved, it is important to note that most patients with this disease are not cured, and thus, further research is imperative. In the current manuscript, we review the clinical landscape for renal cell carcinoma and delve into opportunities to maximize collaborations between community-based practices and academic sites in the hope of promoting more efficient and effective research endeavors. We approach the latter objective in the specific context of City of Hope—a tertiary cancer center that serves the greater Los Angeles area, a catchment that includes approximately 20,000,000 people. City of Hope has within its network 30 community-based satellite clinics, stretching over a radius of 100 miles [9]. With this vast network of community sites and the robust patient population that comes with it, multiple opportunities for collaborative research exist. However, selecting the right research for community versus academic practices is no small feat. Whereas our academic practice at City of Hope is well-staffed, with 5 research nurses and 7 clinical research associates devoted to genitourinary cancers, community sites often have a limited number of research staff who are responsible for managing studies across multiple disease types. These limitations notwithstanding, the integration of academic and community centers has grown into a successful model for conducting clinical and translational research.

2. Renal Cell Carcinoma Incidence and Histology

Renal cell carcinomas are a broad classification referring to tumors originating from the renal pelvis and medulla. The incidence of RCC is increasing, with an estimated 73,750 newly diagnosed cases in 2020 in the United States [10]. The disease now accounts for 5% of cancer diagnoses in men and 3% in women. The rising incidence of RCC can be partially attributed to an increase in the incidental detection of small renal masses during the performance of abdominal imaging for non-specific complaints [11]. Although the majority of incidental findings are small, early-stage masses, these diagnoses have not led to a substantial change in the mortality rate attributed to RCC; in 2020, it is estimated that RCC will account for approximately 15,000 deaths in the United States [10].

The histological variations in RCC have been well-documented [12]. Clear cell RCC (ccRCC) represents the most common subtype, accounting for 80% of diagnoses. ccRCC is pathologically characterized by its clear cell histology and acinar growth patterns. The hallmark molecular alterations of ccRCC include chromosome 3p loss and inactivation of the Von-Hippel Lindau (VHL) gene, which lies at the 3p25 locus [13]. VHL inactivation can occur either somatically or in the germline. Inactivation of *VHL* has been reported in up to 90% of sporadic ccRCC cases [14,15]. Germline inactivations of *VHL* are associated with Von-Hippel Lindau syndrome, which predisposes individuals to bilateral renal masses, as well as hemangioblastomas and retinal angiomas [16]. Other mutations associated with ccRCC are *PBRM1*, *SETD2*, and *BAP1*, all of which also lie on chromosome 3p [15,17].

Non-clear cell RCC (nccRCC) is a heterogenous classification that encompasses the other 20% of RCC diagnoses. Papillary RCC (pRCC) composes the majority of nccRCCs (~15% of total RCC diagnoses). pRCC has historically been subdivided into two classifications based on histology: type 1 involves low-grade nuclei arranged in a single layer, and type 2 encompasses a wide range of morphological presentations that can be further divided into at least three additional subtypes. Type 1 pRCC has been associated with sporadic mutations in the MET protooncogene (10–13% of patients) [18]. Other nccRCCs include chromophobe RCC, MiT translocation RCCs, collecting duct carcinoma, and renal medullary carcinoma. Each of the above-listed subtypes accounts for less than 10% of all RCC diagnoses [19].

As ccRCC represents the overwhelming majority of RCC diagnoses, the remainder of this review will focus primarily on the management of clear cell disease and use RCC interchangeably for ccRCC.

3. Managing Localized Renal Cell Carcinoma

Localized RCC comprises the majority of RCC cases, and in turn, is typically cured with definitive treatment. The standard of care for most localized tumors has been nephrectomy, whether it be partial or radical. Cancer-specific survival rates for localized RCC patients have been estimated to be

84% at five years and 76% at ten years after surgical resection, varying widely with stage. Although these estimates are overwhelmingly positive compared to patients with metastatic disease, one area of research interest has been the potential utility of adjuvant or neoadjuvant therapies to increase disease-free and overall survival (OS). A variety of agents, including IFN-α, IL-2, and chemotherapies, have been trialed as adjuvant therapies for localized RCC, but none demonstrated an improvement in disease-free survival. As the treatment landscape for mRCC has evolved, so too have the investigatory agents for adjuvant and neoadjuvant therapy.

The ASSURE trial and S-TRAC trial both compared adjuvant sunitinib to placebo in patients with high-risk localized RCC [20,21]. ASSURE also contained a third arm (sorafenib). No difference in disease-free survival (5.8 versus 6.1 versus 6.6 years for sunitinib, sorafenib, and placebo, respectively) nor OS was seen in ASSURE, and substantial toxicities were associated with both sunitinib and sorafenib. However, S-TRAC reported a statistically significant increase in disease-free survival with sunitinib versus placebo (6.8 versus 5.6 years) on independent review, but still no difference in OS. Based on the results of S-TRAC, sunitinib was approved for adjuvant use. Although approved, sunitinib is not often leveraged in the adjuvant setting due to the substantial toxicities associated with its use. Various other trials have investigated small molecule inhibitors as adjuvant therapy: PROTECT compared pazopanib to placebo, ATLAS compared axitinib to placebo, and EVEREST compared everolimus to placebo [22–24]. Both PROTECT and ATLAS have reported out and did not demonstrate improved survival with adjuvant therapy, while EVEREST has completed accrual, but results have not yet been reported.

Additional investigation of adjuvant therapy for localized disease has incorporated immune checkpoint inhibitors (CPIs). The recently opened PROSPER RCC trial randomizes patients to receive surgery alone or surgery with perioperative nivolumab (Figure 1) [25]. This study continues to accrue patients. IMmotion 010 also has investigated the role of adjuvant CPI therapy for resected RCC, in this case, comparing atezolizumab to placebo for patients with high-risk of disease recurrence [26]. This trial has not reported results to date. As the disclosed trials have reported minimal or no improvement with adjuvant therapy for localized RCC, systemic therapy is primarily isolated to patients with metastatic disease.

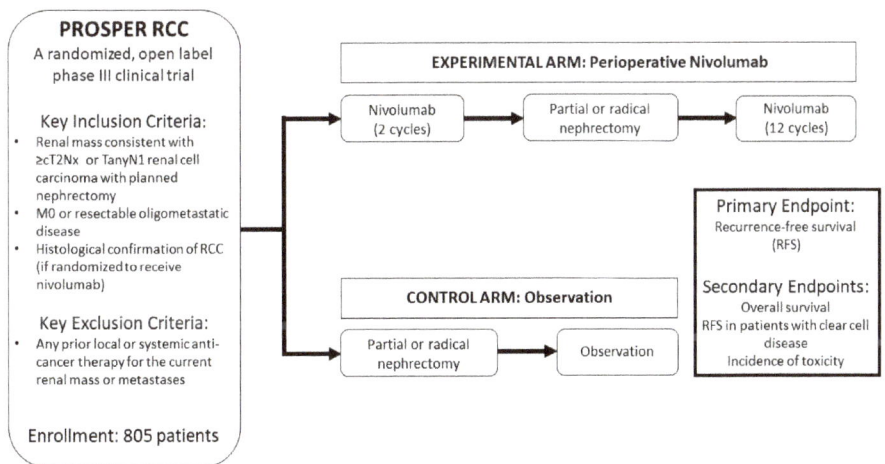

Figure 1. Schema for the phase-III ECOG-ACRIN PROSPER study.

4. The Evolving Management of Metastatic Renal Cell Carcinoma

mRCC carries a relatively poor long-term survival (12% five-year OS) when compared to localized disease (93% five-year OS)—of course, these estimates are changing with emerging therapies.

The systemic therapy landscape for mRCC has rapidly evolved within the last twenty years [27]. At the turn of the century, cytokine-based approaches with high-dose IL-2 and IFN-α represented the best systemic therapeutic option for patients with advanced disease. Both cytokines have been shown in animal and human models to have anti-cancer properties: IL-2 enhances the growth and activation of natural killer cells and CD-8+ T-cells, while IFN-α enhances tumor antigen presentation, among other characteristics [28,29]. While such cytokine approaches promote tumor regression mechanistically, IL-2 and IFN-α both provided limited clinical efficacy, with a median OS of approximately one year and durable responses in the range of only 5–7% [1,30,31]. These agents also posed substantial toxicity profiles, further limiting successful therapeutic outcomes.

4.1. Risk Stratification: MSKCC and IMDC Criteria

Among the most important non-therapeutic advances in the management of mRCC have been the development and implementation of risk classification algorithms. The Memorial Sloan Kettering Cancer Center (MSKCC) Score for renal cell carcinoma represents the first widely-adopted calculation for risk stratification of mRCC patients [31]. The initial MSKCC risk score included five prognostic factors: low Karnofsky performance status, high serum lactate dehydrogenase, low hemoglobin, high serum calcium, and absence of prior nephrectomy. These were used as risk factors to stratify patients into three groups: favorable risk (0 risk factors), intermediate risk (1–2 risk factors), and poor risk (3+ risk factors). Patients with MSKCC favorable risk disease were reported to have a median OS of 20 months, those with intermediate risk had a median OS of 10 months, and poor risk disease carried a median OS of 4 months. The MSKCC model has incorporated various additions into its algorithm over time. The Mekhail extension added two variables: prior radiotherapy and 2+ sites of metastasis [32]. In 2018, the MSKCC risk model was updated to incorporate genomic characteristics, specifically the mutational status of *BAP1*, *PBRM1*, and *TP53* in the stratification algorithm [33]. The MSKCC risk model has been used as an important inclusion criterion and stratification variable for patient randomization in various RCC therapeutic trials [5].

A second prognostic model has been developed and validated for mRCC: the International Metastatic Renal Cell Carcinoma Database Consortium (IMDC) Risk Score. Like the MSKCC model, the IMDC score utilizes clinical variables as prognostic markers to define patient risk. The IMDC model incorporates six prognostic variables: less than one year from the time of diagnosis to onset of systemic therapy, low Karnofsky performance status, low hemoglobin, high calcium, high neutrophil, and high platelet levels [34]. Similar to the MSKCC model, patients are classified into one of three risk groups. Favorable risk (0 factors) carries a median OS of 43.2 months, intermediate risk (1–2 factors) carries a median OS of 22.5 months, and poor risk (3+ factors) carries a median OS of 7.8 months [35]. Like the MSKCC model, the IMDC score has been adopted as a key inclusion criterion and stratification metric for many pivotal RCC trials [6].

4.2. VEGF Tyrosine Kinase Inhibitors, Multi-Kinase Inhibitors, and mTOR Inhibitors

The first shift in the therapeutic approach to mRCC occurred with the advent of small-molecule inhibitors that bind to and inhibit the activity of membranous receptors and intracellular proteins. The primary class of small molecule inhibitors in the mRCC treatment armamentarium are vascular endothelial growth factor–tyrosine kinase inhibitors (VEGF–TKIs). Mechanistically, *VHL* mutations lead to decreased ubiquitinylation of hypoxia-inducible factor (HIF) and upregulation of the circulating VEGF molecule which then binds the VEGF receptor, promoting angiogenesis [36,37]. VEGF–TKIs inhibit the tyrosine kinase domain of the VEGF receptor, and in turn, block the intracellular signaling cascade that promotes angiogenesis and cell division

Multiple VEGF–TKIs have been approved for mRCC. One benchmark phase-III study compared the VEGF–TKI sunitinib to IFN-α in patients with previously untreated mRCC [2]. Sunitinib was demonstrated to prolong progression-free survival (PFS) compared to IFN-α (11 versus 4 months) and was associated with a higher objective response rate (ORR) (31% vs. 6%). The results of this study led to the approval of sunitinib for first-line mRCC patients. Other VEGF–TKI agents approved in mRCC include sorafenib, pazopanib, and axitinib. While these agents have prolonged PFS and produced improved response rates compared to the previous standard-of-care cytokine therapies, VEGF–TKIs are not curative, and patients are susceptible to disease progression upon the development of drug resistance.

An additional class of targeted therapies, so-called multi-kinase inhibitors have also been approved in mRCC. These agents not only act as VEGF–TKIs but also inhibit the tyrosine kinase domains of additional protooncogenes [38]. Cabozantinib is a multi-kinase inhibitor with activity as a VEGF–TKI and also as an inhibitor of MET and AXL, both of which are associated with resistance to VEGF–TKIs. Cabozantinib was first approved for mRCC patients with treatment-refractory disease but was soon trialed as first-line therapy. The phase-II CABOSUN trial compared cabozantinib to sunitinib in the front-line setting [39]. This study met its primary endpoint of improvement in PFS with cabozantinib (8.6 versus 5.3 months) and demonstrated a higher ORR with cabozantinib based on an independent review (20% versus 9%). These results led to the approval of cabozantinib across all lines of therapy for patients with mRCC. However, like sunitinib and other VEGF–TKIs, cabozantinib has limited curative potential. As such, the approach of managing mRCC in the front-line with VEGF–TKIs and multi-kinase inhibitors has been replaced by the recent introduction of immune checkpoint inhibitors.

The mammalian target of rapamycin (mTOR) represents a highly-important intracellular target of mRCC therapy. mTOR is an enzymatic intermediate in the PI3K/AKT/mTOR signaling pathway that regulates the cell cycle [40]. Dysregulation of this pathway is a metabolic feature of many RCC tumors, making the components of its signaling cascade viable targets for pharmacologic inhibition. Two therapies approved for the management of mRCC act in this manner on mTOR: everolimus and temsirolimus. Everolimus is an oral agent that has been approved in combination for mRCC with the VEGF–TKI lenvatinib, following the results of a phase II study comparing the combination to each respective monotherapy [41]. Everolimus with lenvatinib resulted in PFS benefit compared to everolimus alone (14.6 versus 5.5 months) for patients who had received at least one prior VEGF–directed therapy. Temsirolimus, an inhibitory ester analog of mTOR that is applied intravenously, is also approved for mRCC [42]. A phase III trial demonstrated an OS benefit for temsirolimus over IFN-α (10.9 versus 7.3 months) with fewer incidences of serious adverse events [43]. Although no longer a mainstay of early-line therapy, the mTOR inhibitors everolimus and temsirolimus remain important interventions for the management of mRCC. Like VEGF–TKIs and multikinase inhibitors, however, mTOR inhibitors have given way to immune checkpoint inhibitors for the early-line treatment of mRCC.

4.3. Immune Checkpoint Inhibitors

Immune checkpoint inhibition is a relatively recent development in solid tumors, first explored in the context of melanoma [44]. CPIs are synthesized monoclonal antibodies capable of overcoming T-cell inactivation to elicit an anti-tumor response [45]. Approved CPIs exhibit activity on one of two immunoregulatory axes: programmed-death-1/programmed-death-ligand-1 (PD-1/PD-L1) and the cytotoxic-T-lymphocyte-associated protein 4 (CTLA-4). The treatment paradigm for mRCC has advanced greatly since the advent of PD-(L)1 and CTLA-4 inhibitors.

CheckMate-025 was the first study to investigate nivolumab, an anti-PD-1 CPI, in mRCC [5]. This study enrolled patients who had progressed on one or two previous VEGF–TKIs and randomized them to receive nivolumab or everolimus. Nivolumab outperformed everolimus in OS (25 versus 19.6 months) and ORR (25% versus 5%), leading to the approval of nivolumab monotherapy for mRCC patients who had progressed on previous therapy.

The ensuing CheckMate-214 trial compared the combined regimen of nivolumab with ipilimumab, an anti-CTLA-4 CPI, to sunitinib in previously-untreated mRCC [6]. Patients were stratified based on the International Metastatic Renal Cell Carcinoma Database Consortium (IMDC) risk score. In patients with intermediate or poor risk disease, nivolumab + ipilimumab greatly outperformed sunitinib, demonstrating greater ORR (42% versus 27%) and a rate of complete response totaling 9%. However, among patients with favorable risk disease by IMDC criteria, sunitinib was shown to result in prolonged PFS (25.1 versus 15.3 months) and a greater ORR (52% versus 29%). The results from CheckMate-214 established a new treatment algorithm for front-line mRCC, in which dual checkpoint inhibition with nivolumab + ipilimumab form the backbone of therapy for intermediate/poor risk patients but VEGF–TKIs remain a viable first-line option for patients with favorable risk.

4.4. Combination Therapies

Further endeavors have clinically investigated combinations of CPIs with VEGF–TKIs. A myriad of large phase III clinical trials have been undertaken, with three having reported out in early 2019. The IMmotion 151 trial compared the investigatory combination of atezolizumab (an anti PD-L1 CPI) with bevacizumab (an anti-VEGF monoclonal antibody) against sunitinib [46]. This trial met its primary endpoint of improvement in PFS with bevacizumab + atezolizumab (11.2 versus 7.7 months) in the PD-L1+ population. In the intention-to-treat cohort that included all patients regardless of PD-L1 status, PFS favored the combination therapy over sunitinib (11.2 versus 8.4 months). JAVELIN-101 followed a similar design model, comparing the combination of avelumab (an anti-PD-L1 CPI) and axitinib against sunitinib in patients with mRCC who had received no prior therapy [8]. The primary endpoint of improved PFS with axitinib + avelumab in patients who had PD-L1+ disease was met (13.8 versus 7.2 months). Likewise, irrespective of PD-L1 status, axitinib + avelumab was again associated with improved PFS (13.8 versus 8.4 months).

The KEYNOTE-426 trial utilized an experimental arm of pembrolizumab (an anti-PD-1 CPI) with axitinib, which was compared against sunitinib [7]. The axitinib + pembrolizumab combination resulted in a prolonged PFS compared to sunitinib (15.1 versus 11.1 months), and, additionally, ORR was greater in the axitinib + pembrolizumab arm (59% versus 36%). These three trials all reported within the span of two months in 2019. Table 1 summarizes results from trials testing CPIs (in combination with an additional CPI or with VEGF-TKIs) for the first-line treatment of mRCC. A recent press release in April 2020 has also indicated that the CheckMate-9ER trial (NCT03141177) of nivolumab + cabozantinib versus sunitinib for front-line mRCC has met its primary endpoint of improved PFS and secondary endpoints of ORR and OS. The combination of axitinib + pembrolizumab, in particular, has already established a role in the mRCC treatment algorithm for front-line intervention in patients with IMDC good-risk disease [47]. As data from these trials continue to mature and additional trials are undertaken, it is reasonable to believe the approval and usage of combination therapies will expand.

Table 1. Results from four phase-III clinical trials investigating front-line immune checkpoint inhibitor use in metastatic renal cell carcinoma.

Trial	CheckMate-214 (Intermediate + Poor Risk Patients)		IMmotion-151		JAVELIN-101		KEYNOTE-426	
Arms	Nivolumab + Ipilimumab	Sunitinib	Bevacizumab + Atezolizumab	Sunitinib	Axitinib + Avelumab	Sunitinib	Axitinib + Pembrolizumab	Sunitinib
Patients Enrolled	425	422	454	461	442	444	432	429
ORR, % (95% CI)	42 (37–47)	27 (22–31)	37 (32–41)	33 (29–38)	51 (47–56)	26 (22–30)	59 (55–64)	36 (31–40)
Median PFS	11.6	8.4	11.2	8.4	13.8	8.4	15.1	11.1
PFS HR (95% CI)	0.82 (0.64–1.05) *		0.83 (0.70–0.97)		0.69 (0.56–0.84)		0.69 (0.57–0.84)	
OS HR (95% CI)	0.63 (0.44–0.89) †		0.93 (0.76–1.14)		Not Reported		0.53 (0.38–0.74)	
Grade 3/4 Adverse Events, %	46	63	40	54	55	55	63	58

Abbreviations: ORR = overall response rate, CI = confidence interval, PFS = progression-free survival, HR = hazard ratio, OS = overall survival. * 99.1% confidence interval; † 99.8% confidence interval.

4.5. Cytoreductive Nephrectomy for Metastatic Disease: A Continuing Discussion

The utility of cytoreductive nephrectomy as a component of care for mRCC remains a highly-investigated topic. Cytoreductive nephrectomy for removal of the primary tumor in patients with metastatic disease was a standard-of-care for twenty years. However, two recent trials, SURTIME and CARMENA, have changed the paradigm for nephrectomy in mRCC. SURTIME compared immediate nephrectomy (followed by sunitinib therapy) versus deferred nephrectomy (preceded by sunitinib therapy) [48]. The results of this study indicated that deferred nephrectomy did not improve the progression-free rate at 28 weeks compared to immediate nephrectomy (43% versus 42%), but OS was higher in the deferred arm (32.4 versus 15.0 months). These results suggested that initial systemic therapy followed by a potential debulking nephrectomy may be more efficacious for mRCC patients than the former standard of upfront nephrectomy.

CARMENA randomized patients with mRCC to undergo nephrectomy followed by sunitinib or to receive sunitinib alone [49]. Results from this study indicated that sunitinib alone offered a non-inferior alternative to nephrectomy followed by sunitinib, with OS favoring the former (18.4 versus 13.9 months). The results of CARMENA and SURTIME have led to a shift away from cytoreductive nephrectomy as a standard-of-care for mRCC, except in carefully planned cases. However, ongoing trials continue to study the relevance of cytoreductive nephrectomy. The NORDIC-SUN trial (NCT03977571) investigates nephrectomy following therapy with nivolumab + ipilimumab. Patients with IMDC favorable- or intermediate-risk disease are randomized to receive nephrectomy or maintenance nivolumab. Patients who present with poor-risk disease can be randomized within this study as well, so long as their risk classification is adjusted to intermediate-risk following initial therapy with nivolumab + ipilimumab or while on maintenance nivolumab. An additional trial, CYTOSHRINK (NCT04090710), uses stereotactic body radiation therapy (SBRT) as an investigational definitive treatment of the primary tumor site for patients with mRCC. In this trial, patients are randomized to receive the standard-of-care nivolumab + ipilimumab for four cycles, followed by maintenance nivolumab or the experimental arm. The experimental arm consists of one cycle of nivolumab + ipilimumab followed by five fractions of SBRT to the kidney lesion before resuming nivolumab + ipilimumab on the standard schedule. Both these trials are currently open to accrual.

5. Integrating Community and Academic Practices for Renal Cell Carcinoma Research

As RCC incidence continues to grow, the role of the community oncologist has grown increasingly important in the network of care for RCC patients. While clinical and translational research has primarily been led by academic oncologists, a new approach incorporating community practitioners into the research paradigm is now viable. It is important that medical oncologists at academic centers integrate community practitioners, particularly urologists and oncologists, into a collaborative model that promotes exceptional, multi-disciplinary care alongside cutting-edge clinical and translational research. Through the City of Hope network, which encompasses a central academic center and a diffuse network of community sites, we have developed a collaborative model for conducting translational research and clinical trial accrual that integrates academic and community oncologists. Below, we have highlighted our experiences utilizing this integrated structure to advance clinical and translational research and discovery in RCC.

6. Collaborations in Translational Research

As detailed above, the therapies currently in use for mRCC reflect two biological principles, namely, that (1) RCC is driven by angiogenesis and that (2) defects in the immune system can propagate the disease. One of the genomic hallmarks of RCC are defects in the *VHL* gene [15,50]. Mutation of *VHL* (largely sporadic, but possibly hereditary) leads to decreased ubiquitinylation of HIF [51–54]. This, in turn, leads to the upregulation of vascular endothelial growth factor (VEGF), a potent mediator of angiogenesis [55,56]. The interplay of RCC with the immune system is much more complex. Multiple studies have shown varying levels of expression of the immune checkpoint programmed death-ligand 1 (PD-L1) in RCC tissues [7,57,58]. Interaction of PD-L1 with its cognate receptor, programmed death-1 (PD-1), leads to T-cell anergy, which can be overcome with antibodies targeting either entity [59–61].

Interestingly, while VEGF–pathway inhibitors and immune checkpoint inhibitors both reflect "targeted therapies", both are applied in a biomarker-agnostic fashion in patients with mRCC. At City of Hope, a partnership has been forged with TGen, Inc., a company focused on translational genomics. Scientists and clinicians at TGen have developed the Ashion GEM ExTra® platform that allows for both whole-exome sequencing and RNA sequencing [62]. A sample report is shown in Figure 2. In addition to requiring tissue for tumor sequencing, the platform uses blood for germline correction.

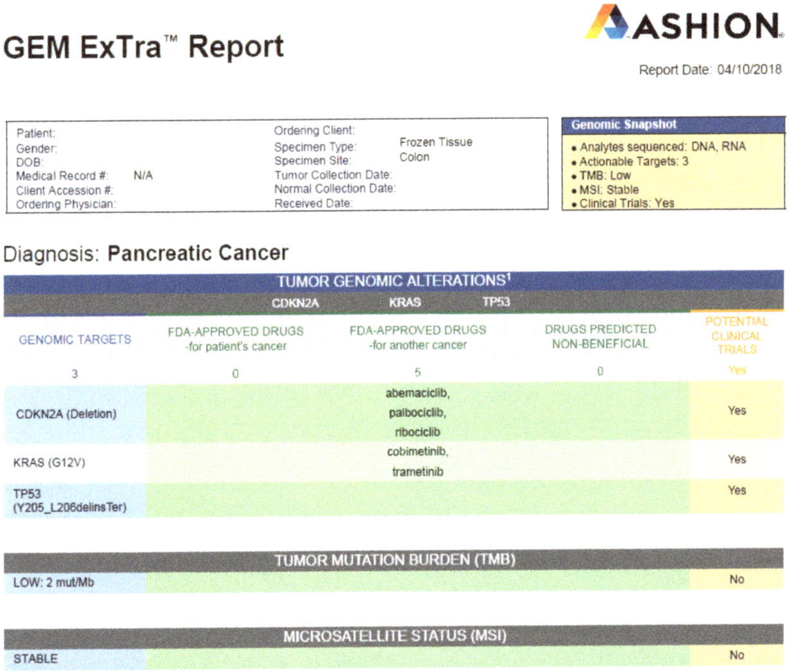

GEM ExTra™ Report

ASHION

Report Date: 04/10/2018

Patient:
Gender:
DOB:
Medical Record #: N/A
Client Accession #:
Ordering Physician:
Ordering Client:
Specimen Type: Frozen Tissue
Specimen Site: Colon
Tumor Collection Date:
Normal Collection Date:
Received Date:

Genomic Snapshot
• Analytes sequenced: DNA, RNA
• Actionable Targets: 3
• TMB: Low
• MSI: Stable
• Clinical Trials: Yes

Diagnosis: **Pancreatic Cancer**

TUMOR GENOMIC ALTERATIONS[1]

CDKN2A KRAS TP53

GENOMIC TARGETS	FDA-APPROVED DRUGS -for patient's cancer	FDA-APPROVED DRUGS -for another cancer	DRUGS PREDICTED NON-BENEFICIAL	POTENTIAL CLINICAL TRIALS
3	0	5	0	Yes
CDKN2A (Deletion)		abemaciclib, palbociclib, ribociclib		Yes
KRAS (G12V)		cobimetinib, trametinib		Yes
TP53 (Y205_L206delinsTer)				Yes

TUMOR MUTATION BURDEN (TMB)

LOW: 2 mut/Mb	No

MICROSATELLITE STATUS (MSI)

STABLE	No

Figure 2. A sample report from the Ashion GEM ExTra test.

A sequencing platform such as Ashion GEM ExTra® offers two benefits in terms of translational research. First and foremost, collecting this data and pooling it across academic and community sites may allow for the development of predictive and prognostic biomarkers. In a recent effort, Salgia et al. reviewed data from 90 patients with mRCC (Salgia et al. ASCO 2020) and examined the association between treatment type and response among those that had received immunotherapy or targeted therapy. Notably, DNA level data suggested that *TERT* promoter alterations were a negative predictor of immunotherapy response, with RNA level data from the study identifying multiple *TERT*-associated pathways that could play a role in immunotherapy resistance.

A further benefit of amassing translational data across community and academic sites is the ability to identify novel opportunities for clinical research. Our pooled data indicate, for instance, a preponderance of mutations in *VHL*, *PBRM1*, *SETD2*, and other mutations in the mammalian target of rapamycin (mTOR) pathway. We have also observed infrequent but clinically significant mutations in genes such as *EGFR*, *MET*, and *ALK* [63,64]. Many phase I and II trials in development focus specifically on these mutations but do so in a tumor agnostic fashion. The genitourinary group physicians at our institution have partnered with community sites and other disease teams to categorize cumulative mutational frequency. By pooling this data across our sites, we can make logical decisions regarding the most appropriate clinical trials to bring into our portfolio.

Biomarker discovery and validation are not isolated to genomics, however. Recent work has elucidated associations between microbiome composition and clinical response to CPIs in mRCC [65]. Additional work from our group and collaborators at TGen, Inc. has investigated the enteric microbiome as a potential biomarker for responses to the above-mentioned therapy regimens in RCC [66]. We have utilized whole genome shotgun metagenomic sequencing to correlate the stool microbiome profile and microbiome diversity of mRCC patients with clinical benefit, both for patients receiving VEGF–TKIs and for patients receiving CPIs (Dizman et al. ASCO 2020). In these studies, we have identified a variety of microbial species (such as *B. Intestihominis* and *B. adolescentis*) that are correlated with clinical benefit in patients receiving systemic therapy for mRCC. The diversification of biomarker pursuits provides another avenue for research collaboration between academic and community partners. Protocols for the collection, storage, and shipment of stool, for example, can be implemented at any site, even those with limited research infrastructure. The clinical volume of community practice sites poses an untapped resource for furthering biomarker discovery and other translational studies in RCC.

7. Collaborations in Clinical Research

7.1. Phase I and II Clinical Trials

Phase I clinical trials have morphed in recent years, moving away from the classical 3 + 3 design [67]. More recent iterations of phase I clinical trials have started with a dose-escalation phase, expanding quickly into phase Ib trial designs, all while seeking validation in disease- or mutation-specific settings. We propose that phase I studies in dose escalation are perhaps most appropriate to remain at academic centers. The dose-escalation phase is one where rigorous oversight is necessary, with multiple visits and correlative studies. Furthermore, this is often the phase in which novel toxicities associated with an agent or combination are recognized and documented. We propose that highly selected phase Ib studies could be conducted in the community (Figure 3). Criteria for site selection in these studies must account for the frequency of study visits and the rigor of correlatives. For instance, if a proposed study requires pharmacokinetic and pharmacodynamic blood assessments on hourly intervals (not unusual in a phase-I protocol), the trial may be challenging in a busy community practice. Similarly, if a study requires repeat biopsies or other invasive assessments, academic centers may be better suited.

Indeed, there are real-world examples of phase I studies that may be too challenging to envision in a community practice setting at this time. For instance, our genitourinary cancers group is heavily invested in studies of chimeric antigen receptor (CAR)–T-cell therapies (Dorff et al. ASCO GU 2020). In addition to the complexities associated with the manufacturing and storage of CAR–T-cells, patients must be kept in an inpatient setting for prompt recognition and treatment of unique side effects of this treatment, such as cytokine release syndrome [68]. At present, commercially available CAR–T-cell therapies are used in a limited subset of patients with hematologic malignancies [69]. Until these therapies are adopted in a much more widespread fashion in the community (with appropriate infrastructure and monitoring), we recommend these studies remain within academic centers.

The phase II study is a vanishing entity, as companies often now move quickly from a large phase Ib effort to phase III. This is true in mRCC space as well—as one example, COSMIC-021 (NCT03170960) is an international study chaired by investigators at our site. This phase Ib study of cabozantinib with atezolizumab enrolled cohorts in RCC, lung cancer, and prostate cancer, as well as more than a dozen other histologies. Based on significant activity in the three noted cohorts, phase III clinical trials have been rapidly launched, including CONTACT-03 (NCT04338269) for mRCC [70]. In general, if phase II studies are to be considered in the community setting, the same factors (visit frequency, correlative studies, and so on) should aid in deciding whether studies are appropriate and should proceed.

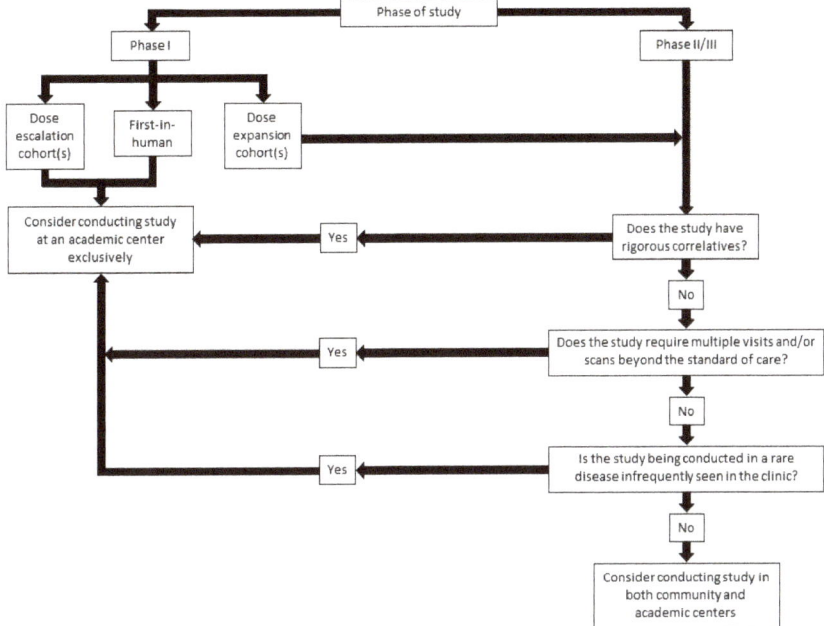

Figure 3. Schema outlining appropriate trial selection for community and academic settings.

7.2. Phase III Clinical Trials

Phase III clinical trials represent an area where collaborations are imperative. These studies often include hundreds (if not thousands) of patients, and to accrue in a rapid fashion, a partnership between academic and community sites is essential. There are two general categories of phase III studies that we consider in our program—one falls under the umbrella of pharmaceutical research, and the other relies upon funding from the National Cancer Institute (NCI), typically through the cooperative group mechanism. The cooperative groups have recently been consolidated—several groups (SWOG, Alliance, NRG, ECOG-ACRIN, and COG) retain members at both academic and community sites.

In general, cooperative group studies have more recently adopted easier thresholds for enrollment and less intensive patient follow-up. An example of this is the phase III PROSPER study, run by ECOG-ACRIN, which we have previously highlighted [25]. This phase III trial compares surgery alone for localized or oligometastatic RCC to surgery with both preoperative and postoperative nivolumab, a PD-1 inhibitor (Figure 1). The study has relaxed eligibility criteria with recent amendments—with randomization possible prior to a histologic diagnosis, and a pretreatment biopsy only required if patients are randomized to perioperative therapy. The study also does not mandate central review.

Such eligibility requirements differ widely from comparable pharmaceutical trials. For example, investigators at our institution led the phase III Immotion010 clinical trial, a study comparing atezolizumab to placebo in patients with completely resected RCC [26]. The study mandated pre-registration assessment of PD-L1 status, and further required central submission of scans. Not only do such measures increase the potential rate of screen failures, but they also increase the complexity of trial administration. Submitting tissue and scans in the pre-registration period (typically 2–3 weeks) is a wieldy task, and community sites must establish whether they have adequate resources to devote to such tasks.

Further, factors such as the study population, in particular tumor histology, must also be carefully considered in the conduct of trials. For example, studies investigating rare tumor histologies (nccRCCs) are challenging to conduct in the community setting due to the infrequency of disease presentation.

One such example is SWOG 1500 (NCT02761057), a study of selective MET-kinase inhibitors for patients with papillary renal cell carcinoma that was chaired by physicians in our genitourinary oncology disease team. Although the study was sponsored by an NCI cooperative group, the relative rarity of papillary histology (~10–15% of metastatic renal cell carcinomas) dictated that the study only be available at the academic center [71]. As patients with rare histologies are often referred from the community to experts at academic centers, consolidation of trial sites in these instances should be considered.

8. Optimizing Partnerships between Community and Academic Sites

As noted previously, the academic cancer center is typically well staffed with multiple research nurses and clinical research associates who work within a single disease space. Each has ownership over a selected number of protocols (typically 2–3), and there are often regular meetings with the principal investigator. These face to face meetings with principal investigators offer an opportunity for education regarding the protocol and, furthermore, allow for a closer degree of oversight of protocol-related activities. At City of Hope, investigators in the genitourinary disease team frequently host didactic sessions for research staff, offering them insight into the current standard management of RCC, bladder, and prostate cancer. As research staff are often charged with screening for enrollment or suggesting toxicity attributions, understanding the underlying disease and associated treatment landscape is critically important.

Models of research in community practices vary but commonly require research staff to manage a much broader swath of clinical protocols across multiple cancer types. Furthermore, the principal investigator for a study may not reside at the community practice site, and thus is unable to engage with clinical and administrative staff on a routine basis. At City of Hope, the vast majority of principal investigators reside at the main campus; thus, elements of study oversight (filing significant adverse events, reporting study deviations) may be somewhat delayed at community sites. In addition, services readily available at the main campus may be less accessible in the community practices; for example, labs may be obtained off-site through third-party vendors. This can create delays in lab reporting, and complicate study protocols that require same-day lab results to issue therapy. Many protocols also embed correlates that require additional processing methods (e.g., centrifugation for separation of plasma aliquots).

Similarly, access to appropriate and timely scans can vary by recruitment location, with an academic center generally able to accommodate access to both standard and novel imaging tests (e.g., fluciclovine or PSMA PET scans for prostate cancer) and not have to rely on third parties to transfer images so that relevant tumor measurements can be obtained. Whereas these may be trivial issues on a main academic campus, access to a centrifuge, processing equipment, and appropriate imaging modalities may be limited at community sites.

Despite these noted limitations, community practices can serve as valuable contributors to clinical research endeavors housed at a main campus. To optimize this relationship and promote successful collaborations, we have implemented several strategies. Firstly, self-nominated community disease team leads are identified to serve as liaisons between the research team on the main campus and oncologists practicing in the community. These individuals also play a role in determining the feasibility of specific clinical trials in the community, taking into account many of the considerations that we have outlined throughout. In addition, these individuals are invited to bimonthly genitourinary disease team meetings, where the group conducts a thorough review of all existing protocols and evaluates new clinical trial proposals. Finally, in recognition of the limited time permitted to community oncologists to learn about existing research endeavors, our genitourinary cancers group has established a newsletter that highlights ongoing and planned clinical trials with only the most salient information—basic eligibility requirements and study schema, for instance. These newsletters have triggered a number of direct referrals for clinical trial enrollment.

One relatively recent development among our community-based satellite clinics is the implementation of a standardized electronic health record (EHR) mirroring that at the main campus, optimizing the process by which physicians can evaluate and triage patients who may be suitable clinical trial candidates.

9. Conclusions

The clinical approach to RCC has drastically changed over the past two decades. The novel therapeutic options introduced to the medical oncologist's armamentarium have leveraged ground-breaking work on angiogenesis and induced hypoxia in addition to the principle of immune checkpoint blockade to overcome T-cell anergy. To maintain the momentum of RCC drug development, rigorous translational research must continue advancing our understanding of RCC biology and clinical trials must continue to accrue patients at a rapid pace. As we have highlighted herein, this can happen effectively and efficiently if community practices are integrated with academic centers in the conduct of translational research and clinical trials. We have proposed a number of strategies to optimize this relationship, with the common theme being enhanced communication. When oncologists at community and academic practices frequently dialogue, gaining a deeper understanding of each other's practice patterns, a portfolio of trials can be developed that optimizes accrual and advances scientific findings more rapidly.

The positive effects of an academic and community collaboration on trial accrual have been evidenced in our network—with our genitourinary cancers group recognized as the top accrual site for the adjuvant EVEREST study, a trial comparing everolimus and placebo in patients with resected localized RCC [24]. Our enrollment was driven in large part by patients seen at our community-based satellite offices. The rapid success of this collaborative effort was used as a foundation for the enrollment of patients into further adjuvant trials (e.g., E2810 and Immotion010), with similar positive outcomes. In sum, a strong collaborative approach between our academic center and affiliated community practices has resulted in a model conducive to high accrual rates across a broad range of clinical trials. This feat, along with the opportunities for collaboration in the translational sciences, underscores the benefit of these partnerships.

Author Contributions: Conceptualization, N.J.S., S.K.P.; Methodology, N.J.S., S.K.P.; Resources, S.K.P.; Data Curation, N.J.S., S.K.P.; Writing—Original Draft Preparation, N.J.S., S.K.P.; Writing—Review & Editing, N.J.S., E.J.P., K.Y., M.Z., S.K.P.; Visualization, N.J.S., S.K.P.; Supervision, S.K.P.; Project Administration, N.J.S., E.J.P., K.Y., M.Z., S.K.P. All authors have read and agreed to the published version of the manuscript.

Funding: This research received no external funding.

Conflicts of Interest: Nicholas Salgia, Errol Philip, Mohammadbagher Ziari, and Kelly Yap have no conflicts of interest that might be relevant to the contents of this manuscript. Sumanta K. Pal, MD—honoraria: Novartis, Medivation, Astellas Pharma; consulting or advisory role: Pfizer, Novartis, Aveo, Myriad; pharmaceuticals: Genentech, Exelixis, Bristol-Myers Squibb, Astellas Pharma; research funding: Medivation.

References

1. Atzpodien, J.; Kirchner, H.; Jonas, U.; Bergmann, L.; Schott, H.; Heynemann, H.; Fornara, P.; Loening, S.A.; Roigas, J.; Muller, S.C.; et al. Interleukin-2- and interferon alfa-2a-based immunochemotherapy in advanced renal cell carcinoma: A Prospectively Randomized Trial of the German Cooperative Renal Carcinoma Chemoimmunotherapy Group (DGCIN). *J. Clin. Oncol. Off. J. Am. Soc. Clin. Oncol.* **2004**, *22*, 1188–1194. [CrossRef] [PubMed]
2. Motzer, R.J.; Hutson, T.E.; Tomczak, P.; Michaelson, M.D.; Bukowski, R.M.; Rixe, O.; Oudard, S.; Negrier, S.; Szczylik, C.; Kim, S.T.; et al. Sunitinib versus interferon alfa in metastatic renal-cell carcinoma. *N. Engl. J. Med.* **2007**, *356*, 115–124. [CrossRef] [PubMed]
3. Sternberg, C.N.; Davis, I.D.; Mardiak, J.; Szczylik, C.; Lee, E.; Wagstaff, J.; Barrios, C.H.; Salman, P.; Gladkov, O.A.; Kavina, A.; et al. Pazopanib in locally advanced or metastatic renal cell carcinoma: Results of a randomized phase III trial. *J. Clin. Oncol. Off. J. Am. Soc. Clin. Oncol.* **2010**, *28*, 1061–1068. [CrossRef] [PubMed]

4. Hutson, T.E.; Al-Shukri, S.; Stus, V.P.; Lipatov, O.N.; Shparyk, Y.; Bair, A.H.; Rosbrook, B.; Andrews, G.I.; Vogelzang, N.J. Axitinib Versus Sorafenib in First-Line Metastatic Renal Cell Carcinoma: Overall Survival From a Randomized Phase III Trial. *Clin. Genitourin. Cancer* **2017**, *15*, 72–76. [CrossRef] [PubMed]
5. Motzer, R.J.; Escudier, B.; McDermott, D.F.; George, S.; Hammers, H.J.; Srinivas, S.; Tykodi, S.S.; Sosman, J.A.; Procopio, G.; Plimack, E.R.; et al. Nivolumab versus Everolimus in Advanced Renal-Cell Carcinoma. *N. Engl. J. Med.* **2015**, *373*, 1803–1813. [CrossRef] [PubMed]
6. Motzer, R.J.; Tannir, N.M.; McDermott, D.F.; Aren Frontera, O.; Melichar, B.; Choueiri, T.K.; Plimack, E.R.; Barthelemy, P.; Porta, C.; George, S.; et al. Nivolumab plus Ipilimumab versus Sunitinib in Advanced Renal-Cell Carcinoma. *N. Engl. J. Med.* **2018**, *378*, 1277–1290. [CrossRef]
7. Rini, B.I.; Plimack, E.R.; Stus, V.; Gafanov, R.; Hawkins, R.; Nosov, D.; Pouliot, F.; Alekseev, B.; Soulieres, D.; Melichar, B.; et al. Pembrolizumab plus Axitinib versus Sunitinib for Advanced Renal-Cell Carcinoma. *N. Engl. J. Med.* **2019**, *380*, 1116–1127. [CrossRef]
8. Motzer, R.J.; Penkov, K.; Haanen, J.; Rini, B.; Albiges, L.; Campbell, M.T.; Venugopal, B.; Kollmannsberger, C.; Negrier, S.; Uemura, M.; et al. Avelumab plus Axitinib versus Sunitinib for Advanced Renal-Cell Carcinoma. *N. Engl. J. Med.* **2019**, *380*, 1103–1115. [CrossRef]
9. Locations, Maps, and Directions. Available online: https://www.cityofhope.org/about-city-of-hope/locations (accessed on 10 April 2020).
10. Siegel, R.L.; Miller, K.D.; Jemal, A. Cancer statistics, 2020. *CA Cancer J. Clin.* **2020**, *70*, 7–30. [CrossRef]
11. Capitanio, U.; Montorsi, F. Renal cancer. *Lancet* **2016**, *387*, 894–906. [CrossRef]
12. Manini, C.; López, J.I. The Labyrinth of Renal Cell Carcinoma. *Cancers* **2020**, *12*, 521. [CrossRef] [PubMed]
13. Signoretti, S.; Flaifel, A.; Chen, Y.B.; Reuter, V.E. Renal Cell Carcinoma in the Era of Precision Medicine: From Molecular Pathology to Tissue-Based Biomarkers. *J. Clin. Oncol. Off. J. Am. Soc. Clin. Oncol.* **2018**, *36*, Jco2018792259. [CrossRef] [PubMed]
14. Sato, Y.; Yoshizato, T.; Shiraishi, Y.; Maekawa, S.; Okuno, Y.; Kamura, T.; Shimamura, T.; Sato-Otsubo, A.; Nagae, G.; Suzuki, H.; et al. Integrated molecular analysis of clear-cell renal cell carcinoma. *Nat. Genet.* **2013**, *45*, 860–867. [CrossRef] [PubMed]
15. Comprehensive molecular characterization of clear cell renal cell carcinoma. *Nature* **2013**, *499*, 43–49. [CrossRef] [PubMed]
16. Mikhail, M.I.; Singh, A.K. Von Hippel Lindau Syndrome. In *StatPearls*; StatPearls Publishing LLC: Treasure Island, FL, USA, 2020.
17. Hakimi, A.A.; Ostrovnaya, I.; Reva, B.; Schultz, N.; Chen, Y.-B.; Gonen, M.; Liu, H.; Takeda, S.; Voss, M.H.; Tickoo, S.K.; et al. Adverse Outcomes in Clear Cell Renal Cell Carcinoma with Mutations of 3p21 Epigenetic Regulators BAP1 and SETD2: A Report by MSKCC and the KIRC TCGA Research Network. *Clin. Cancer Res.* **2013**, *19*, 3259–3267. [CrossRef] [PubMed]
18. Comprehensive Molecular Characterization of Papillary Renal-Cell Carcinoma. *N. Engl. J. Med.* **2015**, *374*, 135–145. [CrossRef]
19. Linehan, W.M.; Srinivasan, R.; Garcia, J.A. Non-clear cell renal cancer: Disease-based management and opportunities for targeted therapeutic approaches. *Semin. Oncol.* **2013**, *40*, 511–520. [CrossRef]
20. Haas, N.B.; Manola, J.; Uzzo, R.G.; Flaherty, K.T.; Wood, C.G.; Kane, C.; Jewett, M.; Dutcher, J.P.; Atkins, M.B.; Pins, M.; et al. Adjuvant sunitinib or sorafenib for high-risk, non-metastatic renal-cell carcinoma (ECOG-ACRIN E2805): A double-blind, placebo-controlled, randomised, phase 3 trial. *Lancet* **2016**, *387*, 2008–2016. [CrossRef]
21. Ravaud, A.; Motzer, R.J.; Pandha, H.S.; George, D.J.; Pantuck, A.J.; Patel, A.; Chang, Y.-H.; Escudier, B.; Donskov, F.; Magheli, A.; et al. Adjuvant Sunitinib in High-Risk Renal-Cell Carcinoma after Nephrectomy. *N. Engl. J. Med.* **2016**, *375*, 2246–2254. [CrossRef]
22. Motzer, R.J.; Haas, N.B.; Donskov, F.; Gross-Goupil, M.; Varlamov, S.; Kopyltsov, E.; Lee, J.L.; Melichar, B.; Rini, B.I.; Choueiri, T.K.; et al. Randomized Phase III Trial of Adjuvant Pazopanib Versus Placebo After Nephrectomy in Patients With Localized or Locally Advanced Renal Cell Carcinoma. *J. Clin. Oncol.* **2017**, *35*, 3916–3923. [CrossRef]
23. Gross-Goupil, M.; Kwon, T.G.; Eto, M.; Ye, D.; Miyake, H.; Seo, S.I.; Byun, S.S.; Lee, J.L.; Master, V.; Jin, J.; et al. Axitinib versus placebo as an adjuvant treatment of renal cell carcinoma: Results from the phase III, randomized ATLAS trial. *Ann. Oncol.* **2018**, *29*, 2371–2378. [CrossRef]

24. Synold, T.W.; Plets, M.; Tangen, C.M.; Heath, E.I.; Palapattu, G.S.; Mack, P.C.; Stein, M.N.; Meng, M.V.; Lara, P.; Vogelzang, N.J.; et al. Everolimus Exposure as a Predictor of Toxicity in Renal Cell Cancer Patients in the Adjuvant Setting: Results of a Pharmacokinetic Analysis for SWOG S0931 (EVEREST), a Phase III Study (NCT01120249). *Kidney Cancer* **2019**, *3*, 111–118. [CrossRef] [PubMed]
25. Patel, H.D.; Puligandla, M.; Shuch, B.M.; Leibovich, B.C.; Kapoor, A.; Master, V.A.; Drake, C.G.; Heng, D.Y.; Lara, P.N.; Choueiri, T.K.; et al. The future of perioperative therapy in advanced renal cell carcinoma: How can we PROSPER? *Future Oncol. (Lond. Engl.)* **2019**, *15*, 1683–1695. [CrossRef] [PubMed]
26. Uzzo, R.; Bex, A.; Rini, B.I.; Albiges, L.; Suarez, C.; Donaldson, F.; Asakawa, T.; Schiff, C.; Pal, S.K. A phase III study of atezolizumab (atezo) vs placebo as adjuvant therapy in renal cell carcinoma (RCC) patients (pts) at high risk of recurrence following resection (IMmotion010). *J. Clin. Oncol.* **2017**, *35*, TPS4598. [CrossRef]
27. Angulo, J.C.; Lawrie, C.H.; López, J.I. Sequential treatment of metastatic renal cancer in a complex evolving landscape. *Ann. Transl. Med.* **2019**, *7*, S272. [CrossRef]
28. Amin, A.; White, R.L. Interleukin-2 in Renal Cell Carcinoma: A Has-Been or a Still-Viable Option? *J. Kidney Cancer Vhl.* **2014**, *1*, 74–83. [CrossRef]
29. Dranoff, G. Cytokines in cancer pathogenesis and cancer therapy. *Nat. Rev. Cancer* **2004**, *4*, 11–22. [CrossRef]
30. Interleukin 2 Gene Therapy for Prostate Cancer: Phase I Clinical Trial and Basic Biology. *Hum. Gene Ther.* **2001**, *12*, 883–892. [CrossRef]
31. Motzer, R.J.; Mazumdar, M.; Bacik, J.; Berg, W.; Amsterdam, A.; Ferrara, J. Survival and Prognostic Stratification of 670 Patients With Advanced Renal Cell Carcinoma. *J. Clin. Oncol.* **1999**, *17*, 2530. [CrossRef]
32. Mekhail, T.M.; Abou-Jawde, R.M.; Boumerhi, G.; Malhi, S.; Wood, L.; Elson, P.; Bukowski, R. Validation and extension of the Memorial Sloan-Kettering prognostic factors model for survival in patients with previously untreated metastatic renal cell carcinoma. *J. Clin. Oncol. Off. J. Am. Soc. Clin. Oncol.* **2005**, *23*, 832–841. [CrossRef]
33. Voss, M.H.; Reising, A.; Cheng, Y.; Patel, P.; Marker, M.; Kuo, F.; Chan, T.A.; Choueiri, T.K.; Hsieh, J.J.; Hakimi, A.A.; et al. Genomically annotated risk model for advanced renal-cell carcinoma: A retrospective cohort study. *Lancet Oncol.* **2018**, *19*, 1688–1698. [CrossRef]
34. Heng, D.Y.; Xie, W.; Regan, M.M.; Warren, M.A.; Golshayan, A.R.; Sahi, C.; Eigl, B.J.; Ruether, J.D.; Cheng, T.; North, S.; et al. Prognostic factors for overall survival in patients with metastatic renal cell carcinoma treated with vascular endothelial growth factor-targeted agents: Results from a large, multicenter study. *J. Clin. Oncol. Off. J. Am. Soc. Clin. Oncol.* **2009**, *27*, 5794–5799. [CrossRef] [PubMed]
35. Heng, D.Y.C.; Xie, W.; Regan, M.M.; Harshman, L.C.; Bjarnason, G.A.; Vaishampayan, U.N.; Mackenzie, M.; Wood, L.; Donskov, F.; Tan, M.-H.; et al. External validation and comparison with other models of the International Metastatic Renal-Cell Carcinoma Database Consortium prognostic model: A population-based study. *Lancet Oncol.* **2013**, *14*, 141–148. [CrossRef]
36. Kaelin, W.G., Jr. The von Hippel-Lindau tumour suppressor protein: O_2 sensing and cancer. *Nat. Rev. Cancer* **2008**, *8*, 865–873. [CrossRef] [PubMed]
37. Kaelin, W.G., Jr. Treatment of kidney cancer: Insights provided by the VHL tumor-suppressor protein. *Cancer* **2009**, *115*, 2262–2272. [CrossRef] [PubMed]
38. Makhov, P.; Joshi, S.; Ghatalia, P.; Kutikov, A.; Uzzo, R.G.; Kolenko, V.M. Resistance to Systemic Therapies in Clear Cell Renal Cell Carcinoma: Mechanisms and Management Strategies. *Mol. Cancer Ther.* **2018**, *17*, 1355–1364. [CrossRef]
39. Choueiri, T.K.; Halabi, S.; Sanford, B.L.; Hahn, O.; Michaelson, M.D.; Walsh, M.K.; Feldman, D.R.; Olencki, T.; Picus, J.; Small, E.J.; et al. Cabozantinib Versus Sunitinib As Initial Targeted Therapy for Patients With Metastatic Renal Cell Carcinoma of Poor or Intermediate Risk: The Alliance A031203 CABOSUN Trial. *J. Clin. Oncol.* **2017**, *35*, 591–597. [CrossRef]
40. Guo, H.; German, P.; Bai, S.; Barnes, S.; Guo, W.; Qi, X.; Lou, H.; Liang, J.; Jonasch, E.; Mills, G.B.; et al. The PI3K/AKT Pathway and Renal Cell Carcinoma. *J. Genet. Genom.* **2015**, *42*, 343–353. [CrossRef]
41. Motzer, R.J.; Hutson, T.E.; Glen, H.; Michaelson, M.D.; Molina, A.; Eisen, T.; Jassem, J.; Zolnierek, J.; Maroto, J.P.; Mellado, B.; et al. Lenvatinib, everolimus, and the combination in patients with metastatic renal cell carcinoma: A randomised, phase 2, open-label, multicentre trial. *Lancet Oncol.* **2015**, *16*, 1473–1482. [CrossRef]
42. Boni, J.P.; Hug, B.; Leister, C.; Sonnichsen, D. Intravenous temsirolimus in cancer patients: Clinical pharmacology and dosing considerations. *Semin. Oncol.* **2009**, *36* (Suppl. 3), S18–S25. [CrossRef]

43. Hudes, G.; Carducci, M.; Tomczak, P.; Dutcher, J.; Figlin, R.; Kapoor, A.; Staroslawska, E.; Sosman, J.; McDermott, D.; Bodrogi, I.; et al. Temsirolimus, interferon alfa, or both for advanced renal-cell carcinoma. *N. Engl. J. Med.* **2007**, *356*, 2271–2281. [CrossRef] [PubMed]
44. Hodi, F.S.; O'Day, S.J.; McDermott, D.F.; Weber, R.W.; Sosman, J.A.; Haanen, J.B.; Gonzalez, R.; Robert, C.; Schadendorf, D.; Hassel, J.C.; et al. Improved Survival with Ipilimumab in Patients with Metastatic Melanoma. *N. Engl. J. Med.* **2010**, *363*, 711–723. [CrossRef] [PubMed]
45. Wei, S.C.; Duffy, C.R.; Allison, J.P. Fundamental Mechanisms of Immune Checkpoint Blockade Therapy. *Cancer Discov.* **2018**, *8*, 1069–1086. [CrossRef] [PubMed]
46. Rini, B.I.; Powles, T.; Atkins, M.B.; Escudier, B.; McDermott, D.F.; Suarez, C.; Bracarda, S.; Stadler, W.M.; Donskov, F.; Lee, J.L.; et al. Atezolizumab plus bevacizumab versus sunitinib in patients with previously untreated metastatic renal cell carcinoma (IMmotion151): A multicentre, open-label, phase 3, randomised controlled trial. *Lancet (Lond. Engl.)* **2019**, *393*, 2404–2415. [CrossRef]
47. Motzer, R.J.; Jonasch, E.; Michaelson, M.D.; Nandagopal, L.; Gore, J.L.; George, S.; Alva, A.; Haas, N.; Harrison, M.R.; Plimack, E.R.; et al. NCCN Guidelines Insights: Kidney Cancer, Version 2.2020. *J. Natl. Compr. Cancer Netw. JNCCN* **2019**, *17*, 1278–1285. [CrossRef]
48. Bex, A.; Mulders, P.; Jewett, M.; Wagstaff, J.; van Thienen, J.V.; Blank, C.U.; van Velthoven, R.; del Pilar Laguna, M.; Wood, L.; van Melick, H.H.E.; et al. Comparison of Immediate vs Deferred Cytoreductive Nephrectomy in Patients With Synchronous Metastatic Renal Cell Carcinoma Receiving Sunitinib: The SURTIME Randomized Clinical Trial. *JAMA Oncol.* **2019**, *5*, 164–170. [CrossRef]
49. Mejean, A.; Ravaud, A.; Thezenas, S.; Colas, S.; Beauval, J.B.; Bensalah, K.; Geoffrois, L.; Thiery-Vuillemin, A.; Cormier, L.; Lang, H.; et al. Sunitinib Alone or after Nephrectomy in Metastatic Renal-Cell Carcinoma. *N. Engl. J. Med.* **2018**, *379*, 417–427. [CrossRef]
50. Linehan, W.M.; Lerman, M.I.; Zbar, B. Identification of the von Hippel-Lindau (VHL) gene. Its role in renal cancer. *JAMA* **1995**, *273*, 564–570. [CrossRef]
51. Ohh, M.; Park, C.W.; Ivan, M.; Hoffman, M.A.; Kim, T.Y.; Huang, L.E.; Pavletich, N.; Chau, V.; Kaelin, W.G. Ubiquitination of hypoxia-inducible factor requires direct binding to the beta-domain of the von Hippel-Lindau protein. *Nat. Cell Biol.* **2000**, *2*, 423–427. [CrossRef]
52. Cockman, M.E.; Masson, N.; Mole, D.R.; Jaakkola, P.; Chang, G.W.; Clifford, S.C.; Maher, E.R.; Pugh, C.W.; Ratcliffe, P.J.; Maxwell, P.H. Hypoxia inducible factor-alpha binding and ubiquitylation by the von Hippel-Lindau tumor suppressor protein. *J. Biol. Chem.* **2000**, *275*, 25733–25741. [CrossRef]
53. Tanimoto, K.; Makino, Y.; Pereira, T.; Poellinger, L. Mechanism of regulation of the hypoxia-inducible factor-1 alpha by the von Hippel-Lindau tumor suppressor protein. *Embo J.* **2000**, *19*, 4298–4309. [CrossRef] [PubMed]
54. Krieg, M.; Haas, R.; Brauch, H.; Acker, T.; Flamme, I.; Plate, K.H. Up-regulation of hypoxia-inducible factors HIF-1alpha and HIF-2alpha under normoxic conditions in renal carcinoma cells by von Hippel-Lindau tumor suppressor gene loss of function. *Oncogene* **2000**, *19*, 5435–5443. [CrossRef] [PubMed]
55. Na, X.; Wu, G.; Ryan, C.K.; Schoen, S.R.; di'Santagnese, P.A.; Messing, E.M. Overproduction of vascular endothelial growth factor related to von Hippel-Lindau tumor suppressor gene mutations and hypoxia-inducible factor-1 alpha expression in renal cell carcinomas. *J. Urol.* **2003**, *170*, 588–592. [CrossRef] [PubMed]
56. Conway, E.M.; Collen, D.; Carmeliet, P. Molecular mechanisms of blood vessel growth. *Cardiovasc. Res.* **2001**, *49*, 507–521. [CrossRef]
57. Choueiri, T.K.; Albiges, L.; Haanen, J.B.A.G.; Larkin, J.M.G.; Uemura, M.; Pal, S.K.; Gravis, G.; Campbell, M.T.; Penkov, K.; Lee, J.-L.; et al. Biomarker analyses from JAVELIN Renal 101: Avelumab + axitinib (A+Ax) versus sunitinib (S) in advanced renal cell carcinoma (aRCC). *J. Clin. Oncol.* **2019**, *37*, 101. [CrossRef]
58. Taube, J.M.; Klein, A.; Brahmer, J.R.; Xu, H.; Pan, X.; Kim, J.H.; Chen, L.; Pardoll, D.M.; Topalian, S.L.; Anders, R.A. Association of PD-1, PD-1 ligands, and other features of the tumor immune microenvironment with response to anti-PD-1 therapy. *Clin. Cancer Res. Off. J. Am. Assoc. Cancer Res.* **2014**, *20*, 5064–5074. [CrossRef]
59. Barber, D.L.; Wherry, E.J.; Masopust, D.; Zhu, B.; Allison, J.P.; Sharpe, A.H.; Freeman, G.J.; Ahmed, R. Restoring function in exhausted CD8 T cells during chronic viral infection. *Nature* **2006**, *439*, 682–687. [CrossRef]

60. Sakuishi, K.; Apetoh, L.; Sullivan, J.M.; Blazar, B.R.; Kuchroo, V.K.; Anderson, A.C. Targeting Tim-3 and PD-1 pathways to reverse T cell exhaustion and restore anti-tumor immunity. *J. Exp. Med.* **2010**, *207*, 2187–2194. [CrossRef]
61. LaFleur, M.W.; Muroyama, Y.; Drake, C.G.; Sharpe, A.H. Inhibitors of the PD-1 Pathway in Tumor Therapy. *J. Immunol.* **2018**, *200*, 375–383. [CrossRef]
62. Nasser, S.; Kurdolgu, A.A.; Izatt, T.; Aldrich, J.; Russell, M.L.; Christoforides, A.; Tembe, W.; Keifer, J.A.; Corneveaux, J.J.; Byron, S.A.; et al. An integrated framework for reporting clinically relevant biomarkers from paired tumor/normal genomic and transcriptomic sequencing data in support of clinical trials in personalized medicine. *Pac. Symp. Biocomput.* **2015**, 56–67. [CrossRef]
63. Pal, S.K.; Sonpavde, G.; Agarwal, N.; Vogelzang, N.J.; Srinivas, S.; Haas, N.B.; Signoretti, S.; McGregor, B.A.; Jones, J.; Lanman, R.B.; et al. Evolution of Circulating Tumor DNA Profile from First-line to Subsequent Therapy in Metastatic Renal Cell Carcinoma. *Eur. Urol.* **2017**, *72*, 557–564. [CrossRef] [PubMed]
64. Pal, S.K.; Bergerot, P.; Dizman, N.; Bergerot, C.; Adashek, J.; Madison, R.; Chung, J.H.; Ali, S.M.; Jones, J.O.; Salgia, R. Responses to Alectinib in ALK-rearranged Papillary Renal Cell Carcinoma. *Eur. Urol.* **2018**, *74*, 124–128. [CrossRef]
65. Routy, B.; Le Chatelier, E.; Derosa, L.; Duong, C.P.M.; Alou, M.T.; Daillère, R.; Fluckiger, A.; Messaoudene, M.; Rauber, C.; Roberti, M.P.; et al. Gut microbiome influences efficacy of PD-1–based immunotherapy against epithelial tumors. *Science (N. Y.)* **2018**, *359*, 91–97. [CrossRef] [PubMed]
66. Pal, S.K.; Li, S.M.; Wu, X.; Qin, H.; Kortylewski, M.; Hsu, J.; Carmichael, C.; Frankel, P. Stool Bacteriomic Profiling in Patients with Metastatic Renal Cell Carcinoma Receiving Vascular Endothelial Growth Factor-Tyrosine Kinase Inhibitors. *Clin. Cancer Res. Off. J. Am. Assoc. Cancer Res.* **2015**, *21*, 5286–5293. [CrossRef]
67. Paoletti, X.; Drubay, D.; Collette, L. Dose-Finding Methods: Moving Away from the 3 + 3 to Include Richer Outcomes. *Clin. Cancer Res. Off. J. Am. Assoc. Cancer Res.* **2017**, *23*, 3977–3979. [CrossRef] [PubMed]
68. Bonifant, C.L.; Jackson, H.J.; Brentjens, R.J.; Curran, K.J. Toxicity and management in CAR T-cell therapy. *Mol. Ther. Oncolytics* **2016**, *3*, 16011. [CrossRef] [PubMed]
69. Gill, S.; Maus, M.V.; Porter, D.L. Chimeric antigen receptor T cell therapy: 25years in the making. *Blood Rev.* **2016**, *30*, 157–167. [CrossRef] [PubMed]
70. Exelixis Partners with Roche to Trial Cancer Combination Therapy. Available online: https://www.clinicaltrialsarena.com/news/exelixis-roche-cancer-trial/ (accessed on 10 April 2020).
71. Cheville, J.C.; Lohse, C.M.; Zincke, H.; Weaver, A.L.; Blute, M.L. Comparisons of outcome and prognostic features among histologic subtypes of renal cell carcinoma. *Am. J. Surg. Pathol.* **2003**, *27*, 612–624. [CrossRef] [PubMed]

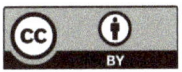

© 2020 by the authors. Licensee MDPI, Basel, Switzerland. This article is an open access article distributed under the terms and conditions of the Creative Commons Attribution (CC BY) license (http://creativecommons.org/licenses/by/4.0/).

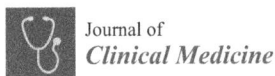

Review

Integrating Academic and Community Cancer Care and Research through Multidisciplinary Oncology Pathways for Value-Based Care: A Review and the City of Hope Experience

Linda D. Bosserman [1,*], Mary Cianfrocca [1], Bertram Yuh [2], Christina Yeon [3], Helen Chen [4], Stephen Sentovich [2], Amy Polverini [5], Finly Zachariah [6], Debbie Deaville [7], Ashley B. Lee [8], Mina S. Sedrak [1], Elisabeth King [9], Stacy Gray [9], Denise Morse [10], Scott Glaser [11], Geetika Bhatt [12], Camille Adeimy [13], TingTing Tan [14], Joseph Chao [1], Arin Nam [1], Isaac B. Paz [5], Laura Kruper [2], Poornima Rao [5], Karen Sokolov [15], Prakash Kulkarni [1], Ravi Salgia [1], Jonathan Yamzon [2] and Deron Johnson [16]

1. Department of Medical Oncology and Therapeutics Research, City of Hope, Duarte, CA 91010, USA; mcianfrocca@coh.org (M.C.); msedrak@coh.org (M.S.S.); jchao@coh.org (J.C.); anam@coh.org (A.N.); pkulkarni@coh.org (P.K.); rsalgia@coh.org (R.S.)
2. Department of Surgery, City of Hope, Duarte, CA 91010, USA; byuh@coh.org (B.Y.); ssentovich@coh.org (S.S.); lkruper@coh.org (L.K.); jyamzon@coh.org (J.Y.)
3. Department of Medical Oncology and Therapeutics Research, City of Hope, South Pasadena, CA 91030, USA; cyeon@coh.org
4. Department of Radiation Oncology, City of Hope, South Pasadena, CA 91030, USA; hechen@coh.org
5. Department of Surgery, City of Hope, South Pasadena, CA 91030, USA; apolverini@coh.org (A.P.); bpaz@coh.org (I.B.P.); porao@coh.org (P.R.)
6. Department Supportive Care Medicine, City of Hope, Duarte, CA 91010, USA; fzachariah@coh.org
7. Department of Enterprise Business Intelligence, City of Hope, Duarte, CA 91010, USA; ddeaville@coh.org
8. Department of Clinical Research Operations, City of Hope, Duarte, CA 91010, USA; ashlee@coh.org
9. Department of Population Sciences in the Division of Clinical Cancer Genomics, City of Hope, Duarte, CA 91010, USA; eking@coh.org (E.K.); stagray@coh.org (S.G.)
10. Department of Quality, Risk and Regulatory Management, City of Hope, Duarte, CA 91010, USA; dmorse@coh.org
11. Department of Radiation Oncology, City of Hope, Duarte, CA 91010, USA; sglaser@coh.org
12. Department of Medical Oncology and Therapeutics Research, City of Hope, Lancaster, CA 93534, USA; gbhatt@coh.org
13. Department of Medical Oncology and Therapeutics Research, City of Hope, Upland, CA 91784, USA; cadeimy@coh.org
14. Department of Medical Oncology and Therapeutics Research, City of Hope, Newport Beach, CA 92660, USA; titan@coh.org
15. Department of Radiation Oncology, City of Hope, Torrance, CA 90503, USA; ksokolov@coh.org
16. Department of Clinical Informatics, City of Hope, Duarte, CA 91010, USA; derjohnson@coh.org
* Correspondence: lbosserman@coh.org

Received: 10 November 2020; Accepted: 29 December 2020; Published: 7 January 2021

Abstract: As the US transitions from volume- to value-based cancer care, many cancer centers and community groups have joined to share resources to deliver measurable, high-quality cancer care and clinical research with the associated high patient satisfaction, provider satisfaction, and practice health at optimal costs that are the hallmarks of value-based care. Multidisciplinary oncology care pathways are essential components of value-based care and their payment metrics. Oncology pathways are evidence-based, standardized but personalizable care plans to guide cancer care. Pathways have been developed and studied for the major medical, surgical, radiation, and supportive oncology disciplines to support decision-making, streamline care, and optimize outcomes. Implementing multidisciplinary oncology pathways can facilitate comprehensive care plans for each cancer patient throughout their cancer journey and across large multisite delivery systems. Outcomes from the delivered pathway-based care can then be evaluated against individual and population benchmarks. The complexity of adoption, implementation, and assessment of multidisciplinary oncology pathways, however, presents many challenges. We review the development and components of value-based cancer care and detail City of Hope's (COH) academic and community-team-based approaches for implementing multidisciplinary pathways. We also describe supportive components with available results towards enterprise-wide value-based care delivery.

Keywords: value-based care; value-based cancer care; oncology pathways; Early Recovery After Surgery (ERAS); team-based care; oncology medical home; integrated cancer care; supportive care pathways; surgical pathways; cancer care plans

1. Introduction: Multidisciplinary Oncology Pathways Are a Foundation of Value-Based Cancer Care

While the majority of cancer care in the US is provided in the community (non-academic) setting, over the past 12 years, the organizational structure of oncology care delivery has shifted to networks of community oncologists partnered with academic centers, hospital systems, or other community practices. Aligned enterprises have evolved from the well-documented closing, merging, or acquisition of community oncology practices since 2008 [1,2]. This change has been driven by two major factors: the move from volume- to value-based payments, requiring more infrastructure management, resources, and market share as well as the rapidly increasing complexity of information needed to provide each cancer patient with the highest quality care while maintaining high patient and staff satisfaction, institutional health, and delivering these at optimal costs [3–5]. Meeting these goals has required innovations and teamwork that was pioneered first in several medical oncology home pilots from practices on the east coast by Dr. Sprandio and on the west coast by Dr. Bosserman as well as other practices across the US [6–11]. In the southwest, Dr. McAneny expanded on her New Mexico medical home model to engage six other US oncology practices in the successful Center for Medicare and Medicaid Innovation (CMMI)-funded COME HOME project [8]. Oncology pathways are a major component of these programs, with studies of implemented pathway programs showing equal or improved outcomes with lower costs in medical oncology [12–17], as well as in other disciplines including surgery, radiation oncology, supportive care, and end of life [18–23]. The evaluation and adoption of oncology pathways were further stimulated by Center for Medicare and Medicaid Services (CMS)'s oncology care MIPPs and Oncology Care Model (OCM) alternate payment programs and private payer pilots with academic and community-based networks and various private payors [24–33].

While multidisciplinary oncology pathway programs have evolved as essential components for evidence-based cancer care delivery within value-based cancer care (VBCC) programs, challenges remain to fully integrate and measure outcomes from multidisciplinary oncology pathways, including when they are combined into care plans across a patient's cancer journey [34–40]. As a practical point, multidisciplinary pathways first must be adopted, implemented, and understood for each specialty before their combined impacts can be evaluated. The processes, teams, and tools to develop, implement, analyze, and iterate multidisciplinary pathway projects throughout a large enterprise remain a work in progress. We detail here the work to date by the City of Hope (COH) academic community network enterprise as an example of the methodology and tools, some well-established and some being pioneered, to implement multidisciplinary oncology pathways and outline many supporting projects that facilitate and optimize their impacts. We share available analytics which continue to evolve and expand in the hope that our work can help others in their transformation to VBCC.

2. Prioritizing Care Model Redesign for Value-Based Cancer Care (VBCC) at City of Hope with Multidisciplinary Oncology Pathways

In response to the City of Hope Enterprise leadership prioritizing the delivery of reportable value-based oncology care, a Value Realization Project (VRP), led by a multidisciplinary group of clinicians, pharmacists, nurses, administrators, informaticists, program managers, quality, data analysts, risk and outcome experts, and our chief medical and administrative officers, was formed. This VRP group developed a Value Framework (VF) with specific projects identified under each of the three pillars of evidence-based care, care management, and care after cancer, as shown in Figure 1. These pillars are derived from the key components identified in the medical oncology home and OCM models as well as several value-based payer initiatives which have shown value [6–8,11,23–33]. A full discussion of our value-based care initiative is beyond the scope of this paper; however, we present our value framework and highlights of several other key projects within the framework to show the interdependence of those projects in advancing the implementation and evolving outcome analytics of multidisciplinary oncology pathways. Interdependent projects include the capture of complete staging data in the electronic health record (EHR), systemic therapy regimen orders built into the EHR, integration of clinical trials and pathway decision support into the EHR, and incorporation of precision medicine, among others. These companion projects support measurable evidenced-based cancer care delivery. We discuss some of the pathways and projects in the other two pillars of VBCC: management of care while on active treatments, and care after active cancer, whether in survivorship or at end of life, as part of our COH supportive care programs. Not shown in Figure 1 are the enterprise-wide initiatives to engage and measure patient and staff satisfaction, institutional health as well as the administrative support needed in informatics, precision medicine, EHR enhancements, care models, and payer contracting to fully meet VBCC goals. As we build each of the identified projects supporting multidisciplinary oncology pathways, we are working on measuring individual pathway use and impacts while working toward measurement of the larger clinical, financial, clinical trial, and quality outcomes. We also continue to iterate methodologies for team-based care and patient engagement trough academic and community staff teams in the evolution toward a mature VBCC model.

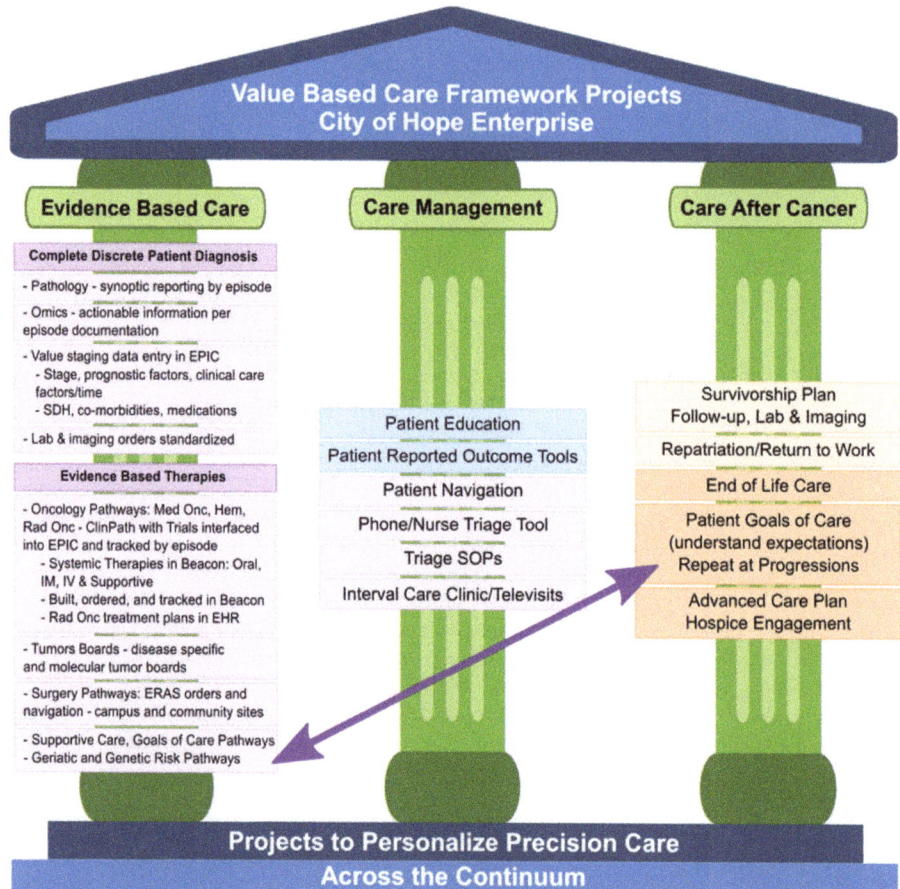

Figure 1. Value-based care framework projects for City of Hope Enterprise: Green represents the three pillars of value-based care: evidence-based care, care management, and care after cancer. The boxes represent categories of projects to facilitate measurable delivery of value-based care. Purple indicates clinician-led projects. Blue indicates patient-focused projects. Orange indicates projects after active therapy or curative therapy, whether in survivorship or end of life. Within the category of complete discrete patient diagnosis are the projects that will help to accomplish this. Omics refers to genomics, proteomics, metabolomics, and microbiome information that impacts a patient's treatment episode choices and potential outcomes. SDH refers to social determinants of health. Med Onc—medical oncology, Hem—hematology, Rad Onc—radiation oncology. ClinPath is the pathway system by Elsevier (formerly called VIA Pathways). EPIC refers to the EHR. IM—intramuscular, IV—intravenous. EHR—electronic health record. ERAS—early recovery after surgery pathways. SOP—standard operating procedures. Televisits—telephone and televideo visits. The purple arrow indicates that goals of care pathways are incorporated during active therapy as well during in advanced end of life care.

3. NCCN Guidelines and Growing Complexity of Evidence-Based Cancer Care Also Stimulated Multidisciplinary Oncology Pathway Development at COH

City of Hope (COH) is a National Cancer Institute (NCI)-designated comprehensive care center and one of the original 13 member institutions that formed the National Comprehensive Cancer Center Network (NCCN) in January of 1995. Within the NCCN, our faculty have participated in and led the development of guidelines for the treatment of cancers for the past 25 years. The COH enterprise now serves patients with cancer and metabolic diagnoses in a region of 25 million residents living in five counties in Southern California as well as more distantly based national and international patients. The COH enterprise includes a central academic, clinical research, hospital and clinical care campus in Duarte, California and a clinically integrated, community practice network of 31 community practices. Approximately 30% of COH physicians practice in the community (either solely or in a mixed hybrid of community/academic practice). Clinicians in the community are mostly general oncology practitioners, while the academic clinicians are disease and disease subtype specialists. Over the past year, we have identified community doctors who have a special interest in a specific cancer and will see patients with that disease preferentially (referred to as disease-leaning), such as breast, thoracic, gastrointestinal, and genitourinary cancers. A single foundation faculty model employs both academic center and community clinicians. The mission of the organization is to develop and bring cutting-edge precision cancer care and clinical research to every patient that is also personalized and delivered with compassion, high quality, and cost consciousness within the value-based cancer care initiative.

Although COH faculty participated in the development of the original eight disease guidelines published by the NCCN in November of 1996 and continue to participate and lead disease guideline committees at NCCN, until the more recent partnership between NCCN and US Oncology and their development of Level 1 Pathways powered by NCCN, the NCCN guidelines were broad and without the detailed pathway approach to better guide individual patient care [32]. COH disease teams regularly discussed narrowing the NCCN guidelines into pathways for specific patient issues and cancer subtypes and some, such as the breast, lung, and renal teams, develop and review pathways that are shared with COH faculty, as described in companion articles in this series [41–43]. With the growth of the COH enterprise, however, the need to more formally establish not only pathways for each disease but the ability to prompt for those choices, keep the pathways up to date, incorporate clinical trials as well as track the use and variations of treatments for each patient (by disease, disease subtype, clinicians, site, and payer), a formal pathway program became a priority. As part of the VBCC initiative, available pathway programs and options were evaluated by a multi-stakeholder group of faculty, staff, nurses, and administrators with campus and community network representatives over a 2-year period. This was led early on by an oncology surgeon who practiced at both the academic center and in the community and understood the practical needs for a tool to guide standardized care for similar patients. Work initially focused on the development of multimodality clinical care pathways, defined as standardized, evidence-based interdisciplinary care management plans, which would identify an appropriate sequence of clinical interventions, timeframes, milestones, and expected outcomes for a comparable patient group, i.e., by diagnosis or surgical procedure. As the work evolved, however, it became clear that the starting point for these larger multimodality care plans should be pathway programs starting with the specialties of medical, radiation, and surgical oncology.

A formal pathway tool became a priority not only to support the measurable delivery of care across the growing COH enterprise but to bring expert input to the point of clinical care for the growing number and complexity of cancer therapies. The continued growth in new Food and Drug Administration (FDA) hematology–oncology drug approvals since 2000 is a telling example of the need to provide real-time expert decision support across an enterprise to aid the delivery of high-quality, high-value cancer care.

The FDA website for oncology–hematology drugs reports that from 2016 through June of 2020, 230 new drug approvals were issued, up from 22 in 2016 to 58 in 2017, 63 in 2018, 46 in 2019, and 41 in the first half of 2020 [44]. These approvals are also increasingly complex and include not only new drugs but new indications for existing drugs. The approval can be under the expedited review process so that the approval could also change with further data. Approvals can include whether the use is approved in early disease, as neoadjuvant, adjuvant therapy, or extended adjuvant or for advanced disease. The approvals can include use only with specific biomarker results from the patient or their tumor, and sometimes only after biomarker testing by specific laboratories. The approvals often specify use only in specific lines of therapy, after previous general or specific therapies, in combination with specific other drugs or drug categories. Biosimilar drugs are also listed in the FDA approvals with their specific uses referenced to the reference drug [44]. Thus, keeping up with the details of the almost weekly new FDA approvals, which individually can impact one or many kinds of cancers, requires increasingly sophisticated and constantly upgraded decision support pathways not only for clinicians but also for patient education to support their participation in shared decision-making and to ensure appropriate use and documentation requirements for authorizations and payer coverage. Financial toxicity has been identified as another growing barrier to patients receiving appropriate cancer therapies, especially targeted, molecular, and immunotherapy-based treatments [45]. Thus, building the workflow infrastructure to support the use of pathway tools which include increasingly higher cost therapies can also support more timely authorization of treatments for patients and can help to engage early patient assistance, when needed, so patients can receive timely care which improves outcomes [46,47]. Several examples of the growing complexity of high-quality care are described in companion articles on colorectal and non-small cell lung cancer by colleagues in this series [48,49].

The development of surgical pathways was driven by the benefits of standardizing surgical type and processes but also by the benefits of reducing morbidity, mortality, and costs by coordinating education and care processes with the many providers involved in a patient's care before, during, and after surgery [50–53]. These comprehensive care plans have come to be known as Early Recovery after Surgery (ERAS) pathways [54–57]. At City of Hope, ERAS pathway work began in the early 2000s by the urology faculty with the development and implementation of a successful ERAS pathway for cystectomies showing lower length of stay, complications, and readmission rates that were confirmed by outside groups as well [19,58,59]. This stimulated the development of further urology ERAS pathways as well as ongoing work on ERAS pathways for other surgical subspecialty departments for the COH academic campus and at regional hospitals where COH faculty practice.

Given these many drivers toward standardizing care in all specialties that could provide better care, better outcomes, and potentially lower costs, City of Hope's Value Realization Project identified a Value-Based Core (VBC) team of experts to meet regularly and work with a multidisciplinary physician VBC group team, using the Value Framework projects noted in Figure 1 above, to engage disease leaders in medical oncology, surgery, and radiation oncology along with administrators, information technology (IT) and informatics and EHR experts to evaluate, implement, and iterate oncology pathways for the enterprise. Insights and outcomes from this work follow and add to the work of other academic community network enterprises working together to improve the quality of care for cancer patients [60,61].

4. Medical Oncology, Radiation Oncology, and Hematology Subspecialty Pathways

4.1. Evaluation and Adoption Process for Pathway Processes and Tool for the Enterprise

Initial meetings identified medical oncology pathways as the starting point for a formal oncology pathway tool. Available oncology pathway programs, their implementation, and integration abilities were evaluated during regular multi-stakeholder meetings. In 2016, a decision was made to use the VIA Oncology Pathways developed at the University of Pittsburg Medical Center (UPMC) Hillman Cancer Center (now ClinPath by Elsevier and will be referred to as such going forward) which met the criteria of the January 2015 ASCO Policy Statement on Clinical Pathways in Oncology as well as their criteria for high-quality pathway programs shown in Figure 2 [62,63]. The ClinPath pathways were then evaluated and approved by each medical oncology disease team for a 1 January 2017 go live date. The ClinPath system was chosen because it addressed the most common tumor types with readily available evidence summaries for clinician review and prioritized pathways by efficacy, toxicity, and cost [64]. The pathways were being recognized by payers as part of growing value-based payer initiatives [16,17,30–32]. The ClinPath Pathway program also welcomed our faculty to actively participate and, when appropriate, lead pathway disease committees. The regular disease committee meetings, made up of national pathway disease experts and interested users, work to keep pathways updated regularly. In addition, pathways were available for hematology and radiation oncology, with plans for further expansion of pathways for additional solid tumors, hematology, radiation, and possibly surgical pathways. A computer icon tool could be launched from campus and community computers on different EHR platforms for the January 2017 go live with the capability to be later integrated into the planned enterprise wide EHR change to the EPIC system (EPIC systems, Verona WI) in December of 2017.

ASCO Criteria for High-Quality Pathway Programs

Pathway Development	Implementation and Use	Analytics
Expert Driven Reflects Stakeholder Input	Clear and Achievable Expected Outcomes	Efficient and Public Reporting of Performance Metrics
Transparent, Evidence-Based Clinically Driven Up-to-Date	Integrated Cost-Effective Technology and Decision Support	Outcomes Driven Incentives
Comprehensive and Promotes Participation in Clinical Trials	Efficient Processes for Communication and Adjudication	Promote Research and Continuous Quality Improvement

Figure 2. ASCO's criteria for high-quality oncology pathway programs under pathway development, implementation and use, and analytics as described by Zon et al., J Oncol Prac 13:207–210, 2017 [63].

4.2. Initial Medical Oncology ClinPath Adoption Processes and Definitions

Following the decision in 2016 to implement ClinPath pathways, starting with medical oncology, teaching decks were built by the COH pathway and education teams to share the rationale, clarify the diseases for initial navigation at go live 1 January 2017, and share use and development expectations. On-pathway vs. off-pathway treatment decisions were defined. On-pathway decisions were decisions that adhered to the pathway's decision algorithm for that specific stage of disease. Clinical trials and secondary treatments for alternate patient scenarios were still considered to be on-pathway, as were any decisions to not treat or to take a patient off active treatment. Off-pathway decisions that did not align with pathway recommendations on review were typically driven by new data not yet incorporated into the pathway (indicated as physician disagrees with pathway choice or a free texted comment to that effect, reports not shown), unique patient presentations, specific patient preferences, and on occasion by physician discretion. It was emphasized that while it was expected that for most cancers, on-pathway choices would be in the range of 80% or more, there would never be an expectation of a specific pathway compliance percentage by doctor or by disease type. It was also recognized that in these times of rapid new drug discovery and molecular targeting, the best therapy for an individual patient may not yet be in the pathway tool. All clinicians were encouraged to join one or more pathway disease committees to participate in the ongoing development process, review the latest evidence, and share best practices.

4.3. Key Milestones and Practical Time Implementations for ClinPath Pathways across the COH Enterprise

January 2017: Medical Oncology go live for six disease types: Medical oncologists at the academic campus and community sites were trained and instructed to use the pathway tool over 6–8 weeks prior to go live for all new medical oncology therapies including both initial therapy and subsequent therapies in six disease categories: breast, lung, genitourinary (GU), gastrointestinal (GI), gynecologic (GYN), and head and neck. Educational tip sheets and training team personnel were available on an ongoing basis for individual support as well. Other solid tumor types and some hematology diseases were available in the tool but optional for use and not assessed as part of our initial metrics. COH had two EHR systems when the VIA pathways went live: Allscripts on campus and Touch Works in the community. Both were interfaced to pull patient demographic and physician schedule information into the pathway tool. After that, however, clinicians would navigate pathways by entering discrete staging and prognostic or clinical care feature elements to reach the recommended pathway choice or choices. Physicians were required to enter a reason when an off-pathway decision was chosen. After making a therapy choice, clinicians then went back to their EHR to order the chosen therapy. Clinicians were made aware of plans for future EPIC integration, addition of clinical trials into the pathways, and expansion of tracking and reporting for other disease types and specialties. Although formal surveys were not done, clinicians expressed frustrations from the double entry of data from their EHR notes into the pathway system, having to use the system when they were confident and familiar with the appropriate pathway choice as well as skepticism on future upgrades and benefits to their disease programs (personal communications).

2 December 2017: Enterprise-wide transition to Epic: Treatment protocols were built in Beacon by the disease teams based on the regimens used in the previous systems and a review of those in the pathway system before go live. Additional COH-specific regimen preferences and many clinical trials were also built. Oral chemotherapy regimens were not prioritized. Standardized nausea regimens based on NCCN emetogenic levels were added for each regimen as well as hypersensitivity premedication regimens and they were integrated when needed to avoid overuse of steroid medications. All documentation, data entry, and ordering were then done in the EPIC EHR across the enterprise.

January 2018: OnCore clinical trial management system went live. Its benefit to the pathway program is discussed below.

August 2018 and ongoing: Clinical trials were formally added into the ClinPath pathway tool by disease teams starting with the most commonly seen cancers in the community. Additional solid tumor clinical trials have been added and closed trials removed as noted below.

March 2019: Radiation oncology clinicians on campus and community sites went live on ClinPath radiation pathways with integration of COH radiation oncology clinical trials as described below.

20 July 2019: The one-way integration between the Epic EHR and the pathway tool was started and is described below.

August 2020: Hematology pathways had been available in the ClinPath system but their formal evaluation by disease leads began as well as identification of clinical trials to be added to the ClinPath pathways. As reviews are being completed, trials are being added and formal launch of enterprise-wide use and measurement of ClinPath for the common hematology diagnoses is scheduled to start December 2020 as described below.

6 October 2020: The two-way integration between the EPIC EHR and the ClinPath tool went live in the EHR for 11 disease subtypes (breast, bladder, colorectal, gastroesophageal, melanoma, mesothelioma, ovary, prostate, testicular, small cell lung, and thyroid). With two-way integration, we expect that most if not all discrete staging elements from the EPIC staging forms will be interfaced to auto-populate into the ClinPath tool over time and as elements are added to the EPIC system. Any additional or missing discrete data elements in the EHR system would still have to be entered into the pathway tool to trigger a pathway prompt. At go live, tumor types fell into three categories from this pioneering work: fully mapped tumors (breast, colorectal, gastroesophageal, melanoma, mesothelioma, bladder, ovary, sarcoma, small-cell lung cancer, testicular, thyroid, and uterus), partially mapped tumors (head and neck, prostate), and pending mapped tumors (anal, non-small cell lung, neuroendocrine, pancreatic, renal). When clinicians navigate within the EHR to the ClinPath system, the data elements entered into the EPIC staging forms are then shown on a field next to the ClinPath data entry choices. For fully mapped tumors, one click of an APPLY button automates the entry of the EPIC data into the ClinPath system. The doctor then continues navigating to the pathway choices. For a partially mapped tumor, those elements that are mapped will auto-populate in ClinPath and the others will have to be manually entered. For non-mapped tumors, the EPIC data are there to see but each element has to be manually clicked before continuing the navigation. Whether or not a tumor is fully, partially, or not yet mapped, however, after a pathway choice is made, whether for a clinical trial or a standard regimen, the user is then taken back to the EPIC Beacon regimen for completing the order or ordering a clinical trial team evaluation. This two-way integration will continue to expand by matching additional data elements captured in EPIC to the pathway decision trees to more efficiently guide pathway choices. In addition, the EHR system is working to include data elements that more fully describe a patient's disease status as required by decision support tools. It is expected that ongoing work will continuously reduce duplicate data entry requirements, including for the growing number of actionable genomic results, while ensuring that the primary clinical information remains in the enterprise EHR [65]. A survey of provider experience, time savings (if any), and satisfaction was built and, pending team approval, will be sent to all faculty who use the ClinPath system in November of 2020 to further inform this work.

4.4. Clinical Trials Incorporated into ClinPath System and Integrated with Clinical Trials Management System Can Prompt for Available Trials and Track Adoption

Studies have shown improved clinical trial assessment and accruals for clinical trials incorporated into pathway tools that are routinely used, including by multisite organizations [66,67]. The ability to add clinical trials available at and through our COH enterprise was another key reason the ClinPath pathway system was chosen in 2016 [68]. Prior to incorporating clinical trials into our pathway tool, though, COH implemented the OnCore clinical trials management system (CTMS) in January 2018. This system provides faculty and clinical research teams with a comprehensive integrated system that supports virtually all aspects of clinical trial offerings including features for managing studies, electronically capturing protocol and patient data, creating custom reports, and supporting financial activities. Having it fully linked into the decision support pathway tool enhances clinician notification of available clinical trial options, especially timely notices of pending, open, on hold, or closed trials to maximize clinical efficiencies.

The OnCore tool integrated with the EHR will hopefully enhance the value of the pathways tool through bi-directional data flows indicating protocol status and patient demographics. Phase I of the project included the decommissioning of the legacy clinical trials management system (MIDAS) and migration of protocol status and data. Phase II of the project linked detailed subject management activities enabling COH to track patient visits, enhance charge segregation, and payment reconciliation. OnCore was also integrated with City of Hope's regulatory committee management platform, iMEDRIS to provide greater efficiency and data integrity. Phase III, which is going live Q3 of 2020, involves migrating and making available to investigators the IRB-approved versions of the protocol-related documents and informed consent forms in OnCore and decommissioning our current Clinical Trials On Line (CTOL) system, where these documents are currently. This will reduce the number of systems which investigators will need to navigate.

A major goal of an integrated decision support pathway tool is the incorporation of clinical trials prompted by the patient's disease information. After the initial pathway tool launched in January of 2017, training was reinforced, navigations increased but both campus and community faculty were eager to have clinical trials placed into the pathways. The pathway team PharmD (DJ) collected a list of clinical trials from each disease lead, worked with them to place each trial in the appropriate pathway branch points, then submitted the information to the pathway company for inclusion in the tool for all faculty at all COH sites. This process took 4–5 weeks for each disease. The schedule and disease types for availability of the clinical trials in the pathway tool went as follows: GI: 8/2018, 15 trials; Lung: 2/2019, 15 trials; GYN: 5/2019, 5 trials; Breast: 7/2019, 18 trials; GU: 9/2019, 20 trials'; Head and Neck: 4/2020, 12 trials.

Still pending disease types for adding clinical trials in solid tumors are melanoma, sarcoma, and neurologic tumors. With the hematology division now actively engaged in finalizing their adoption of the ClinPath hematology disease pathways, disease leads are working with the pathway PharmD lead to have their clinical trials added into the pathway tool for the planned launch of enterprise-wide use of the hematology pathways in December of 2020. Doctors, APPs, and disease leads have informally but almost universally expressed anticipated value in improving clinical trial identification for their patients as they navigate their therapies in the pathway tool.

Pathway reports show 4.5% of patients by individual medical record number were on a past or present clinical trial from the start of our pathway use in January of 2017 until June of 2020 for the six originally monitored cancers (GI, Lung, Breast, GU, GYN, and Head and Neck). The per quarter percent of patients on a trial varied from 2% to a high of 7–8% in Q4 of 2018 and Q1 of 2019 after the GI and lung cancer trials were added to the pathways. The impact of the full integration of clinical trials into the pathway tool will not be fully assessable until additional programs are matured during 2021–2022. These include the ongoing expansion of clinical trial hubs into regional community sites, which started in 2020 and will cover most of the network regions in the next 2 years. Figure 3 shows that our overall accrual numbers remained similar overall in the community sites and the academic center between 2017 and 2019. The academic accruals include community patients referred to the center who entered a clinical trial. The overall numbers for 2020 reflect only 9 months of data which are promising, given the reported major decreases in clinical trial accruals across the US since the COVID-19 pandemic began in March 2020. As the community network clinical trials programs expand with regional trial directors and trial hubs, plans to open more trials for eligible patients in the community, and the addition of hematology trials for the common hematology diseases frequently seen in the community sites, we expect that the inclusion of clinical trials in the ClinPath pathways will stimulate increased assessments and accruals for community network patients over the next 2 years. The expansion of the discrete data capture in the EHR system and pathway navigation reports will also be fed back regularly to disease teams and the clinical trial leadership so that they can better track the impact of assessments and accruals for clinical trials across the enterprise. The ability to track every patient who goes on a systemic therapy in hematology and medical oncology as well as a radiation oncology treatment plan will allow trial leads to more quickly identify gaps in referrals that can then be addressed. Additional issues are reviewed by colleagues in an accompanying article in this series [69].

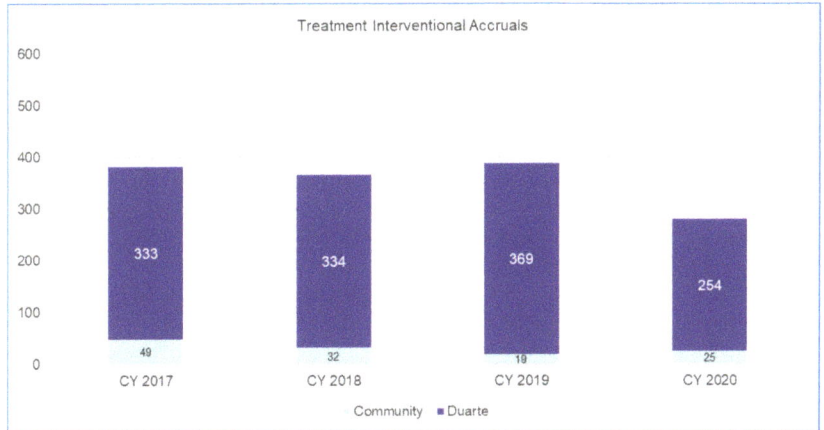

Figure 3. Clinical trial accrual at Duarte and community sites 2017 through September 2020. Light blue bars are the number of patients accrued to treatment trials at community sites where some trials were available. Dark blue bars are number of patients accrued to treatment trial at the Duarte academic campus.

4.5. Oversight and Insights from ClinPath System Pathways Use in Medical, Hematology, and Radiation Oncology at COH

The ClinPath pathways program at COH was and is overseen by an interdisciplinary team which continues to meet two or more times per month. This team reviews and directs data analytics, gathers feedback from clinicians and administrators, directs dashboard and interface development, sharing of reports to individual clinicians, site and disease leads as well as administrative and contracting leadership. They oversee and encourage ClinPath disease committee and leadership participation as well as ongoing clinical trial and EHR integration with expansion of pathway adoption across diseases and disciplines. The group reviews monthly pathway compliance rates to identify outliers, leading to further study of clinical issues, patient issues, or individual faculty issues that alter compliance rates, most often because new data have not yet been incorporated or there is not a pathway for an individual's episode of care need. COH faculty's participation and, for some, leadership of disease committees has been essential in supporting timely updates of practice changing information as well as sharing back information and the national perspectives on care standards.

Utilization of the pathways by COH clinicians has increased over time and serves as one of the performance metrics for members in medical oncology. These metrics are reviewed by the leadership (including the chairs, senior medical director of community practices, and regional medical directors of community practices) as well as the COH pathway and the value-based leadership teams to maximize standardization, quality, and value of clinical care across the enterprise.

Clinicians, especially those in the community, report that the availability of the pathways has improved clinician efficiency and time management. With the knowledge that these are standardized pathways, agreed upon by the entire institution, with the added benefit of integrated clinical trials, there is less need to contact disease team academic leader(s) for many opinions, even in these times of increasing availability of newer therapies and clinical trials.

While doctors are navigating new therapy starts consistently in the pathway tool, the COH pathway team was asked to track the correlation between indicating a pathway choice in the tool and ordering the regimen in the EHR as a quality control measure. A Variation of Care report was designed in 2019 and reports the monthly rates of any difference between what was navigated in the ClinPath system and what was ordered in the EPIC EHR through the Beacon module. The data from May to December of 2019 showed that the difference varied from a low of 0 variations from 871 navigations in 11/2019 to a maximum of 18 variations from 688 (2.6%) navigations in October of 2019. Overall, discrepancies were rarely over 3%. A random chart evaluation noted that these discrepancies occurred when patients or providers changed their treatment plan based on additional work-up, most often when additional disease was found. They then ordered the therapy in the EPIC EHR Beacon treatment orders but did not go back into the ClinPath tool to change the navigation information in the pathway tool. This also happened for rare patient preference for an alternate therapy after the initial ClinPath navigation was done.

Since our ClinPath go live in January of 2017 until early Q3 2020 when data were reported for this manuscript, clinicians had done 28,271 total navigations, including 16,034 navigations from the academic clinicians and 12,190 navigations from the community clinicians, including 47 at our newest Newport Beach site, opened in January of 2020. The percentage of therapies ordered in Beacon that were navigated in the pathway tool by enterprise, community, and campus doctors since implementation is shown in Figure 4. Pathway navigation was higher on the academic campus except for two quarters. The reasons are under further evaluation.

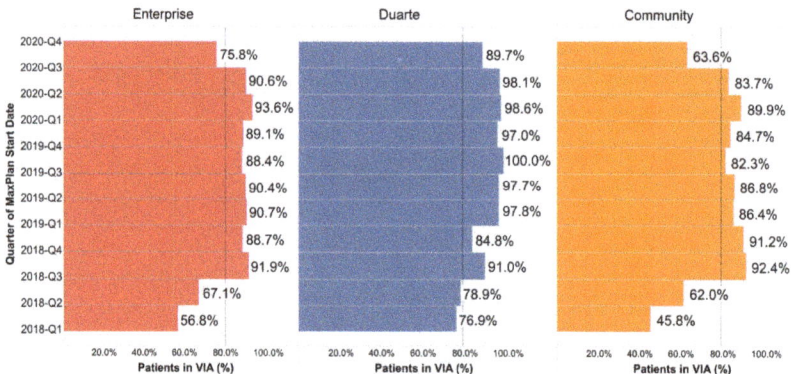

Figure 4. Percentage of new EPIC Beacon starts that were navigated in ClinPath by medical oncologists for solid tumors since go live for enterprise overall then by Duarte campus site and all community sites. Note Q3 data were incomplete at time of manuscript data collection in May 2020, so the final% of patients in Q3 who were navigated in ClinPath is likely higher, as is seen in other recent quarters.

Simply having a pathway system does not ensure the use, usefulness, or production of informative analytics. A multidisciplinary pathway team of clinicians, analytic, quality, her, and informatics experts meets every 2 weeks to evaluate pathway use, compliance by disease type and clinician, track low compliance issues to understand if a new therapy not yet incorporated into the pathway or other reason is increasing off-pathway choices, use of clinical trials, and whether the indicated therapy in the pathway system is, in fact, the ordered therapy in the EHR. An enterprise-wide incentive program to capture pathway use and choices for medical oncology was launched in 2020 and final percent navigations in the pathway for all medical oncology therapies in the EHR trends have risen significantly. Disease leads have also requested regular reporting of every patient who meets specific disease, stage, and other criteria for an available trial as to whether or not the trial was considered and if a trial evaluation and ultimate accrual occurred. Several leads are asking for real-time reports so that they can more proactively reach out to network clinicians to resolve any barriers for patient accrual to an available clinical trial. Ultimately, by tracking specific clinical trial eligibility and accrual by site, disease, and trial type across the enterprise, the trial team can optimize which types of trials are opened at which sites to maximize clinical trial resources.

Having a pathway tool enables the tracking of the percentage of patients who are treated on-pathway (including clinical trials) and off-pathway across the enterprise and by academic vs. community network sites as shown in Figure 5. Academic clinicians consistently see more patients treated off-pathway, which, on reviews, has been explained by the higher number of patients seen where a pathway does not exist for the patient presentation or where a different treatment is recommended due to new molecular findings or emerging data are not yet incorporated into the pathway. After reviewing data, the pathway committee has identified and recommended to the pathway vendor that they add that additional reason as an option in the dropdown list when entering a reason for choosing an off-pathway therapy. Such a new choice for going off-pathway, "new information not yet incorporated into the pathway" could then be tracked for each tumor type and stage during six month intervals over twelve to twenty four month periods to see if and when such a therapy choice is added to the pathway. This could also better inform clinicians about how rapidly new, practice-changing therapies that experts agree should be used become available for prompting in the ClinPath decision support pathway tool.

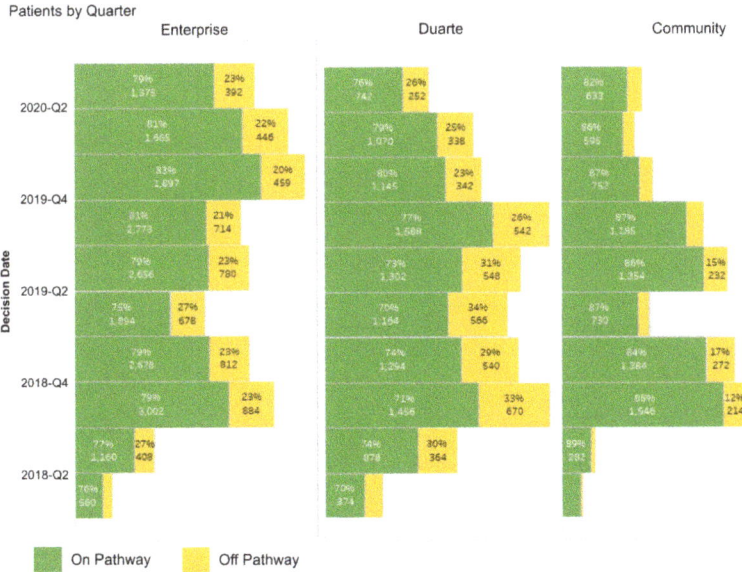

Figure 5. Pathway compliance percentage over time for medical oncology patients navigated in pathway tool (ClinPath) for enterprise, Duarte academic campus, and community sites for new therapy regimens ordered in the EPIC-BEACON EHR from January 2019 through June of 2020. Green bars are on-pathway choices (including clinical trials) and yellow bars are off-pathway choices. Note that the scale of the x-axis representing the numbers of patients is different for each group to show the comparison percentages in one graph. The combined number of patients navigated in Duarte and community sites is reflected in the number totals described on the enterprise graph.

4.6. Pathways for Radiation Oncology Using ClinPath Program

As with medical oncology pathways, radiation therapy pathways were piloted by the University of Pittsburgh Medical Center (UPMC) group, who led the development of the ClinPath (then called VIA) pathways for radiation oncology based on the same principles used for the development of medical oncology pathways to standardize care for the most common radiation treatments, prioritizing efficacy then toxicity then costs. Studies by their group showed that using the pathways with a peer review process appeared to encourage compliance with clinical pathway recommendations [70]. Specific studies included one showing increased community practice physicians' adoption of hypofractionated regimens for whole breast radiation [71].

This is significant as several studies have shown slow and or poor adoption of evidence-based use of shorter course radiation treatments which have lower costs and shorter treatment times for patients with equivalent outcomes. Hypofractionation for breast cancer is a good example. While the majority of women undergoing radiation therapy for early breast cancer have equal disease control with equal or better cosmetics and a shorter course for patients has been adopted by UK and Canadian clinicians for the majority of patients, it has been much slower to be adopted in the US despite positive long-term outcomes in studies and expanded guidelines for use by the American Society for Radiation Therapy (ASTRO) [72–75]. As in medical oncology and hematology, the growing options for the use of different radiation techniques such as 3D conformal, intensity-modulated radiation therapy (IMRT), proton beam, and other methods of localized radiation therapies along with shorter treatment courses have led to increasing use of radiation therapy pathways to support busy clinicians through their prioritizing efficacy, toxicity, and safety as another component of value-based care [76,77].

As the COH enterprise expanded with many satellite sites delivering convenient local radiation therapy treatments, the radiation oncology department chose to implement and use ClinPath radiation pathways at all sites in March 2019. COH has the largest single institution radiation oncology network in California, comprised of 46 physicians practicing at 20 satellite sites. ClinPath pathways were integrated into the day-to-day clinical practice for 35 radiation oncologists at 16 sites as four outside hospital site doctors are not yet on the system. Radiation oncologists with specific disease interests contributed to the development of some of the pathways and some faculty now co-lead some radiation oncology disease pathway committees. Clinical trial options were also integrated into the pathway options customized to our institution.

The radiation oncologists use the EPIC EHR for all care, except the specific radiation therapy planning, which is done in the radiation-specific modules of MOSAIQ or ARIA EHRs at different sites. The pathways have had a launch button integrated in the EPIC EHR and the radiation oncologists are looking forward to the two-way integration in progress so that the staging in EPIC will be pulled into the pathway system which is on the planning agenda for 2021–2022.

The pathways, besides giving case-by-case feedback regarding treatment options to clinicians, also give detailed recommendations regarding the technical aspects of radiation (i.e., dose constraints, fractionation options), which is useful at the time of actual radiation treatment planning. The pathways cover the most common disease sites and scenarios. There are still complex or rare cases that do not fit into any of the existing pathways, where the radiation oncologist notes "no pathway", and there is an option to add a narrative comment.

In general, the pathways program has been well received. There has been >90% participation rate by COH radiation oncologists in using the pathway tool to capture their treatment decisions, with most physicians using it to indicate 100% of their decisions. Physicians are also sent auto-generated weekly reminders listing any patients where pathways data about their treatment choice were not entered. COH does not require strict adherence to the pathway's preferred choice, but the analytic team gives physicians feedback which can show clinicians where their choices fall and how they compare to their peers. On- and off-pathway rates are tracked for feedback to individual clinicians, disease, and regional site leads. Pathway compliance remains high after initial launch and has been at or above the generally accepted 80% pathway compliance benchmark, which is an accepted standard in the radiation oncology quality assurance program as defined by the quality assurance review center (QARC), which established an 80% rate based on clinical trial standards [78]. The COH on-pathway rates for the combined enterprise and the separate Duarte and community sites are available but we share in Figure 6 how available additional reporting can further detail the types of therapy or trial as well as who has just completed a therapy plan or who is off therapy by quarter for all patients seen. This same graphic can be constructed separately for Duarte campus radiation therapy, for all as well as for individual sites and by doctor.

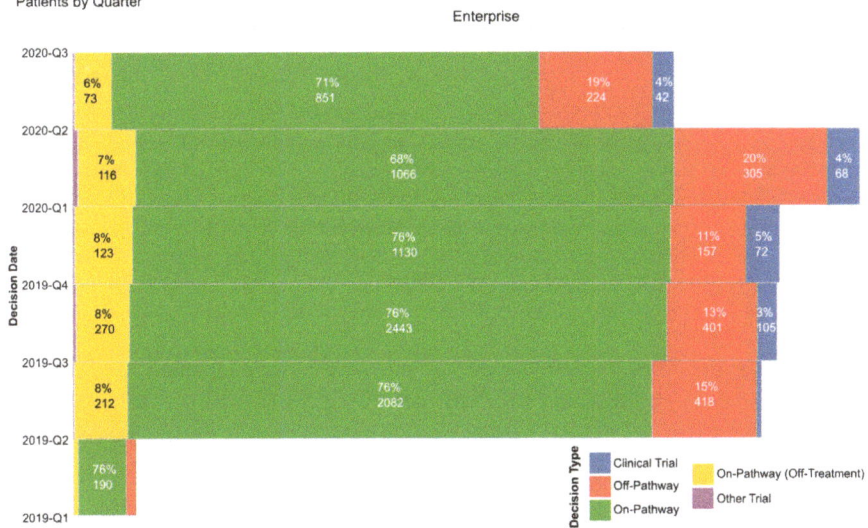

Figure 6. Individual patients seen by radiation oncologists by the enterprise per quarter since ClinPath pathways were initiated for radiation therapy in Q1 of 2019. The numbers represent the number of individuals with a decision made each quarter who are: on therapy with a non-pathway diagnosis, shown as "other trial" (purple), were on a pathway but went off treatment (yellow) that quarter, on a pathway treatment (green), are off treatment (light blue), are on an off-pathway treatment, (red) or on a clinical trial (dark blue) for an on-pathway disease.

Individual radiation oncologists informally report at leadership meetings that they have found the pathway information regarding various fractionation options helpful. Feedback and questions regarding pathways content are welcomed at all levels but formal feedback from radiation oncologists has not been solicited. COH faculty working at the main medical center and satellites engage via many regularly scheduled virtual meetings both before and exclusively after the COVID-19 pandemic from March 2020 forward. They have weekly peer review of patient new starts, monthly didactic sessions regarding a specific disease site where a COH attending reviews a case and asks residents questions, anyone can contribute, and is extremely well-attended. They also have weekly breast and head and neck tumor boards and include community physicians on disease teams. The entire radiation oncology department has previously gotten together for a yearly in-person one-day science and clinical care retreat, which will be held virtually during the pandemic. Although no single physician has time to participate in every discussion, the regular meetings are available with technology support. Clinical leaders note that it remains challenging to engage and include new and distant satellites as they continue to be added to the COH network, but this is an identified priority.

The COH radiation oncology department has also created an internal Microsoft Teams messaging system where anyone can share case questions and message the entire department. It has yet to be regularly utilized but doctors are in the process of being trained on the Microsoft Teams functionalities. E-mail, therefore, is still the most utilized form of communication department-wide. Overall, pathway compliance is high for the enterprise, as shown in Figure 6 above. Reasons for off-pathway choices are captured as for other specialties, reported and reviewed by the disease teams. Any recommendations for pathway updates are communicated to the appropriate ClinPath disease committees.

4.7. Additional Multidisciplinary Pathways for VBCC: Geriatric Oncology and Genetic Counseling/Risk Assessment

Geriatric oncology is an established field pioneered by the late COH faculty member, Dr. Arti Hurria. Dr. Hurria's goal was to bring the principles of geriatric oncology into practice through standards and pathways to improve the care of older adults with cancer. Given that one in three Americans aged 60 years or older will be diagnosed with cancer in their lifetime and the population of older adults is growing rapidly with the aging of the U.S. and worldwide populations, cancer incidence is expected to rise by 67% for individuals aged 65 or older between 2010 and 2030. Although older adults represent the majority of individuals with cancer, they are severely under-represented in clinical trials and research. Hence, the majority of evidence that sets the standards of care for oncology treatment pathways is derived from younger individuals.

To address these unmet needs, COH formed the Cancer and Aging program in 2006, under the leadership of Dr. Hurria, which ultimately led to the formation of the Center in Cancer and Aging (CCA) in 2017. The mission of the CCA is to join investigators from all cancer disciplines to study the biology, treatment, and survivorship issues of older adults with cancer. Over the last decade, COH staff have led over 30 studies in cancer and aging, enrolled more than 5000 patients on studies, disseminated research findings through more than 250 publications, and received competitive grants from the NIH as well as philanthropic funding. CCA is one of the elite centers in cancer and aging in the nation.

With this background work, COH's CCA is now leading the way in expanding pilot pathway projects into community sites, starting with standardizing geriatric assessments (GA), which can help to guide personalized care for our increasingly aging population while achieving their best health outcome. For example, an ongoing implementation study of an APP-led multidisciplinary team telehealth intervention is being conducted in one of COH's 31 community cancer sites. This Antelope Valley regional site is in a remote area of high need and limited resources. Learnings from this pilot will be used to expand geriatric pathways for assessments and care planning across our enterprise.

Colleagues at COH have also examined the multifaceted barriers hindering participation of older adults in cancer trials. They offer strategies to improve the participation of older adults in clinical trials in an accompanying article in this series [79]. It is expected that many of the projects outlined in COH's Value Framework, such as the complete discrete staging and collection of social determinants of health along with geriatric assessments with clinical trial integrations into the pathway navigation tool for systemic therapies in medical oncology, hematology, and radiation oncology, will help to support the piloting of these strategies.

Clinical cancer genomics has been an expertise at COH since the department was established in 1996 which has grown to provide training, research, and consultative services overseen now by the division of clinical cancer genomics (CCG). A counseling, research, and professional teaching program, internationally recognized for its onsite and telehealth training of healthcare providers worldwide, continues with ongoing professional conferences open to trainees and the COH faculty at all sites. At the academic center, the department provides consultations for individual cancer risk assessments, genetic testing and result interpretation, risk reduction counseling, and clinical trial enrollment. The CCG division is also engaged in the support of COH's enterprise precision medicine initiative to expand somatic and germline testing with associated counseling on results, integration of results into care pathways and into research teams to power new discoveries. Work to standardize these processes through discrete data entry in EPIC on the upgraded staging forms is in progress, along with ways to present clinically actionable results of expanding somatic and germ line genomic testing to clinicians within the data for each patient's episode of cancer throughout their journey. Having relevant clinically actionable data for integration into decision support pathway tools and molecular tumor boards while having the larger dataset easily accessible for analytics and discovery by the research teams is a current priority of the precision medicine, genomics, informatics, value-based care, and disease specialty teams informed by input from faculty at both the academic and community sites.

Genomics pathway work is in the earlier stages of development and will be informed by the expansion of CCG services to the enterprise through academic community faculty and staff teamwork. Pathway work has started with one day per week onsite genetic counseling consultations at one local network site. This has now expanded to one day per week of genetic counseling services being available now by telehealth to patients at all community sites. MD geneticist counseling is offered 2 days per month for the community sites after an initial pilot at one community site. Another pilot pathway for genetic assessments is underway with two breast surgeons, trained and supported by the academic CCG team to provide genetic cancer risk assessment (GCRA) to their breast cancer patients with referral to campus for additional genetic counseling or genetics MD for complicated cases as needed. A breast surgeon at another community site is being trained and will provide GCRA services to her patients as well as to other affected and unaffected patients seen by faculty at that site as well as any external referrals. That surgeon also plans to develop a high-risk screening clinic for all cancer types at that community site. Two additional medical geneticists and two additional genetic counselors are being recruited for our second academic campus site in Orange County to provide precision medicine and clinical cancer genomics initiatives.

Standardizing the collection and validated data entry of discrete multigenerational family histories and incorporating these data into individual patients' cancer or cancer risk data is another project in the planning stages in the value-based framework. It is being worked on in sequential pilots and projects toward enabling our EHR database to capture relevant family and patient histories that can prompt the development of genomics pathways to trigger precision medicine and clinical cancer genomic services as well as personalized therapies within the ClinPath pathway tool. The opportunity to leverage the expertise of the genomics division, working as a team with the community faculty and COH informaticists, holds the promise of developing more pathways for automating risk assessments, genomic counseling, testing, and interpretation as well as clinical trials as part of each patient's comprehensive care plan. Pathways at COH in other disciplines as described in this manuscript are serving as models to build these to better serve patients across our enterprise.

4.8. Expansion of ClinPath Pathways Use for Hematology Diseases

While our acute leukemia teams are working to develop comprehensive care plans and pathways to include diagnosis, therapy, trials, and follow-up for acute myelogenous leukemia (AML) and acute lymphoblastic leukemia (ALL), which is primarily treated on the campus, they have developed referral trees to ease access to campus leukemia experts and their pathways by community faculty and outside providers. For the other major hematology diseases, lymphomas, myeloma, myelodysplastic diseases, and benign idiopathic thrombocytopenic purpura (ITP), which are commonly treated in the community and can involve years of sequenced therapies with growing costs, the ClinPath system has expert hematology disease committees and pathways available in the ClinPath tool alongside the medical and radiation oncology pathways.

The growth of value-based contracting, where payers track metrics on compliance with disease pathways for commonly treated diseases, made adding hematology disease team engagement and enterprise-wide clinical use of the ClinPath hematology pathways a priority for Q4 2020. Since many of these diseases are seen and treated by community faculty, the pathway oversight team reviewed and found that 983 navigations had been done for five types of hematology diseases using the ClinPath tool without any requirement or specific training for their use. While a formal survey was not done, members of the pathway team talked to community faculty and several reported that when they have a question, they use the pathway for hematologic diseases to rapidly inform them of the latest therapies and regimen details for patients with these diseases, especially for the most common diagnoses. They report saving more complex cases for individual campus faculty expert discussions, tumor boards, or second opinion referrals. On the campus side, informal discussion with disease experts raised concerns that clinical trials be more widely disseminated as well as nuanced strategies adopted by campus disease experts who meet weekly to standardize their approaches. While academic faculty welcome calls, referrals, and interactions with the growing community network faculty, they felt that hematology care could be enhanced by hematology pathway adoption.

With the March 2020 California-wide COVID-19 pandemic slowdown in onsite clinical care, the value, staging, and pathway leadership engaged the department chair of hematology in demonstrations of the current EHR, ClinPath pathway tool, and pending interfacing capabilities for the hematologic diseases with clinical trials available in the ClinPath system. Five initial academic and community-based disease leads for diffuse large B-cell lymphoma (DLBCL), chronic lymphocytic leukemia (CLL), Hodgkin's disease, multiple myeloma, and immune thrombocytopenia (ITP) were identified and those for chronic myelogenous leukemia (CML), myelodysplastic syndromes (MDS), and the other lymphoma subtypes followed. For each disease or subtype of the lymphomas, a video meeting was scheduled, ClinPath pathways and EHR staging data element capture on the current EHR staging forms were shared, and feedback solicited. Disease leads identified additional discrete data elements that track to pathway prompts and a list of those recommended for addition as part of an EHR staging upgrade program was captured and shared with the staging form upgrade build team. Hematology faculty were signed up on the pathway system, made aware of the disease committee meeting timing, and encouraged to participate in adding COH expertise to the pathway regimen discussions. A major drawing point is the ability to add the clinical trials to the flow sheet nodes in the pathway tool as we did for medical and radiation oncology. The disease leads anticipate that this will expand awareness, screening, and ultimately accrual to clinical trials in hematology. The leads have also requested real-time in-basket messaging for patients with specific disease features who would be eligible for a trial and reporting on whether or not a trial was chosen so they could reach out to their colleagues in real time to gain a deeper understanding and to address any barriers to accruals. Having the expanded datasets of disease data and therapy choices will also better inform disease leads on populations served at various sites to better inform opening of targeted clinical trials. After 9 months of meetings, trainings, and engagement, the hematology pathways in ClinPath will be tracked for use and on-pathway compliance starting in December of 2020 with planned ongoing engagement with disease leads and faculty who see hematology patients and build out of more comprehensive analytic reports.

5. Oncology Surgery Pathways with ERAS and COH Experience

5.1. ERAS Pathways for Value-Based Surgical Care

While pathway work in medical oncology expanded during the early 2000s, surgical pathways, referred to as "early recovery after surgery", or ERAS pathways were developed out of early work by Professor Henrik Kehlet in Denmark on multidisciplinary care approaches to standardize colorectal cancer surgical care that improved outcomes [51,56]. An international ERAS study group was formed in 2001 to "develop perioperative care and to improve recovery through research, education, audit and implementation of evidence-based practice." The group later formed an ERAS society in 2010 and a US branch, ERAS@USA in 2016, as data accumulated that orders alone were not enough to improve outcomes but comprehensive approaches to pre, day of, and postoperative (post op) care could improve outcomes in growing numbers of cancer surgeries [80]. The goals of ERAS pathways are to decrease practice variability, lessen morbidity and mortality, and lower costs through education, care coordination, and specific orders before, during, and after cancer surgeries. These are built into care plans on paper or in EHRs to prompt for all agreed upon steps across the surgical journey. Clinical, quality, clinical trial, and financial outcomes can then be analyzed and benchmarked as in other oncology disciplines.

Depending on the surgery, the preoperative (pre-op) processes might include performing an American College of Surgeons developed National Surgical Quality Improvement Program (NSQIP) risk score. This tool predicts the risk of post-op complications "using data from a large number of patients who had a surgical procedure similar to the one the patient may have" [80,81]. This tool is available online and is allowed to be opened from EHRs. Geriatric risk indicators based on data from patients >age 65 were added in 2019 [82]. Using such calculations, for example, post-op nausea and vomiting risks can inform tailored nausea and vomiting prevention education and mediation orders to improve outcomes. The pre-op orders can include breathing training, drain training, smoking cessation, and education on limiting alcohol. They include a review of home medications and any modifications recommended during the pre and postoperative periods. Other goals include improving pain control with limited opioid use through education and standardized orders as well as increasing early mobility to minimize length of stay and enhance the patient experience. The clinical, quality, clinical trial, and financial outcomes of these standardized approaches for specific cancer patients undergoing specific cancer surgeries can then be benchmarked. Teams can use these data for continuous improvement for cancer surgery patients and to better prepare and care for patients at multiple sites. Another key opportunity is standardizing direction of specific high-risk surgeries to high-volume centers where extensive subspecialty surgical expertise has been shown to lower morbidity and mortality and often improve survival across multiple cancer types, systems, and countries despite ongoing controversies on methodologies and the retrospective data reviews [83–90]. Having teams of academic center and community network clinicians working closely together can ease the transitions and the teamwork between academic- and community-based surgical specialists, help to ensure that patients can be easily referred to the academic center for appropriate surgeries per the group pathways while providing continuity and standardization of care using the general and disease-specific ERAS order sets.

City of Hope's urologic oncologic surgeons started adopting ERAS pathways for cystectomy back in 2008 and garnered a large database on outcome benefits published in 2016 [19]. City of Hope's academic-based surgeons have the most substantial experience worldwide in performing robotic cystectomy. These patients were an ideal population to design further care improvements around due to the high-risk patient demographic (elderly, many comorbid conditions), complexity of surgery (5–8-h surgeries mixing together multiple organ systems), and challenges of baseline post-surgery recovery (>80% complication rates, >30% major complication rates, and >30% readmission rates). The evolution of a pathway that became the cystectomy ERAS pathway started when the campus urologists began using almivopan to assist with bowel recovery as bowel resection is a key recovery factor in cystectomies. The academic urologists oversaw their high volume of surgeries while integrating teams to deliver standardized care at COH's academic specialty cancer hospital. They adopted standard orders for pre-op preparation, operative intervention, and post-op management to facilitate recovery for patients. In collaboration with the supportive medicine department, they developed a multidisciplinary rounding team specifically for cystectomy patients that provided an organized plan of care for each patient daily and kept patients actively involved in understanding and participating in their care. Their pathway details the order components for medical management, symptom management, patient education, supportive care, and case management from the operative day through the day of discharge and specifies the follow-up visit order. Adopting a coordinated care program led to several improvements: the hospital length of stay after surgery decreased from 8 days to 6 days, the 30-day complication rate decreased from 68% to 50%, multiple late-stage patients were primarily referred by urology to hospice (in contrast to prior practice where all poor prognosis patients were referred to medical oncology), and some patients and caregivers reported in Press Ganey surveys that they felt much more informed and empowered in their care [19].

5.2. Expanding Cystectomy ERAS Pathways to Regional Hospitals and for Prostate Cancer Surgeries

After establishing a successful ERAS program at COH, urology teams rolled out the cystectomy pathway with similar principles to surrounding community hospitals where faculty practiced. Although outcome data show that surgeries of this complexity ideally should be conducted at specialized care centers [59,91], the realities of where our patients reside, their insurance company restrictions, and distributed care delivery necessitate being able to deliver the same standard of care outside COH. Thus, the academic community team faculty partnership built a general ERAS pathway in the order system of the Cerner EHR for a regional hospital where faculty practiced. Over the course of 6 months, they conducted numerous meetings with hospital leadership, nursing leadership, pharmacy, social work, case management, operating room, and nutrition to replicate the model created for the COH campus. At the central academic campus and community sites, teams continue to make iterative implementation improvements using the dedicated pathway functionalities within the EPIC EHR system that incorporates standardized care to reduce variation and cost, organize day-by-day care coordination and documentation, and prompt for discrete capture of outcomes to build robust reporting of outcome and quality measurements.

The urology group next adopted ERAS pathways to drive same day discharges after robotic prostatectomy. Historically, there was a disincentive in fact to discharge these patients the same day as they were considered inpatient only surgeries. However, CMS rule changes have now considered this an outpatient surgery. The group adopted prehabilitation, usage of regional transverse abdominis plane (TAP) anesthesia blocks, early ambulation and feeding, and use of non-narcotic pain medication. This significantly reduced the need for patients to use narcotics, which is beneficial to them individually and in combatting the opioid crisis. Internal data review showed that patients returned home sooner to recover in the comfort of their family and returned to baseline functional and dietary levels much sooner as well.

5.3. Expanding ERAS Pathways for Breast Cancer, Colorectal, GYN, Thoracic, and Other Cancer Surgeries

Other surgical oncology teams at COH have worked to develop ERAS pathways for on-campus surgeries as well as for many regional hospitals where our faculty work to achieve similar goals of standardizing surgical care, improving outcomes, and lowering healthcare costs while more actively engaging patients [91–94]. In one regional hospital, a generalized ERAS pathway was developed and built into their hospital's EHR to fast-track postoperative mastectomy recovery and minimize narcotic use. At COH, the EPIC EHR has an ERAS breast surgery pathway that incorporates pre-op education, a visit with occupational therapy, and a tailored medication order set. The educational component involves a one-on-one session with a breast team nurse that is performed during the patient's pre-anesthesia testing visit. Patients receive information on nutrition, exercise, and alcohol/smoking cessation. The information is aimed at preparation for surgery, as well as post-op and long-term recovery strategies. The patients then have an appointment with an occupational therapist to learn about recommended post-op exercises and lymphedema precautions. This "prehabilitation" visit has been found to expedite return to baseline function for patients following breast cancer surgery. Finally, the dedicated breast surgery order set includes medications shown to improve postoperative pain control and minimize intractable postoperative nausea and vomiting [95,96]. The importance of non-narcotic pain control is twofold, as opioids lead to a host of troublesome side effects and COH is focused on combatting the current opioid epidemic [97]. Additionally, the medications given to minimize post-op nausea and vomiting are especially important in breast surgery, as these patients are more likely to develop significant post-op symptoms that prohibit early hospital discharge [98].

The COH ERAS breast surgery pathway can also be tailored to fit an individual surgeon's preferences or patient needs. The COH breast team has an internal (available on request) detailed mastectomy ERAS pathway order set which details the orders on pre-op education, patient preparation, prehabilitation with physical therapy (PT), or occupational therapy (OT) if needed, educate and order specific medicine prescriptions for post-op care before surgery, and ensures that patients understand the post-op caregiving needs before surgery. On the day of surgery, the anesthesia team is actively involved both at campus and at any of the regional hospitals in their part of optimizing enhanced recovery strategies including as appropriate: intraoperative administration of anti-emetics, intravenous (as opposed to inhalational) anesthetic agents, maintenance of euvolemia, and minimization of opioids. These orders have been aligned with studies showing lessened nausea and vomiting and minimizing post-op opioid requirements, which facilitates faster patient recovery and lessens length of stay [99]. Following surgery, post-op visits, nursing care, and care coordination have helped to lower readmission rates while reducing suffering and promoting faster recoveries. We have surgical specialty teams developing, piloting, or using ERAS pathways in the breast, colorectal, thoracic, and gynecologic surgery programs. As they are developed and implemented with structured orders in the EHR from paper orders, the informatics, analytic, and finance teams are getting engaged to develop outcome reports.

Although expanding comprehensive ERAS pathways to every site our patients are seen in remains in process, other departments at COH and various regional hospitals have reported having benefited from involvement in the ERAS pathway work and order set development. Faculty and staff in the anesthesia department were engaged to align perioperative and intraoperative patient management which, once adopted, were embraced for other surgeries. Surgical faculty have reported informally that some outside anesthesia groups have also eagerly participated in ERAS approaches in our community hospital network to improve the care for patients on and off ERAS pathways.

5.4. Challenges with ERAS Pathway Use

While COH surgical specialists uniformly report that they are very successful in getting together and developing clinical agreement and alignment with each other and with other community oncology surgeons at outside hospitals when needed, full implementation of the pathways for all cancer surgeries at COH campus and in all community hospital sites remains a work in progress. A review of the example of the process steps for our mastectomy ERAS pathway is shown in Table 1 and illustrates the complexity of ERAS pathways. To achieve optimal surgical outcomes for cancer surgery patients, ERAS pathways have shown that many different participants in different locations with specific timing, educational, procedural, medication, or care-related tasks need to be facilitated and remain an active focus of our care and quality improvement efforts [92–99]. A model template showing the temporal and detailed types of order considerations for ERAS pathways for cancer surgeries demonstrating this is shown in Table 1.

Table 1. Detailed timing and order categories to address in ERAS pathways cancer surgeries.

Pre-Operative Orders Weeks Ahead Addressing:	Intra-Operative Orders Addressing:
Education visit and potential handouts	Fluid management
Assess post-op n/v risks and educate	IV/inhalational anesthetics
NSQIP surgery risk calculator	Regional anesthesia
Smoking and alcohol cessation	Deep Venus Thrombosis prophylaxis
Breathing exercise teaching	
Diet and activity guidance	**Post-Anesthesia Care Unit:**
Prehabilitation OT/PT teaching	Pain guidelines
Lab orders	Catheter guidelines
Medication education for pre-op and post-op	
Bathing instructions	**Extended Stay Orders:**
	Nursing care
Pre-Operative Orders Days or Day Before Surgery:	Medications
Patient instructions prior to surgery	DVT prophylaxis
Nasal and skin disinfection	As needed medications
Medication fills for post-op needs	
Prehabilitation OT/PT teaching	**Post-Op Orders Addressing:**
Pre-anesthesia testing	Follow-up nurse triage call
Pre-op fasting	Post-op visit scheduling
Pre-op medications	
Pre-op DVT prophylaxis	

Our ERAS pathway leaders report an easy process in determining alignment for patient and nursing educational needs and process steps and tracking goals for ERAS pathways among team members. Operationalizing multidisciplinary at home, in clinic, in hospital, and post-hospital steps flawlessly, however, remains challenging. Coordinating the different disciplines with staff internally is slightly easier but made more difficult with the many hospital outpatient and freestanding hospital facilities where our patients receive care. Our surgical lead for the value-based care ERAS development reported that the most challenging aspects of implementation have been related to nursing education, engagement, and data tracking. While there was consensus on the content of both preoperative and postoperative education, identifying the resources and a workflow that could be seamlessly incorporated into each patients' journey for different cancer surgeries at different sites and in different EHRs outside of our enterprise EPIC system remains a work in progress. With respect to tracking compliance and patients' clinical outcomes related to the different ERAS pathways, one group plans to pilot a third-party application with an EPIC EHR incorporation. Others are working on various internal EHR tools and the patient portal tools to improve scheduling and prompting of patient education and follow-up care as well as early symptom reporting and triage. In addition to compliance with the pathways, other endpoints being evaluated are length of stay, post-op pain, complications, and survival. Formal measurement of staff satisfaction has not been done but is discussed at surgical department meetings. Patient satisfaction is measured for their overall care by standardized Press Ganey surveys, which consistently report high satisfaction scores but do not evaluate the impact of ERAS pathways alone.

6. Supportive Care Pathways

As with other oncology care pathways, those in supportive care have also been shown to be effective in improving care quality and lowering costs based on many trials evaluating care navigation, emotional support for patients and their families with cancer, electronic patient-reported outcomes integrated into care models that address identified symptoms regularly as well as those formalizing goals of care discussions and advanced care planning [20,21,100–105].

COH, like many large academic centers, has a palliative care department focused on clinical care and research. Projects have been done in pain management, regular biopsychosocial assessments, and care coordination as well as in end of life care. The larger enterprise focus on value-based care has worked to engage the many expert providers and research teams to more formally identify the projects in supportive care that are essential in the value-based framework to provide interval care, care navigation, and care after cancer with the goals of improving care quality as well as clinical outcomes while optimizing the patient and staff experience. The expansion of several ongoing or supportive care pilots was underway before the COVID-19 pandemic expanded our use of telehealth for patient visits across the enterprise. Support services at COH had discussed pilots to expand social work, nutrition counseling, and other projects or pilots were in discussion to expand supportive care pathways to all enterprise sites. With the launch of telehealth technology enterprise-wide after March 2020 that included an iterative EPIC EHR integration and expansion of telehealth coverage by payers, some of these projects are being expedited and optimized through hybrid in-person and telehealth service pathways. Highlights of some of the pathways in our supportive care programs are:

Expanding Goals of Care Discussions as part of shared decision-making can help to avoid ineffective care, especially at the end of life, and help patients to achieve their broad life goals. While there are numerous other services provided by the Department of Supportive Care Medicine at COH, we will highlight three distinct efforts: the integrated care service, Hospice in the Village, and a goals of care pilot in poor prognosis patients.

The Integrated Care Service is a dedicated supportive care team comprised of a palliative care hospitalist, advance practice provider, social worker, chaplain, and pharmacist who provides intensive interdisciplinary inpatient and outpatient care to patients with multiple complex care needs, including high symptom burden, advanced disease, and challenging psychosocial concerns. In the last year, the team has cared for approximately 300 medical oncology and hematology inpatients, with over 50 being cared for in a primary capacity. As processes and results are studied, they will serve as potential models to deploy in partnering with community hospitals where COH faculty practice to build unique faculty outside hospital and clinician partnerships to achieve pathways for similar care improvements for patients hospitalized outside of the academic campus hospital.

City of Hope's Hospice in the Village on the Duarte campus has furnished apartment units with full amenities, specially designed for hospice care. Hospice in the Village allows patients to receive hospice care, from their preferred provider, in a private and comfortable home-like environment, when home is not an option. For the last year and a half, overall, 100 patients were cared for in the village, representing over 550 avoided inpatient days. A pilot in a community site for a similar home-based hospice and higher-level care (below acute level) is being explored.

A collaborative hematology, oncology, and supportive care pilot is underway utilizing various means to identify high-risk patients, including supervised machine learning, which triggers a supportive care pathway that includes patient screening (including assessing patient perception of prognosis), advance care planning, training on communication, structured goals of care documentation, and engages supportive care disciplines based on patient and family identified needs. The structure of the patient and family meeting pathway is shown in Figure 7, with further information available at the COH website [106].

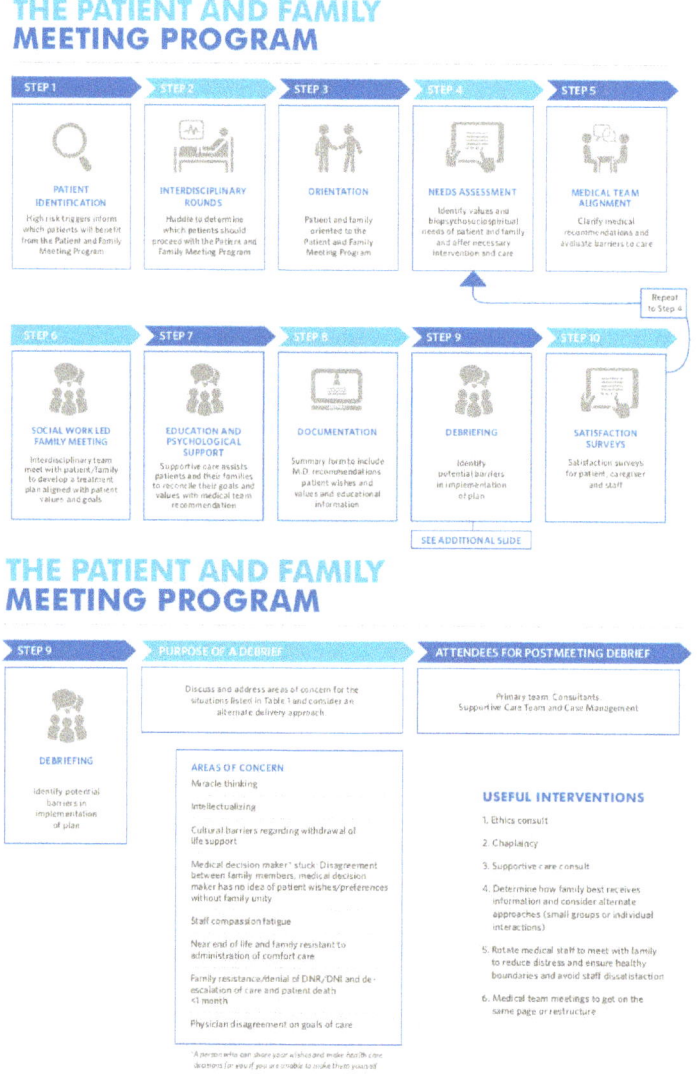

Figure 7. Ten-step supportive care patient and family meeting program pathway with expanded details about step 9 in second section of diagram to improve end of life care at COH.

Implementing Advanced Care Planning Pathways across the enterprise is another key component of our value project's care after cancer pillar. Advance care planning is often poorly incorporated in oncology practices, with reported advance directive (AD) rates generally less than 50% [107]. Concerted efforts were made to improve the overall number of ADs in new patients across the enterprise and specifically for patients undergoing hematopoietic stem cell transplantation (HSCT). The Department of Supportive Care Medicine at COH, in collaboration with medical faculty and administrative support, created a patient-centered ACP pathway program.

The first two years (2013 and 2014) broadly focused on all new COH patients. The last two years (2015 and 2016) included a specific focus on patients undergoing HSCT. The primary goal was a completed AD in the electronic medical record before day 0 of transplant. In addition to provider and transplant team engagement, major time points for supportive care integration to facilitate AD completion were identified, including: (1) registration, (2) new patient orientation, (3) the clinical visit when transplant was decided, (4) pre-transplant education class, (5) clinical social work psychosocial assessment visit, and (6) the pre-transplant hospital days. Between 2012 and 2016 at COH, 1784 transplants were performed. For HSCT patients in 2012, baseline AD capture rate before day 0 of transplant was 28.6%. With the institutional AD program, the AD capture rate before day 0 of transplant was 31.6% for 2014, compared with 2012 (odds ratio, 1.17(95% CI, 0.85–1.60); $p = 0.33$).

With both institutional and hematology-specific programs, the AD capture rate before day 0 was 69.5% for 2016, compared to 2014 (odds ratio, 4.30 (95% CI, 3.14–5.91); $p < 0.001$). While the institutional AD program in 2014 insignificantly impacted HSCT AD completion rates, improving the rate of AD completion from 28.6% to 69.5% in HSCT patients required both institutional AD efforts and a targeted pathway program [108].

After this progress, the team's advance care planning efforts returned to focus on building a scalable advance care planning pathway to support the advanced care planning and AD completions in our 31 network clinics. While advance directives in California can be finalized by two witnesses or a notary, at COH, for our predominantly cancer-focused population, we have opted to not solicit witnesses and elected to offer complimentary notarization services for healthcare documents to minimize a major identified barrier to AD completion. Presently, a pilot pathway is under way, leveraging the Prepare for Your Care advance directive developed by the University of California San Francisco (UCSF) and having these advance directives notarized electronically. Several staff advance directives have been successfully completed and initial patient tests are under way to ensure ease of use, feasibility, and adoption. Building the structured steps and documents into the EHR is on the project roadmap so the AD pathway tools can be available enterprise-wide and outcomes can be tracked and reported for targeted improvements. Additional information regarding City of Hope's advance care planning program is available on the website [109].

Pathways to address, prevent, and treat cancer symptoms through standardizing assessments, triage, and treatments is not only a key component of our value framework's management of patients on therapy pillar, it is a key component of ASCO's Quality Oncology Practice Initiative (QOPI) metrics and Center for Medicare and Medicaid Services' (CMS) Merit-Based Incentive Payment System (MIPS) measures, which we track for compliance [110,111]. Standardized use of patient reported outcome tools has also been shown to improve survival as well as relieve suffering [20,112,113].

Phone Triage Pathways: Our EHR regimens are all built to include evidence-based nausea, vomiting, and hypersensitivity medications that can then be obtained pretreatment and discussed at the chemotherapy teaching visit. The medications are based on the NCCN low, minimal, moderate, and high emetogenic risk of the regimen, which automates a major quality metric to ensure appropriate pre- and post-medications.

Support Screen Pathways: Our management of care pillar for value-based care also uses pathways for phone triage, biopsychosocial, and per visit symptom assessments and care. We implemented the triage pathway as a pilot in 2018 with the campus breast disease team, which was expanded to campus medical oncology clinics in 2019 and is now being prepared for piloting in the community sites using the EPIC phone triage tool with embedded Schmidt Thompson evidence-based assessment pathways and per disease team or site standard operating protocols for triaging patients with cancer symptoms. We are expanding the nationally recognized work of the supportive care faculty's biopsychosocial Support Screen tool with validated questionnaires and integrated support materials or referrals in a pilot at two community sites. Patients, at specific visits or remotely, can respond to questions on iPads in clinic or through our EPIC MyChart portal. Ongoing work that will be informed by the community pilots will work to address the challenges of addressing complex biopsychosocial needs through hybrid models using community resources supplemented by academic experts. Challenges of identifying resources and activating them based on individual patient needs across an enterprise remains an active project to expand these well validated supportive care pathways for biopsychosocial symptom monitoring and interventions across the enterprise.

Oncology Review of System Pathways: We have also built a multidisciplinary community developed oncology review of symptoms (ONC-ROS) questionnaire into a patient-reported outcome questionnaire available to patients through the EPIC MyChart portal before each visit or in clinic within the EPIC rooming questionnaire that medical assistants can complete with patients prior to visits. The 39 questions cover the most common toxicities for cancer patients receiving medical oncology, surgical oncology, and radiation oncology therapies. Community doctors preferred one questionnaire that medical assistants, who help multiple doctors, could be trained and become familiar with for efficient use. The 39 symptoms are divided into systems which require answering only the positive symptoms; then, with one click, the remaining symptoms can be noted as negative. For the nine symptoms that are monitored for the ASCO-QOPI and CMS-MIPS metrics (n/v, diarrhea, constipation, anxiety, depression, pain, fatigue, falls, and shortness of breath), a positive response opens additional questions to assess patient acceptance of that toxicity or desire for interventions that can be addressed at the visit. The questionnaire responses integrate into the EPIC visit note template as the review of systems for clinician review and editing to ensure symptoms are addressed, which has been shown to lessen hospital and ER visits while speeding up complex documentation to support appropriate billing levels and providing mineable data [20]. The use of the ONC ROS after teachings on capturing a pain score and pain plan of care in EPIC after the December 2017 go live numerically improved the capture of the pain plan of care QOPI metric average or the three reporting periods (Fall 2016, Spring and Fall 2017) before our EPIC transition compared to the four reporting periods (Spring and Fall 2018 and Spring and Fall 2019) after the EPIC transition. This occurred in both the campus (64% pre-EPIC to 93% post) and community sites (39% pre-EPIC to 86% post) as shown in Figure 8. COH's quality team, who collect and report the QOPI scores from the EHR, reported that increased symptom-reporting data from use of the ONC ROS questionnaire in patient visit notes as well as having the NCCN nausea risk level medication orders built into the chemotherapy orders in our EPIC EHR were the main reasons for our improved enterprise QOPI scores for the reporting periods after EPIC compared to those before EPIC implementation. As shown in Figure 9, the score improved from 84% pre-EPIC without the OncROS and nausea regimens built into regimens to 87.6% post-EPIC with the use of the OncROS and nausea medications built into chemotherapy regimens for the enterprise. Ongoing work evaluating which patient-reported outcome tool might work with our triage pathways, multidisciplinary pathways, the EPIC EHR, and our diverse patients is in progress toward a standardized PRO tool for all services. Our criteria for choosing an enterprise-wide tool include patient and provider satisfaction for ease of use, efficacy to improve clinical care, and integration of the PRO tool into care pathways to improve value-based outcomes and ease documentation to support team-based triage communication and provide mineable data to support quality assessments.

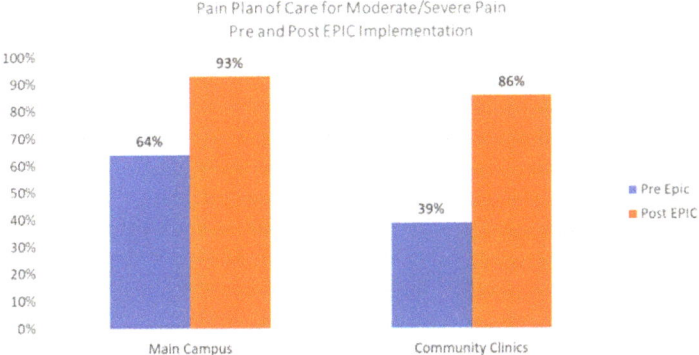

Figure 8. Pain plan of care compliance for those reporting moderate to severe pain. Blue represents results from the 3 QOPI reporting quarters (Fall 2016, Spring and Fall 2017) from the previous EHRs (Allscripts on campus and TouchWorks in community sites) prior to the EPIC implementation. Orange represents results from the 4 QOPI reporting quarters (Spring and Fall 2018 and Spring and Fall 2019) after the December 2017 EPIC transition for both the campus and community sites.

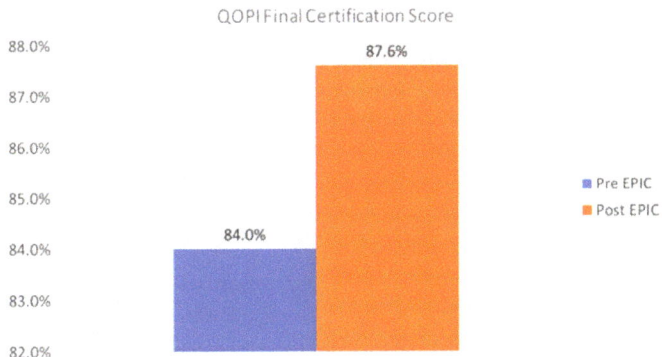

Figure 9. COH enterprise QOPI final certification scores. Blue represents the 3 reporting quarters (Fall 2016, Spring 2017 and Fall 2017) before the -EPIC implementation. Orange represents the 4 QOPI reporting quarters (Spring and Fall 2018 and Spring and Fall 2019) after the EPIC go live December 2017.

7. Other Enterprise Academic Community Teamwork Supporting Personalized Pathways for Value-Based Care Delivery

Disease team meetings include academic and community doctors and APPs who get to know and develop respect for each other. They discuss the newest science, clinical trials, and care opportunities that are not yet in pathways, pending disease committee reviews and the 6–12-month processes. Disease teams maintain internal pathway flow diagrams with some modifications embraced before they are formally available in national pathway tools.

New pre-ClinPath pathway update tool for practice changing therapies in development: COH has identified the need for a new tool to capture and share in a standardized monthly update format new practice changing updates agreed to by disease teams. Tracking analytics are being developed concurrently to track the sharing of new practice changing knowledge with the agreement to add to pathways, the availability in the pathway tool, and the uptake by faculty across the enterprise for long-term quality improvement work. Baseline studies in three tumor types are underway to inform this new process.

Tumor boards: These are all now done for tumor types by teleconferencing so the multidisciplinary teams of campus and community faculty actively participate. Some community doctors report that they are submitting at least one case to each tumor board and regularly submit to the tumor board of 1–2 cancers which they may be particularly focused on. They report that the move to tele-tumor boards for all faculty has increased participation and feel that they are sharing and learning more from the entire multidisciplinary team in very open and collegial discussions. This is true for the weekly molecular tumor board as well.

Joint clinics: Many academic faculty have agreed to cover or see patients from time to time in different community clinics and some community doctors spend regular time in academic campus clinics. The academic faculty appreciates the tight knit and efficient teamwork at community sites who evolved to be very efficient in a highly managed care world. Academic experts get to share one-on-one the latest molecular or other discoveries during real-time patient encounters with their community faculty colleagues and observe the use of ClinPath and other pathways at community sites. Friendships and increased collegiality have blossomed, which encourages ongoing sharing that offers every patient access to cutting-edge knowledge. A system to facilitate second opinions between the campus and community faculty has also helped to increase patient peace of mind while allowing them to receive care at the site closest to their home.

Regional, disease team and campus symposia and lectures are shared with all faculty. The medical oncology department holds quarterly half-day symposia where campus and community faculty present the latest science and care pathways as well as sharing clinical trial, value-based care, and programmatic updates. Disease teams also hold retreats to share the latest disease-specific knowledge and clinical trials, which is another helpful format for networking and building of collegial relationships. The pandemic restrictions on in person meetings led the medical oncology department to hold their sixth symposia in October of 2020, where 118 members participated in a 5-h update on science and clinical programs. The feedback was enthusiastic for the format, where there was active engagement and extensive group and interpersonal sharing of ideas in the chat function while members avoided having to travel from family on a weekend.

8. Other Value-Based Care Framework Projects Integrated with the Pathways Programs

Development of enterprise disease trees is a newer initiative being done to aid further in the standardization process of developing personalized multidisciplinary care plans throughout the enterprise. Community disease and regional leaders are closely involved with academic-based colleagues in building the initial decision tree for breast cancer. Next up in the queue are GI and GU multispecialty decision tree builds. The campus disease trees include locations for complex surgeries or other cancers as well as timing and genomic testing for both somatic and germline mutations. Within these disease trees is an enterprise-wide initiative to extend germline and somatic genomic testing to all patients as well as the integration of the results into the disease pathways. This will be piloted in one site (South Pasadena) close to the academic center and then expand to all sites by 2021. Pulling in the disease-specific pathways from medical oncology, hematology, radiation oncology, and surgical oncology, along with supportive care pathways, nutrition, genetic counseling, and testing as well as other rehabilitative services, will help to define when in a patient's course of care is provided and in which sites by which experts.

Increased interoperability of EHRs, especially EPIC, is an ongoing project. An advantage of EPIC, which, in CA, is the primary EHR for major university cancer centers (COH and Stanford) as well as the UC system hospitals (UCLA, UCI, UCSD, UC Merced, UCR, and UCSF), as well as the Kaiser Permanente Health System, which serves 40% of California residents, is the ability to review past records, therapies, and diagnoses, which can better inform current care plan development. Continued regulatory pressure to improve the interoperability of all EHR systems and the laboratory, imaging, and diagnostic companies is important to ensure that accurate patient data are available to treating clinicians to facilitate proper care plan development.

Improved functionality of EHRs to capture data more efficiently and support customized care planning is an ongoing focus for most oncologists to empower value-based care initiatives. The goal that we started with at COH, to develop personalized multidisciplinary CARE PLANS for each patient, continues to advance as disease and discipline-specific pathways are implemented, which can be then be made for each patient with our fast and frugal tree approach (described above). Getting to the point where every patient can be given a comprehensive, multidisciplinary care plan that can be navigated and managed remains a top priority for COH and other organizations focused on actualizing all the elements of VBCC.

Staging initiative for discrete data elements engages faculty in defining the data elements needed for decision support and downstream outcomes for each type of cancer. The AJCC has identified components for staging diseases that now include three categories: traditional staging elements, prognostic features, and clinical care features [114]. While the latest, AJCC 8, which became active in the US for staging in January of 2018, expanded these ideas in breast and some other cancers, most cancers do not have these details defined by the AJCC [114]. These are the growing number of discrete disease and patient-specific data components that track to pathway prompting when the patient goals and other comorbidities make it likely that a standard evidence-based pathway will have the best outcome [115]. Capture of these discrete elements facilitates the interfacing of data entry in the main EHR for an organization, then linking those features into decision support tools to minimize duplicate data entry and improve practice efficiencies, as we have pioneered and described above. Our initial 10-month, enterprise-wide 2020 staging initiative showed that 92% of all new patients seen in medical surgical and radiation oncology between January and September 15 of 2020 had required staging data elements entered in the EHR. The next steps for 2021 will be expanding the required data elements for entry and dashboard reporting to clinicians to include elements that are capturable in the EHR that can map to decision support in the pathway tool while we simultaneously expand the tumor types we have full mapping of EHR data elements into the pathway tool and back to therapy orders for medical and radiation oncology, as discussed above.

Oral hemotherapy drugs are built into the EHR as regimens: In preparation for further integration between our EHR and the ClinPath pathway tool, we identified 58 oral cancer drugs which had not been built into our chemotherapy ordering system (Beacon for EPIC). These are included in 96 protocols which will be prompted from the pathway program, so both academic and community medical oncologists then hematologists were recruited, agreed to build specific protocols including the references, associated NCCN nausea level, dosing, visit, lab, and specific drug guidance using a standardized Excel tool. Examples of current protocols were shared at individual or small group teaching sessions held through video visits. The builds for all but the last 25 protocols have been completed, including validation by an oncology Pharm D since April 2020, which was stimulated by the March 2020 COVID-19 pandemic work from home emphasis. We anticipate that the remaining 25 regimens will be built and validated by December of 2020 and have a goal that all of the 96 regimens will be available in the EPIC Beacon ordering system by Q1 2021.

Once completed, we will launch a best practice alert if a clinician orders an oral chemotherapy agent in the stand-alone prescription system of the HER rather than ordering it in the fully integrated chemotherapy order section in the EPIC Beacon system. The advantage of the build in the specific chemotherapy order system is the tie into the pathway, prompting the ability to standardize chemotherapy teaching visits in each order, support for the authorization processes, and integration into our recently launched specialty pharmacy program. With these integrations, any additional coverage needs for high-cost specialty and other cancer therapies can be identified and addressed early on while also facilitating analytic reporting on specific patient tumor types and disease features treated by specific regimens over measurable time periods for clinical and financial outcomes.

Outreach to community hospitals and ambulatory surgery centers is ongoing to share ERAS and other supportive care pathway work and engage diverse teams in meeting the care steps. Working across systems remains a challenge as noted. There is a clear focus, however, on developing these so that, wherever the patient chooses to get their care, the same high-quality care standards will be incorporated into the care processes and embraced by all staff, whether they work for our enterprise, a partnered entity, or a standalone facility. An advantage of our academic community faculty team model is the easy sharing and customization abilities of our clinicians and administrators so that the additional tools and processes developed at our NCI designated comprehensive cancer center can be shared with community-based hospitals and clinicians outside our enterprise.

The COH Enterprise data warehouse collects data elements from all digital platforms used by the enterprise and supports VBCC as well as research and other initiatives. It is overseen by a governance committee with clinical informatics, precision medicine, and information technology experts, who make data available to empower care and insights. From the data warehouse, Tableau dashboards can be created for feedback to clinicians and administrators along with many other informatic formats to process large datasets for study, some of which are shown as figures in this manuscript. The digital framework to turn information into real-world data is described in Figure 10.

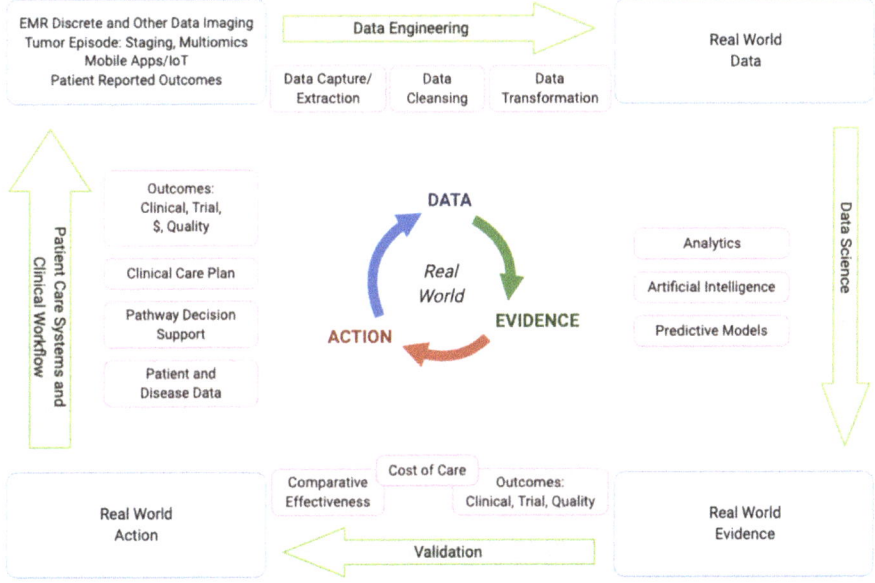

Figure 10. City of Hope's overriding digital framework to empower value-based care and real-world insights.

9. Challenges of Keeping Pathways Updated and Minimizing Burnout

Among the many workstreams we have discussed here, two other challenges should be highlighted: the challenge to keep decision support tools up to date in real time and the importance of engaging physicians in the design and efficient implementation of value-based projects as team members to minimize burnout. Our enterprise has recognized and is addressing methods to keep pathway tools up to date and engage clinicians in the many value-based project processes. These challenges are both minimized by the integrated academic community faculty foundation teamwork, which not only gains from the diverse experiences and wisdom of the faculty but can help to reduce the growing burnout rates and earlier retirement events for cancer clinicians. Three components of burnout described by the AMA Steps Forward highlight a culture of wellness, personal resilience, and practice efficiencies as the major areas contributing to burnout [116]. Internal COH faculty surveys identified practice efficiencies as the most important factor contributing to burnout in our faculty as collected and shared at regular faculty meetings. These surveys have prioritized work to address efficiencies and teamwork as we implement VBCC projects with academic and community team inputs.

Implementing multidisciplinary pathways across an enterprise and expanding to outside organizations faces the ongoing challenge of keeping pathway and decision support tools up to date in real time so that clinicians can deliver value-based care across the enterprise. Oncology is fortunate to have so many continuing new discoveries that can improve outcomes, but they require real-time tools and programming to bring practicing changing diagnostic and therapeutic knowledge to clinicians. Doing this with academic disease team leads working with integrated academic community disease teams helps to share the knowledge and build real-time enterprise tool updates until the larger pathway decision tools are updated. This can also improve workflows that can enhance patient and practitioner satisfaction [116]. It can also help to reduce burnout from extended work hours from individual clinicians having to individually evaluate the copious amounts of detailed new cancer information for the many kinds of cancer patients that they see.

A second challenge is to engage clinicians and staff teams in pathways and value-based initiative work so that the data entry, programming of digital tools, and workflow processes align to minimize their contribution to burnout while empowering evidence-based care delivery. Faculty who are encouraged and rewarded by leadership to participate in their passion for cutting-edge care and clinical research, while contributing to enterprise and professional initiatives, can lessen the sense of loss of meaning in work and a feeling they are a replaceable robot in an assembly line of patient care. Dashboard feedback that engages doctors and their teams with the results of discrete data entry and clinical trial outcomes can fuel pride in their and their care team's work with patients as well as in their role in the success of the larger enterprise. While many clinicians expressed initial push back on the increased workloads to enter discrete staging and pathway navigation data, as familiarity with the systems increased and the integration of the tools as well as the clinical trials expanded, there was a growing sense, which has not been formally measured, that the time spent entering defined, discrete data once is likely offset by time savings from authorization clerks, searching for patient information to inform clinical trial prioritization, expanded efficiencies in database-related clinical research, improved inter-specialty communication of the patient's disease and course, and, as sequences of disease descriptions build across a patient journey, markedly speeding up the ability of clinicians to gain a rapid understanding of what a patient has had, what they were treated with, and where the next steps in diagnostics, follow-up, or subsequent therapies should be. All of these tradeoffs would benefit from formal study that might also help to inform new pilots about return on investments regarding who and when on the team with what training are optimal for specific data entry if not the doctors or APPs [116].

This work can also be informed by many experts outside of medicine as we continue to iterate and learn from pioneering efforts. Dr. Etienne Wenger, PhD is one such globally recognized thought leader in the field of learning theory and its application to business who is a pioneer of "community of practice" research. Especially relevant to our work is his statement that "Communities of practice are important to the functioning of any organization, but they become crucial to those that recognize knowledge as a key asset" [117].

COH as an enterprise is addressing these two challenges along with the many others discussed. The pathways and care plan development programs benefit with leadership supporting active clinician engagement across our academic and community cancer center sites, which addresses several major components to minimize burnout: improving work place efficiencies, reducing social isolation at work, and the sense of loss of meaning in work that care standardization without engagement can bring. This has helped clinicians and staff to embrace the shift to value-based care through personalized precision medicine with integrated clinical research. The addition of teamwork across the enterprise by clinicians, managers, nurses, pharmacists, administrators, quality and informatics experts with our IT teams also iterates improvements in EHR functionalities, allowing more patient-reported input and team-based data entry, which can free up clinician time to analyze data and engage patients in developing a personalized, multidisciplinary care plan. The many projects outlined with multidisciplinary oncology pathways as a key component towards enterprise delivery of high-quality cancer care can be done with thoughtful attention to methodologies and team engagement so that value-based care, defined as the combination of high-quality care, patient satisfaction, provider satisfaction, and enterprise health at the appropriate costs, can be achieved.

10. Conclusions

Patients, clinicians, patients' families, employers, and payers want to have the best care plan available, discussed and implemented seamlessly with ongoing patient support to achieve the best cancer care outcome, whether this is a cure or improved quality of life. Diagnostic testing, genomics, imaging, and clinical assessments have increasingly complex discrete data elements that need to be transformed into actionable information and decision support. This knowledge also needs to be communicated effectively in the shared decision-making process with patients and payers. Pathway programs with decision support tools integrated into the clinical workflows can inform high-quality clinical trial, treatment, and supportive care decisions efficiently when overseen and supplemented by disease teams informed by integrated academic community faculty partnerships. This knowledge, integrated into EHRs and digital tools, can empower true VBCC throughout a fully integrated, multisite enterprise.

Thus, while many see oncology pathways as focusing only on medical oncology and hematology regimens, they are just as important for specific patient populations such as geriatrics, clinical cancer genetics, AYA, and pediatric populations as well as for surgical oncology, radiation oncology, and supportive care. Combining pathways personalized to each patient can then build the evidence-based comprehensive care plans to optimize each patient's cancer journey for their best health outcome. Foundational work on multidisciplinary oncology pathways, which started with COH's early engagement and leadership with the NCCN, has progressed to the development and implementation of disease-specific, supportive care, subpopulation-specific (i.e., geriatrics), and multidisciplinary pathways toward our goal of comprehensive, individual patient care plans. This work, coordinated under our Value Realization enterprise project, is overseen by faculty and administrative teams with diverse scientific and practical operational knowledge as well as academic and community expertise. The partnered teams have facilitated this pioneering work as an enterprise to develop, implement, and analyze the methodology and infrastructure to care for each cancer patient with a personalized care plan based on their cancer diagnosis, detailed and evolving molecular diagnostics, clinical trials, and bio-psychosocial needs with tools to support engagement in shared decision-making at initial diagnosis and any subsequent recurrences.

As more community oncology practitioners with practical implementation and local cultural expertise join local, regional, and national networks with experts who maintain the intense, detailed focus in subspecialty areas of oncology care, this combined knowledge and perspective can be shared through standardized decision support oncology pathway tools supplemented with real-time, team-led modifications as new knowledge helps us to achieve better outcomes with less toxicity for patients, regardless of where they live. Our COH enterprise commitment to one standard of high-quality care for every patient led to the pilots and multidisciplinary oncology pathway programs using tools, teams, and processes that can serve to inform others as network affiliations grow. While this work is empowered by the team-based, one faculty, one standard of care philosophy across our enterprise, there are many operational and implementation steps to deliver and measure this care standard. The work has benefitted from the combined strength of the academic faculty's deep scientific knowledge and focus with the community faculty's deep clinical and operational knowledge in partnership with administrators, project leads, informaticists, IT experts, and committees.

Implementing and integrating multidisciplinary oncology pathway programs also benefits from other partnered projects with subspecialty groups, IT interfaces, EHR functionalities, care teams, and analytic reporting as reviewed. While multidisciplinary oncology pathways are key components in the delivery of high-quality cancer care, they are only one of the many important component projects of VBCC. Achieving measurable delivery of all component projects within the three VBCC pillars of evidenced-based care, care management, and care after cancer with high levels of patient satisfaction, clinician satisfaction, and institutional health with optimized costs remains a work in progress. Early reports of COH's successes and the successes reported by others can serve to inform and inspire ongoing work in VBCC [8,11,26,27,30,34].

Author Contributions: Conceptualization: L.D.B., B.Y., S.S., H.C., S.G. (Stacy Gray), F.Z., E.K., S.G. (Scott Glaser), R.S., D.J. Formal Analysis: L.D.B., F.Z., D.D., A.B.L., D.M., S.G.(Scott Glaser), J.C., A.N., D.J. Data Curation: L.D.B., B.Y., S.S., A.P., F.Z., D.D., A.B.L., M.S.S., E.K., S.G.(Scott Glaser), D.M., A.N., D.J. Writing—original draft preparation: L.D.B., B.Y., C.Y., H.C., S.S., A.P., F.Z., A.B.L., M.S.S., E.K., S.G. (Stacy Gray), S.G. (Scott Glaser), T.T., A.N., I.B.P., P.K., D.J. Writing—review and editing: L.D.B., M.C., B.Y., C.Y., H.C., S.S., A.P., F.Z., D.D., A.B.L., M.S.S., E.K., S.G. (Stacy Gray), D.M., S.G. (Scott Glaser), G.B., C.A., T.T., J.C., A.N., I.B.P., L.K., P.R., K.S., A.N., P.K., R.S., J.Y., D.J. All authors have read and agreed to the published version of the manuscript.

Funding: This research received no external funding. The work was conducted as quality improvement projects under institutional programs.

Conflicts of Interest: Linda Bosserman serves as an unpaid member and co-chair of the breast cancer pathway committee for Elsevier's Clinical Pathways and serves as an unpaid member of the adult oncology steering board for the EPIC electronic health record. Chao disclosed he has financial relationships in the last 36 months with Merck, Amgen, Macrogenetics, Ono Pharmaceutical, Foundation Medicine and Daiichi-Sankyo. Elisabeth King is a member of a Pfizer advisory board and on AstraZeneca's speaker's bureau. No conflicts were reported by other coauthors related to this manuscript.

References

1. Kirkwood, M.K.; Hanley, A.; Bruinooge, S.S.; Garrett-Mayer, E.; Levit, L.A.; Schenkel, C.; Seid, J.E.; Polite, B.N.; Schilsky, R.L. The State of Oncology Practice in America, 2018: Results of the ASCO Practice Census Survey. *J. Oncol. Pract.* **2018**, *14*, e412–e420. [CrossRef] [PubMed]
2. Community Oncology Alliance, 2018 Community Oncology Practice Impact Report. 2 April 2018. Available online: https://communityoncology.org/2018-community-oncology-practice-impact-report/ (accessed on 23 June 2020).
3. Levit, L.; Balogh, E.; Nass, S. *Delivering High-Quality Cancer Care: Charting a New Course for A System in Crisis*; Ganz, P., Ed.; Committee on Improving the Quality of Cancer Care: Addressing the Challenges of an Aging Population; Board on Health Care Services; Institute of Medicine; National Academies Press (US): Washington, DC, USA, 2013.
4. Bosserman, L.D. Benefits and Challenges of Growing Oncology Networks in the United States. *J. Oncol. Pract.* **2018**, *14*, 761–762. [CrossRef] [PubMed]
5. Albanese, C.; Aaby, D.; Platchek, T. *Advanced Lean in Healthcare*; CreateSpace Independent Publishing Platform: Scotts Valley, CA, USA, 2014; ISBN 149614189X.
6. Sprandio, J.D. Oncology patient-centered medical home and accountable cancer care. *Commun. Oncol.* **2010**, *7*, 565–572. [CrossRef]
7. Bosserman, L.D.; Verrilli, D.; McNatt, W. Partnering with a payer to develop a value-based medical home pilot: A West Coast practice's experience. *Am. J. Manag. Care* **2012**, *18*, SP189–SP190. [CrossRef]
8. Waters, T.M.; Kaplan, C.M.; Graetz, I.; Price, M.M.; Stevens, L.A.; McAneny, B.L. Patient-Centered Medical Homes in Community Oncology Practices: Changes in Spending and Care Quality Associated with the COME HOME Experience. *J. Oncol. Pract.* **2019**, *15*, e56–e64. [CrossRef]
9. Piana, R. *Integration across the Spectrum: Community Perspective on the Medical Oncology Home Model*; The ASCO Post: Huntington, NY, USA, 2015.
10. Thompson, G. The Oncology Medical Home: Embodiment of the American Pioneering Spirit. *Oncol. Pract. Manag.* **2012**, *2*, 6.
11. Page, R.D.; Newcomer, L.N.; Sprandio, J.D.; McAneny, B.L. The Patient-Centered Medical Home in Oncology: From Concept to Reality. *Am. Soc. Clin. Oncol. Educ. Book* **2015**, e82–e89. [CrossRef]
12. Neubauer, M.A.; Hoverman, J.R.; Kolodziej, M.; Reisman, L.; Gruschkus, S.K.; Hoang, S.; Beveridge, R.A. Cost effectiveness of evidence-based treatment guidelines for the treatment of non-small-cell lung cancer in the community setting. *J. Oncol. Pract.* **2010**, *6*, 12–18. [CrossRef]

13. Hoverman, J.R.; Cartwright, T.H.; Patt, D.A.; Espirito, J.L.; Clayton, M.P.; Garey, J.S.; Pyenson, B. Pathways, outcomes, and costs in colon cancer: Retrospective evaluations in two distinct databases. *J. Oncol. Pract.* **2011**, *7* (Suppl. 3), 52s–59s. [CrossRef]
14. Weese, J.L.; Shamah, C.J.; Sanchez, F.A.; Perez Moreno, A.C.; Mitchell, D.; Sessa, T.; Amy, B. Use of treatment pathways reduce cost and decrease ED utilization and un-planned hospital admissions in patients (pts) with stage II breast cancer. *J. Clin. Oncol.* **2019**, *37* (Suppl. 15), e12012. [CrossRef]
15. Jackman, D.M.; Zhang, Y.; Dalby, C.; Nguyen, T.; Nagle, J.; Lydon, C.A.; Jacobson, J.O. Cost and survival analysis before and after implementation of Dana-Farber clin-ical pathways for patients with stage IV non-small-cell lung cancer. *J. Oncol. Pract.* **2017**, *13*, e346–e352. [CrossRef] [PubMed]
16. Newcomer, L.N.; Gould, B.; Page, R.D.; Donelan, S.A.; Perkins, M. Changing Physician Incentives for Affordable, Quality Cancer Care: Results of an Episode Payment Model. *J. Oncol. Pract.* **2014**, *10*, 322–326. [CrossRef]
17. Doyle, C. Anthem's Clinical Pathways Demonstrate Value: The Payer Perspective. *Am. Health Drug Benefits* **2015**, *8*, 28. [PubMed]
18. Scott, J.A.; Milligan, S.; Wong, W.; Winn, D.; Cooper, J.; Schneider, N.; Parkes, S.; Feinberg, B.A. Validation of observed savings from an oncology clinical pathways program. *J. Clin. Oncol.* **2013**, *31*, 6553. [CrossRef]
19. Kardos, S.V.; Chan, K.G.; Yuh, B.E.; Yamzon, J.; Ruel, N.; Zachariah, F.; Lau, C.S.; Crocitto, L.E. Recovery after surgery and care coordination pathway at City of Hope: Length of stay, readmissions, and complications. *J. Clin. Oncol.* **2016**, *34*, 410. [CrossRef]
20. Basch, E.; Deal, A.M.; Dueck, A.C.; Scher, H.I.; Kris, M.G.; Hudis, C.; Schrag, D. Overall Survival Results of a Trial Assessing Patient-Reported Outcomes for Symp-tom Monitoring During Routine Cancer Treatment. *JAMA* **2017**, *318*, 197–198. [CrossRef] [PubMed]
21. Koprowski, C.; Petrilli, N.; Johnson, E.J.; Sites, K. The Supportive Care of Oncology Patients (SCOOP) Pathway: A novel Ap-proach to Improving the Patient Experience in the Curative Treatment of Cancer. *J. Clin. Pathw.* **2019**, *5*, 39–43.
22. Grant, M.; Ferrell, B.R.; Rivera, L.M.; Lee, J. Unscheduled readmissions for uncontrolled symptoms. A health care challenge for nurses. *Nurs. Clin. N. Am.* **1995**, *30*, 673–682.
23. Quality Payment Program Executive Summary, MACRA. 16 October 2016. Available online: https://qpp.cms.gov/docs/QPP_Executive_Summary_of_Final_Rule.pdf (accessed on 12 October 2020).
24. Findlay, M.; Rankin, N.M.; Shaw, T.; White, K.; Boyer, M.; Milross, C.G.; Lourenço, R.D.A.; Brown, C.; Collett, G.; Beale, P.; et al. Best Evidence to Best Practice: Implementing an Innovative Model of Nutrition Care for Patients with Head and Neck Cancer Improves Outcomes. *Nutrients* **2020**, *12*, 1465. [CrossRef]
25. Smith, T.J.; Hillner, B.E. Ensuring Quality Cancer Care by the Use of Clinical Practice Guidelines and Critical Pathways. *J. Clin. Oncol.* **2001**, *19*, 2886–2897. [CrossRef]
26. Lederman, L. Are Medical Homes and ACOs the Future of Cancer Care? Oncology Business Review. September 2012 Edition, Volume 11, Issue 9. Available online: https://obroncology.com/article/are-medical-homes-and-acos-the-future-of-cancer-care-2/ (accessed on 7 October 2020).
27. Kuznar, W. Patient-Centered Oncology Medical Home Improves Health Outcomes at Lower Costs to Patients and Payers. *Value Based Cancer Care* **2014**, *5*, 1579. Available online: http://valuebasedcancer.com/issues/2014/october-2014-vol-5-no-8/1579-patient-centered-oncology-medical-home-improves-health-outcomes-at-lower-costs-to-patients-and-payers (accessed on 7 October 2020).
28. Bunkhead, C. Achieving Higher Quality, Lower Cost through Oncology Medical Homes. *Oncol. Pract. Manag.* **2015**, *5*, 6. Available online: http://oncpracticemanagement.com/issues/2015/september-2015-vol-5-no-6/550-achieving-higher-quality-lower-cost-through-oncology-medical-homes (accessed on 7 October 2020).
29. Patel, M. The Oncology Care Model: Aligning Financial Incentives to Improve Outcomes. *Oncology Practice Manag.* **2016**, *6*, 12. [CrossRef]
30. Colligan, E.M.; Ewald, E.; Ruiz, S.; Spafford, M.; Cross-Barnet, C.; Parashuram, S. Innovative Oncology Care Models Improve End-Of-Life Quality, Reduce Utilization And Spending. *Health Aff.* **2017**, *36*, 433–440. [CrossRef]

31. Hoverman, J.R.; Neubauer, M.A.; Jameson, M.; Hayes, J.E.; Eagye, K.J.; Abdullahpour, M.; Verrilli, D.K. Three-Year Results of a Medicare Advantage Cancer Management Program. *J. Oncol. Pract.* **2018**, *14*, e229–e237. [CrossRef]
32. Neubauer, M. Clinical pathways: Reducing costs and improving quality across a network. *Am J Manag. Care* **2020**, *26*, SP60–SP61.
33. Walker, B.; Frytak, J.; Hayes, J.; Neubauer, M.; Robert, N.; Wilfong, L. Evaluation of Practice Patterns Among Oncologists Par-ticipating in the Oncology Care Model. *JAMA Netw. Open* **2020**, *3*, e205165. [CrossRef]
34. Ellis, P.G. Development and Implementation of Oncology Care Pathways in an Integrated Care Network: The Via Oncology Pathways Experience. *J. Oncol. Pract.* **2013**, *9*, 171–173. [CrossRef]
35. Miller, B. How the First Oncology ACO Achieves Savings Every Year, Advisory Board: Oncology Rounds. 1 March 2016. Available online: https://www.advisory.com/research/oncology-roundtable/oncology-rounds/2016/03/miami-cancer-institute (accessed on 12 October 2020).
36. Frois, C.; Howe, A.; Jarvis, J.; Grice, K.; Wong, K.; Zacker, C.; Sasane, R. Drug Treatment Value in a Changing Oncology Landscape: A Literature and Provider Perspective. *J. Manag. Care Spec. Pharm.* **2019**, *25*, 246–259. [CrossRef]
37. Cox, J.V.; Ward, J.C.; Hornberger, J.C.; Temel, J.S.; McAneny, B.L. Community Oncology in an Era of Payment Reform. *Am. Soc. Clin. Oncol. Educ. Book* **2014**, e447–e452. [CrossRef]
38. Avalere Health. Clinical Pathways: Overview of Current Practices and Potential Implications for Patients, Payers, and Providers. July 2015. Available online: https://www.phrma.org/report/clinical-pathways-overview-of-current-practices-and-potential-impliationsor-patients-payers-and-providers (accessed on 12 October 2020).
39. Rocque, G.B.; Williams, C.; Kenzik, K.; Jackson, B.E.; Halilova, K.I.; Sullivan, M.M.; Rocconi, R.P.; Azuero, A.; Kvale, E.; Huh, W.K.; et al. Where Are the Opportunities for Reducing Health Care Spending Within Alternative Payment Models? *J. Oncol. Pract.* **2018**, *14*, e375–e383. [CrossRef] [PubMed]
40. Neubauer, M. Clinical Pathways Can Lead to Cost Savings, Better Care. *Onc. Bus Rev. Green* **2014**, *11*. Available online: https://obroncology.com/article/clinical-pathways-can-lead-to-cost-savings-better-care-2/ (accessed on 12 October 2020).
41. Mortimer, J.E.; Kruper, L.; Cianfrocca, M.; Lavasani, S.; Liu, S.; Tank-Patel, N.; Yeon, C. Use of HER2-Directed Therapy in Metastatic Breast Cancer and How Com-munity Physicians Collaborate to Improve Care. *J. Clin. Med.* **2020**, *9*, 1984. [CrossRef] [PubMed]
42. Salgia, R.; Mambetsariev, I.; Tan, T.; Schwer, A.; Pearlstein, D.P.; Chehabi, H.; Baroz, A.; Fricke, J.; Pharaon, R.; Romo, H.; et al. Complex Oncological Decision-Making Utilizing Fast-and-Frugal Trees in a Community Setting—Role of Academic and Hybrid Modeling. *J. Clin. Med.* **2020**, *9*, 1884. [CrossRef]
43. Salgia, N.J.; Philip, E.J.; Ziari, M.; Yap, K.; Pal, S.K. Advancing the Science and Management of Renal Cell Carcinoma: Bridging the Divide between Academic and Community Practices. *J. Clin. Med.* **2020**, *9*, 1508. [CrossRef]
44. FDA. Hematology/Oncology (Cancer) Approvals and Safety Notifications. 2016–June 2020. Available online: https://www.fda.gov/drugs/resources-information-approved-drugs/hematologyoncology-cancer-approvals-safety-notifications (accessed on 23 June 2020).
45. Tran, G.; Zafar, S.Y. Financial toxicity and implications for cancer care in the era of molecular and immune therapies. *Ann. Transl. Med.* **2018**, *6*, 166. [CrossRef] [PubMed]
46. Zafar, S.Y.; Peppercorn, J.M.; Schrag, D.; Taylor, D.H.; Goetzinger, A.M.; Zhong, X.; Abernethy, A.P. The financial toxicity of cancer treatment: A pilot study assessing out-of-pocket expenses and the insured cancer patient's experience. *Oncologist* **2013**, *18*, 381–390. [CrossRef] [PubMed]
47. Zafar, S.Y. Financial Toxicity of Cancer Care: It's Time to Intervene. *J. Natl. Cancer Inst.* **2016**, *108*, djv370. [CrossRef]
48. Karimi, M.; Wang, C.; Bahadini, B.; Hajjar, G.; Fakih, M. Integrating Academic and Community Practices in the Management of Colorectal Cancer: The City of Hope Model. *J. Clin. Med.* **2020**, *9*, 1687. [CrossRef] [PubMed]

49. Rajurkar, S.; Mambetsariev, I.; Pharaon, R.; Leach, B.; Tan, T.; Kulkarni, P.; Salgia, R. Non-Small Cell Lung Cancer from Genomics to Therapeutics: A Frame-work for Community Practice Integration to Arrive at Personalized Therapy Strategies. *J. Clin. Med.* **2020**, *9*, 1870. [CrossRef]
50. Basse, L.; Hjort Jakobsen, D.; Billesbølle, P.; Werner, M.; Kehlet, H. A clinical pathway to accelerate recovery after colonic re-section. *Ann. Surg.* **2000**, *232*, 51–57. [CrossRef]
51. Kehlet, H.; Mogensen, T. Hospital stay of 2 days after open sigmoidectomy with a multimodal rehabilitation programme. *BJS* **1999**, *86*, 227–230. [CrossRef] [PubMed]
52. Fearon, K.C.; Ljungqvist, O.; Von Meyenfeldt, M.; Revhaug, A.; DeJong, C.H.C.; Lassen, K.; Nygren, J.; Hausel, J.; Soop, M.; Andersen, J.P.; et al. Enhanced recovery after surgery: A consensus review of clinical care for patients undergoing colonic resection. *Clin. Nutr.* **2005**, *24*, 466–477. [CrossRef] [PubMed]
53. Ljungqvist, O. ERAS–enhanced recovery after surgery: Moving evidence-based perioperative care to practice. *JPEN J. Parenter. Enteral Nutr.* **2014**, *38*, 559–566. [CrossRef] [PubMed]
54. Carmichael, J.C.; Keller, D.S.; Baldini, G.; Bordeianou, L.; Weiss, E.; Lee, L.; Steele, S.R. Clinical Practice Guidelines for Enhanced Recovery After Colon and Rectal Surgery From the American Society of Colon and Rectal Surgeons and Society of American Gastrointestinal and Endo-scopic Surgeons. *Dis. Colon Rectum* **2017**, *60*, 761–784. [CrossRef] [PubMed]
55. Ljungqvist, O.; Scott, M.; Fearon, K.C. Enhanced Recovery after Surgery: A Review. *JAMA Surg.* **2017**, *152*, 292–298. [CrossRef]
56. Kehlet, H. Enhanced Recovery Protocols (ERP): Need for Action. *Ann Surg.* **2018**, *268*, e85. [CrossRef]
57. Brindle, M.E.; Nelson, G.; Lobo, D.; Ljungqvist, O.; Gustafsson, U.O. Recommendations from the ERAS®Society for standards for the development of enhanced recovery after surgery guidelines. *BJS Open* **2019**, *4*, 157–163. [CrossRef]
58. Chenam, A.; Chan, K.G. Enhanced Recovery after Surgery for Radical Cystectomy. *Cancer Treat. Res.* **2018**, *175*, 215–239. [CrossRef]
59. Scarberry, K.; Berger, N.G.; Scarberry, K.B.; Agrawal, S.; Francis, J.J.; Yih, J.M.; Abouassaly, R. Improved surgical outcomes following radical cystectomy at high-volume centers influence overall survival. *Urol. Oncol.* **2018**, *36*, 308.e11–308.e17. [CrossRef]
60. Ellis, P.G.; O'Neil, B.H.; Earle, M.F.; McCutcheon, S.; Benson, H. The usefulness of clinical pathways (CP) in managing quality and cost in oncology networks. *J. Clin. Oncol.* **2016**, *34* (Suppl. 4), 715. [CrossRef]
61. Chiang, A.C.; Lake, J.; Sinanis, N.; Brandt, D.; Kanowitz, J.; Kidwai, W.; Tara, H. Measuring the Impact of Academic Cancer Network Development on Clinical Inte-gration, Quality of Care, and Patient Satisfaction. *J. Oncol. Pract.* **2018**, *14*, e823–e833. [CrossRef] [PubMed]
62. Zon, R.T.; Frame, J.N.; Neuss, M.N.; Page, R.D.; Wollins, D.S.; Stranne, S.; Bosserman, L.D. American Society of Clinical Oncology Policy Statement on Clinical Pathways in Oncology. *J. Oncol. Pract.* **2016**, *12*, 261–266. [CrossRef] [PubMed]
63. Zon, R.T.; Edge, S.B.; Page, R.D.; Frame, J.N.; Lyman, G.H.; Omel, J.L.; Wollins, D.S.; Green, S.R.; Bosserman, L.D. American Society of Clinical Oncology Criteria for High-Quality Clinical Pathways in Oncology. *J. Oncol. Pract.* **2017**, *13*, 207–210. [CrossRef]
64. McCutcheon, S.; Ellis, P.G.; Hess, R.; Krebs, M.; Lokay, K. Frequency of efficacy, toxicity and cost as the deciding factor when determining clinical pathways. *J. Clin. Oncol.* **2016**, *34*, e18169. [CrossRef]
65. Ersek, J.L.; Black, L.J.; Thompson, M.A.; Kim, E.S. Implementing Precision Medicine Programs and Clinical Trials in the Community-Based Oncology Practice: Barriers and Best Practices. *Am. Soc. Clin. Oncol. Educ. Book* **2018**, *38*, 188–196. [CrossRef]
66. Shamah, C.J.; Saphner, T.J. Effect on clinical trial participation by integration of a clinical pathway program into an electronic health record (EHR). *J. Clin. Oncol.* **2016**, *34*, 167. [CrossRef]
67. Saphner, T.; Thompson, M.A.; Planton, S.; Singh, M.; Glandt, N.; Robinson, L.; DeBartolo, J. Insights from Building a New National Cancer Institute Community On-cology Research Program Site. *WMJ* **2016**, *115*, 191–195.

68. Ellis, P.G.; Weese, J.L. Clinical pathways as a platform to support clinical research. In Proceedings of the 107th Annual Meet-ing of the American Association for Cancer Research, New Orleans, LA, USA, 16–20 April 2016.
69. Kim, D.J.; Otap, D.; Ruel, N.; Gupta, N.; Khan, N.; Dorff, T.B. NCI–Clinical Trial Accrual in a Community Network Affiliated with a Designated Cancer Center. *J. Clin. Med.* **2020**, *9*, 1970. [CrossRef]
70. Gebhardt, B.J.; Heron, D.E.; Beriwal, S. A peer review process as part of the implementation of clinical pathways in radiation oncology: Does it improve compliance? *Pract. Radiat. Oncol.* **2017**, *7*, 332–338. [CrossRef]
71. Rajagopalan, M.S.; Flickinger, J.C.; Heron, D.E.; Beriwal, S. Changing practice patterns for breast cancer radiation therapy with clinical pathways: An analysis of hypofractionation in a large, integrated cancer center network. *Pract. Radiat. Oncol.* **2015**, *5*, 63–69. [CrossRef] [PubMed]
72. Haviland, J.S.; Owen, J.R.; Dewar, J.A.; Agrawal, R.K.; Barrett, J.; Barrett-Lee, P.J.; Mills, J. The UK Standardisation of Breast Radiotherapy (START) trials of radiotherapy hypofractionation for treatment of early breast cancer: 10-year follow-up results of two randomised controlled trials. *Lancet Oncol.* **2013**, *14*, 1086–1094. [CrossRef]
73. Koulis, T.A.; Phan, T.; Olivotto, I.A. Hypofractionated whole breast radiotherapy: Current perspectives. *Breast Cancer Targets Ther.* **2015**, *7*, 363–370. [CrossRef] [PubMed]
74. Whelan, T.J.; Pignol, J.-P.; Levine, M.N.; Julian, J.A.; MacKenzie, R.; Parpia, S.; Shelley, W.; Grimard, L.; Bowen, J.; Lukka, H.; et al. Long-Term Results of Hypofractionated Radiation Therapy for Breast Cancer. *N. Engl. J. Med.* **2010**, *362*, 513–520. [CrossRef] [PubMed]
75. Smith, B.D.; Bellon, J.R.; Blitzblau, R.; Freedman, G.; Haffty, B.; Hahn, C.; Patton, C. Radiation therapy for the whole breast: Executive summary of an American Soci-ety for Radiation Oncology (ASTRO) evidence-based guideline. *Pract. Radiat. Oncol.* **2018**, *8*, 145–152. [CrossRef]
76. Rodríguez-Lopéz, J.L.; Ling, D.C.; Heron, D.E.; Beriwal, S. Lag Time Between Evidence and Guidelines: Can Clinical Pathways Bridge the Gap? *J. Oncol. Pract.* **2019**, *15*, e195–e201. [CrossRef]
77. Heron, D.E.; Beriwal, S.; Benson, H.; Lorinc, Z.; Barry, A.; Lokay, K. The benefits of clinical pathways (CP) for radiation oncology in a large cancer care network. *J. Clin. Oncol.* **2016**, *34*, 148. [CrossRef]
78. Fitzgerald, T.; Urie, M.; Ulin, K.; Laurie, F.; Yorty, J.; Hanusik, R.; Kessel, S.; Jodoin, M.B.; Osagie, G.; Cicchetti, M.G.; et al. Processes for Quality Improvements in Radiation Oncology Clinical Trials. *Int. J. Radiat. Oncol.* **2008**, *71*, S76–S79. [CrossRef]
79. Liu, J.; Gutierrez, E.; Tiwari, A.; Padam, S.; Li, D.; Dale, W.; Pal, S.K.; Stewart, D.; Subbiah, S.; Bosserman, L.; et al. Strategies to Improve Participation of Older Adults in Cancer Research. *J. Clin. Med.* **2020**, *9*, 1571. [CrossRef]
80. ERAS Society Mission and History. Available online: https://erassociety.org/about/history/ (accessed on 29 October 2020).
81. Bilimoria, K.Y.; Liu, Y.; Paruch, J.L.; Zhou, L.; Kmiecik, T.E.; Ko, C.Y.; Cohen, M.E. Development and Evaluation of the Universal ACS NSQIP Surgical Risk Calculator: A Decision Aid and Informed Consent Tool for Patients and Surgeons. *J. Am. Coll. Surg.* **2013**, *217*, 833–842.e3. [CrossRef]
82. Cohen, M.E.; Liu, Y.; Ko, C.Y.; Hall, B.L. An Examination of American College of Surgeons NSQIP Surgical Risk Calculator Accuracy. *J. Am. Coll. Surg.* **2017**, *224*, 787–795. [CrossRef] [PubMed]
83. NSQIP Surgical Risk Score Calculator. Available online: https://riskcalculator.facs.org/RiskCalculator/PatientInfo.jsp (accessed on 19 October 2020).
84. Begg, C.B.; Cramer, L.D.; Hoskins, W.J.; Brennan, M.F. Impact of Hospital Volume on Operative Mortality for Major Cancer Surgery. *JAMA* **1998**, *280*, 1747–1751. [CrossRef] [PubMed]
85. Halm, E.A.; Lee, C.; Chassin, M.R. Is volume related to quality in health care. A systematic review and methodologic cri-tique of the research literature. *Ann. Intern. Med.* **2002**, *137*, 511–520. [CrossRef] [PubMed]
86. Birkmeyer, J.D.; Siewers, A.E.; Finlayson, E.V.; Stukel, T.A.; Lucas, F.L.; Batista, I.; Welch, H.G.; Wennberg, D.E. Hospital Volume and Surgical Mortality in the United States. *N. Engl. J. Med.* **2002**, *346*, 1128–1137. [CrossRef] [PubMed]
87. Birkmeyer, J.D.; Skinner, J.S.; Wennberg, D.E. Will Volume-Based Referral Strategies Reduce Costs Or Just Save Lives? *Health Aff.* **2002**, *21*, 234–241. [CrossRef]
88. Ihse, I. The volume-outcome relationship in cancer surgery: A hard sell. *Ann. Surg.* **2003**, *238*, 777–781. [CrossRef]

89. Birkmeyer, J.D.; Sun, Y.; Wong, S.L.; Stukel, T.A. Hospital Volume and Late Survival after Cancer Surgery. *Ann. Surg.* **2007**, *245*, 777–783. [CrossRef]
90. Finlayson, E.V.A.; Goodney, P.P.; Birkmeyer, J.D. Hospital Volume and Operative Mortality in Cancer Surgery. *Arch. Surg.* **2003**, *138*, 721–725. [CrossRef]
91. Hillner, B.E.; Smith, T.; Desch, C.E. Hospital and physician volume or specialization and outcomes in cancer treatment: Im-portance in quality of cancer care. *J. Clin. Oncol.* **2000**, *18*, 2327–2340. [CrossRef]
92. Carli, F.; Gillis, C.; Scheede-Bergdahl, C. Promoting a culture of prehabilitation for the surgical cancer patient. *Acta Oncol.* **2017**, *56*, 128–133. [CrossRef]
93. Forsmo, H.M.; Erichsen, C.; Rasdal, A.; Tvinnereim, J.M.; Kørner, H.; Pfeffer, F. Randomized Controlled Trial of Extended Perioperative Counseling in Enhanced Recovery After Colorectal Surgery. *Dis. Colon Rectum* **2018**, *61*, 724–732. [CrossRef] [PubMed]
94. Hoag Hospital ERAS Video for Patient Education. Available online: https://www.hoag.org/about-hoag/videos/enhanced-recovery-after-surgery-eras-/ (accessed on 23 June 2020).
95. Wesmiller, S.W.; Sereika, S.M.; Bender, C.M.; Bovbjerg, D.; Ahrendt, G.; Bonaventura, M.; Conley, Y.P. Exploring the multifactorial nature of postoperative nausea and vomiting in women following surgery for breast cancer. *Auton. Neurosci.* **2017**, *202*, 102–107. [CrossRef] [PubMed]
96. Conway, B. Prevention and Management of Postoperative Nausea and Vomiting in Adults. *AORN J.* **2009**, *90*, 391–413. [CrossRef] [PubMed]
97. Benyamin, R.; Trescot, A.; Datta, S.; Buenaventura, R.; Adlaka, R.; Sehgal, N.; Glaser, S.E.; Vallejo, R. Opioid complications and side effects. *Pain Physician* **2008**, *11*, S105–S120. [PubMed]
98. Jacobs, A.; Lemoine, A.; Joshi, G.P.; Van De Velde, M.; Bonnet, F.; Pogatzki-Zahn, E.; Schug, S.; Kehlet, H.; Rawal, N.; Delbos, A.; et al. PROSPECT guideline for oncological breast surgery: A systematic review and procedure-specific postoperative pain management recommendations. *Anaesthesia* **2020**, *75*, 664–673. [CrossRef]
99. Practice Guidelines for Preoperative Fasting and the Use of Pharmacologic Agents to Reduce the Risk of Pulmonary As-piration: Application to Healthy Patients Undergoing Elective Procedures: An Updated Report by the American Society of Anesthesiologists Task Force on Preoperative Fasting and the Use of Pharmacologic Agents to Reduce the Risk of Pulmonary Aspiration. *Anesthesiology* **2017**, *126*, 376–393.
100. Wagner, E.H.; Ludman, E.J.; Bowles, E.J.A.; Penfold, R.; Reid, R.J.; Rutter, C.M.; Chubak, J.; McCorkle, R. Nurse Navigators in Early Cancer Care: A Randomized, Controlled Trial. *J. Clin. Oncol.* **2014**, *32*, 12–18. [CrossRef]
101. Temel, J.S.; Greer, J.A.; Muzikansky, A.; Gallagher, E.R.; Admane, S.; Jackson, V.A.; Dahlin, C.M.; Blinderman, C.D.; Jacobsen, J.; Pirl, W.F.; et al. Early Palliative Care for Patients with Metastatic Non–Small-Cell Lung Cancer. *N. Engl. J. Med.* **2010**, *363*, 733–742. [CrossRef]
102. Zimmermann, C.; Swami, N.; Krzyzanowska, M.; Hannon, B.; Leighl, N.; Oza, A.; Donner, A. Early palliative care for patients with advanced cancer: A clus-ter-randomised trial. *Lancet* **2014**, *383*, 1721–1730. [CrossRef]
103. Rummans, T.A.; Clark, M.M.; Sloan, J.A.; Frost, M.H.; Bostwick, J.M.; Ms, P.J.A.; Johnson, M.E.; Gamble, G.; Richardson, J.; Brown, P.; et al. Impacting Quality of Life for Patients With Advanced Cancer With a Structured Multidisciplinary Intervention: A Randomized Controlled Trial. *J. Clin. Oncol.* **2006**, *24*, 635–642. [CrossRef]
104. Rabow, M.W.; Dibble, S.L.; Pantilat, S.Z.; McPhee, S.J. The comprehensive care team: A controlled trial of outpatient palliative medicine consultation. *Arch. Intern. Med.* **2004**, *164*, 83–91. [CrossRef] [PubMed]
105. Bakitas, M.; Lyons, K.D.; Hegel, M.T.; Balan, S.; Brokaw, F.C.; Seville, J.; Ahles, T.A. Effects of a palliative care intervention on clinical outcomes in patients with ad-vanced cancer: The Project ENABLE II randomized controlled trial. *JAMA* **2009**, *302*, 741–749. [CrossRef] [PubMed]
106. Patient and Family Meeting Program Pathway. Available online: https://www.cityofhope.org/education/health-professional-education/supportive-care-medicine-professional-education/supportive-care-clinical-programs/patient-and-family-meeting (accessed on 23 June 2020).
107. Yadav, K.N.; Gabler, N.B.; Cooney, E.; Kent, S.; Kim, J.; Herbst, N.; Courtright, K.R. Approximately One In Three US Adults Completes Any Type Of Advance Di-rective For End-Of-Life Care. *Health Aff.* **2017**, *36*, 1244–1251. [CrossRef] [PubMed]

108. Zachariah, F.; Popplewell, L.; Forman, S.J.; Gorospe, G.; Wong-Toh, J.; Morse, D.; Emanuel, L.; Ito-Hamerling, G.; Garcia, N.; Horak, D.; et al. The advance directive completion rates in the hematopoietic stem cell transplant population in a major transplant cancer center. *J. Clin. Oncol.* **2017**, *35*, 16. [CrossRef]
109. Information on City of Hope's Advanced Care Planning Program. Available online: https://www.cityofhope.org/education/health-professional-education/supportive-care-medicine-professional-education/supportive-care-clinical-programs/advance-care-planning (accessed on 23 June 2020).
110. ASCO QOPI-Related Measures and Certification Standards Manual. Available online: http://practice.asco.org/quality-improvement/quality-programs/quality-oncology-practice-initiative/qopi-related-measures (accessed on 30 October 2020).
111. The Quality Payment Program-CMS. Available online: https://qpp.cms.gov/ (accessed on 30 October 2020).
112. Handley, N.R.; Schuchter, L.M.; Bekelman, J.E. Best Practices for Reducing Unplanned Acute Care for Patients with Cancer. *J. Oncol. Pract.* **2018**, *14*, 306–313. [CrossRef]
113. Barkley, R.; Soobader, M.-J.; Wang, J.; Blau, S.; Page, R.D. Reducing Cancer Costs Through Symptom Management and Triage Pathways. *J. Oncol. Pract.* **2019**, *15*, e91–e97. [CrossRef]
114. Edge, S.B.; Hortobagyi, G.N.; Giuliano, A.E. New and important changes in breast cancer TNM: Incorporation of biologic factors into staging. *Expert Rev. Anticancer. Ther.* **2019**, *19*, 309–318. [CrossRef]
115. Amin, M.B.; Greene, F.L.; Edge, S.B.; Compton, C.C.; Gershenwald, J.E.; Brookland, R.K.; Meyer, L.; Gress, D.M.; Byrd, D.R.; Winchester, D.P. The Eighth Edition AJCC Cancer Staging Manual: Continuing to build a bridge from a population-based to a more "personalized" approach to cancer staging. *CA Cancer J. Clin.* **2017**, *67*, 93–99. [CrossRef]
116. AMA Web Site: Redesign Your Practice. Reignite Your Purpose. AMA's Practice Improvement Strategies. Available online: https://www.ama-assn.org/amaone/practice-support (accessed on 6 November 2020).
117. Wenger, E. Communities of Practice: Learning as a Social System. Systems Thinker. 9:5 June/July 1998. Available online: https://thesystemsthinker.com/communities-of-practice-learning-as-a-social-system/ (accessed on 23 June 2020).

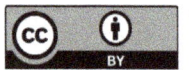

© 2021 by the authors. Licensee MDPI, Basel, Switzerland. This article is an open access article distributed under the terms and conditions of the Creative Commons Attribution (CC BY) license (http://creativecommons.org/licenses/by/4.0/).

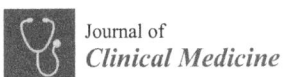

Review

Frontline Management of Epithelial Ovarian Cancer—Combining Clinical Expertise with Community Practice Collaboration and Cutting-Edge Research

Edward Wenge Wang [1,*], Christina Hsiao Wei [2], Sariah Liu [1], Stephen Jae-Jin Lee [3], Susan Shehayeb [4], Scott Glaser [5], Richard Li [5], Siamak Saadat [1], James Shen [1], Thanh Dellinger [3], Ernest Soyoung Han [3], Daphne Stewart [1], Sharon Wilczynski [2], Mihaela Cristea [1] and Lorna Rodriguez-Rodriguez [3]

1. Department of Medical Oncology and Therapeutics Research, City of Hope National Medical Center, Duarte, CA 91010, USA; sarliu@coh.org (S.L.); ssaadat@coh.org (S.S.); jashen@coh.org (J.S.); dapstewart@coh.org (D.S.); MCristea@coh.org (M.C.)
2. Department of Pathology, City of Hope National Medical Center, Duarte, CA 91010, USA; cwei@coh.org (C.H.W.); swilczyn@coh.org (S.W.)
3. Department of Surgical Oncology, City of Hope National Medical Center, Duarte, CA 91010, USA; stelee@coh.org (S.J.-J.L.); tdellinger@coh.org (T.D.); ehan@coh.org (E.S.H.); lorrodriguez@coh.org (L.R.-R.)
4. Department of Population Sciences, City of Hope National Medical Center, Duarte, CA 91010, USA; sshehayeb@coh.org
5. Department of Radiation Oncology, City of Hope National Medical Center, Duarte, CA 91010, USA; sglaser@coh.org (S.G.); rli@coh.org (R.L.)
* Correspondence: edwang@coh.org; Fax: +1-626-301-8233

Received: 21 July 2020; Accepted: 28 August 2020; Published: 1 September 2020

Abstract: Epithelial ovarian cancer (EOC) is the most common histology of ovarian cancer defined as epithelial cancer derived from the ovaries, fallopian tubes, or primary peritoneum. It is the fifth most common cause of cancer-related death in women in the United States. Because of a lack of effective screening and non-specific symptoms, EOC is typically diagnosed at an advanced stage (FIGO stage III or IV) and approximately one third of patients have malignant ascites at initial presentation. The treatment of ovarian cancer consists of a combination of cytoreductive surgery and systemic chemotherapy. Despite the advances with new cytotoxic and targeted therapies, the five-year survival rate for all-stage EOC in the United States is 48.6%. Delivery of up-to-date guideline care and multidisciplinary team efforts are important drivers of overall survival. In this paper, we review our frontline management of EOC that relies on a multi-disciplinary approach drawing on clinical expertise and collaboration combined with community practice and cutting edge clinical and translational research. By optimizing partnerships through team medicine and clinical research, we combine our cancer center clinical expertise, community practice partnership, and clinical and translational research to understand the biology of this deadly disease, advance therapy and connect our patients with the optimal treatment that offers the best possible outcomes.

Keywords: epithelial ovarian cancer; frontline treatment; surgical debulking; adjuvant chemotherapy; maintenance therapy; PARP inhibitor; genetics counseling; clinical research; team medicine

1. Introduction

Epithelial ovarian cancer (EOC) is the most common histology of ovarian cancer, defined as epithelial cancer derived from the ovaries, fallopian tubes, or primary peritoneum [1]. It is the fifth most common cause of cancer-related death in women in the United States, with an estimated 21,750 new cases and 13,940 deaths in 2020 [2]. Because of a lack of effective screening [3] and non-specific symptoms, EOC is typically diagnosed at an advanced stage (FIGO stage III or IV) and approximately one third of patients have malignant ascites at initial presentation. The treatment of ovarian cancer is primarily limited to cytoreductive surgery and systemic chemotherapy. Despite the advances with new cytotoxic and targeted therapies, the five-year survival rate for all-stage EOC in the United States is 48.6% [4]. The delivery of up-to-date guideline care and multidisciplinary team efforts are important drivers of overall survival [5].

The City of Hope National Medical Center (COH) is an NCI-designated Comprehensive Cancer Center based in Duarte, California. Its service area includes Los Angeles, San Bernadino, Riverside, and Orange Counties. Together, these four counties are home to 46% of California's total population. COH delivers high quality cancer care to this sizable demographic through its large network of community oncology practice clinics in the area. In this paper, we review the frontline management of EOC and how we combine our cancer center clinical expertise, community practice partnership, and clinical and translational research to understand the biology of this deadly disease and advance therapy.

2. Surgical Management

Cytoreductive surgery (debulking) plays a fundamental role in managing EOC. Studies show that survival is inversely correlated with the volume of residual disease after cytoreductive surgery [6–13]. Thus, the goal of surgery is to remove all visible disease [6,9,12,14–18]. In a 2011 meta-analysis of 11 retrospective studies of primary cytoreduction for advanced EOC, there was improved survival with optimal (residual disease ≤ 1 cm in maximum tumor diameter) versus suboptimal (residual disease > 1 cm in maximum tumor diameter) cytoreduction (hazard ratio (HR) 1.36, 95% CI 1.10–1.68), and further improved survival with no gross residual disease (HR 2.20, 95% CI 1.90–2.54) [19]. In a 2013 meta-analysis of 18 studies (retrospective and prospective) of women with stage IIB or higher EOC who underwent cytoreduction and platinum/taxane chemotherapy, each 10% increase in the proportion of patients undergoing complete cytoreduction was associated with a 2.3 month increase in median survival compared with a 1.8 month increase for optimal cytoreduction [14].

Furthermore, improved outcomes in advanced EOC have been shown in high volume hospitals (≥20 cases/year) and high-volume surgeons (≥10 cases/year) [20]. Given the importance of the extent of cytoreduction and volume of cases on outcome and the potential morbidity with an extensive major abdominal surgery, predicting which patients will be able to have at least an optimal cytoreduction is valuable. This is primarily performed through physical examination and computed tomography (CT) of the chest, abdomen, and pelvis. Diagnostic laparoscopy can also be utilized to help triage patients with primary debulking or neoadjuvant chemotherapy [21–23]. It is of utmost importance that a gynecologic oncologist experienced in extensive cytoreductive surgeries evaluates the patient to determine resectability, as achieving no gross residual disease or optimal cytoreduction largely depends on the judgment, experience, skill, and aggressiveness of the surgeon. Additionally, patient factors, such as age, performance status, medical comorbidities, and preoperative nutritional status, are important considerations, as some patients may not be able to tolerate an extensive cytoreduction. The commonly accepted criteria for unresectability include mesenteric root involvement, diffuse involvement of the stomach and/or large parts of the small or large bowel, extra-abdominal disease, infiltration of the duodenum and/or parts of the pancreas (not limited to the pancreatic tail), or involvement of the large vessels of the hepatoduodenal ligament, celiac trunk, or behind the porta hepatis [24].

Our strong partnership with community practices provides a large number of patients in Los Angeles and the Greater Los Angeles area with access to a high volume, high complexity cancer center. In addition to hysterectomy, bilateral salpingo-oophorectomy, and omentectomy, additional procedures can include small bowel resection, large bowel resection, stoma formation, diaphragm peritonectomy plus/minus segmental full-thickness diaphragm resection, splenectomy plus/minus distal pancreatectomy, segmental liver resection, cholecystectomy, partial stomach resection, and partial bladder/ureteral resection. We advocate against routine lymphadenectomy (pelvic, para-aortic) in patients undergoing cytoreduction for stage III or IV disease as it has not been shown to improve overall survival and results in increased postoperative morbidity [25]. However, we do resect suspicious or enlarged lymph nodes to achieve a complete or optimal cytoreduction. An intraperitoneal (IP) catheter for IP delivery of adjuvant chemotherapy may be placed in select patients who have obtained optimal primary cytoreduction, as combination treatment with intravenous (IV) and IP chemotherapy has been shown to prolong overall survival [26–28]; although newer trials have advocated for IV delivery of chemotherapeutics that may have similar outcomes but less morbidity than IP chemotherapy [29].

Patients referred to COH from our community clinics for the surgical management of EOC are assessed by our gynecologic surgical oncologist team and we perform primary cytoreduction for EOC in selected patients (those medically fit to undergo an extensive surgery and in whom it is deemed a resection to no gross residual disease or at least in whom an optimal debulking can be achieved) followed by adjuvant chemotherapy. Other patients deemed unresectable may undergo neoadjuvant chemotherapy and then re-evaluation for possible interval cytoreduction. We perform heated intraperitoneal chemotherapy (HIPEC) in a clinical trial setting for translational purpose toward personalized medicine. We collect biospecimens including peritoneal samples with and without tumor cells, blood samples before and after HIPEC. Paired tumor/normal whole exome sequencing (WES) and whole transcriptome sequencing (RNAseq) is performed for analyses of germline and somatic genomic landscapes, as well as gene expression phenotypes before and after treatment, including the assessment of driver mutations, mutation signatures, tumor mutation burden, and immune signatures. Hyperthermia increases the penetration of chemotherapy and increases the chemosensitivity of the cancer by impairing DNA repair. Additionally, hyperthermia induces apoptosis and activates heat-shock proteins that serve as receptors for natural killer cells, inhibits angiogenesis, and has a direct cytotoxic effect by promoting the denaturation of proteins. In a 2018 randomized trial, van Driel et al. reported a nearly 12-month survival benefit in those receiving HIPEC versus no HIPEC after undergoing at least an optimal interval cytoreduction with a similar rate of grade 3 or 4 adverse events between the two groups [30]. It is unclear if the IP administration, the heat, or the additional dose of chemotherapy is responsible for the benefit as all three interventions were utilized. These results are encouraging; however, further studies are needed before there is widespread adoption of this technique, which requires additional technical expertise [31,32].

Pressurized intraperitoneal aerosol chemotherapy (PIPAC) is another approach we are evaluating in the clinical trial setting. PIPAC is a novel minimally-invasive drug delivery system in which normothermic chemotherapy is administered into the abdominal cavity as an aerosol under pressure [33,34]. This approach uses the advantage of the physical properties of gas and pressure by generating an artificial pressure gradient and enhancing tissue uptake of the aerosolized chemotherapy. Due to high local bioavailability during PIPAC, lower concentrations of chemotherapy can be utilized, thus minimizing side effects and toxicity.

3. Gynecologic Pathology: Diagnostic Evaluation

Accurate pathologic diagnosis is the cornerstone of our treatment approach. When patients come to COH with a diagnosis of EOC made in the community, their surgical pathology is reviewed by our gynecologic pathology team. There are four major histologic types of ovarian epithelial tumors—serous, mucinous, endometrioid, and clear cell. High grade serous carcinoma (HGSC) is the most common, and lethal histologic subtypes of all ovarian epithelial malignancies are diagnosed, often presenting at an advanced stage. A subset of these patients carry germline mutations in double-strand DNA repair genes, such as BRCA1, BRCA2, RAD51c, and PALB2. Therefore, diagnosis of HGSC carries specific prognostic, therapeutic, and genetic implications. The ovarian cancer TCGA study showed that HGSC is characterized by a near universal p53 mutation [35]. Most of the p53 mutations lead to the overexpression or deletion of the protein, and these can be detected using immunohistochemistry.

In morphologically ambiguous cases, performing a p53 mutation analysis may be helpful, and p53 mutation status can be used to temporally track patients' tumors over time. Knowledge about the clinical and functional consequences of various p53 mutations is emerging. We perform whole-exome and RNA sequencing using the next generation sequencing platform for HGSC tumors. This allows us to define the p53 mutation profile in tumors and helps us to better understand clinical and treatment significance.

HGSC also displays genomic instability with high copy-number variations across the genome [36]. This unstable genomic landscape is a collective reflection of high tumor replication rate and the tumor cells' underlying defective DNA repair mechanisms, specifically homologous recombination repair (HRR) [37]. In HGSC, which displays homologous recombination deficiency (HRD), tumors rely on alternative but error-prone pathways, including non-homologous end-joining and single-strand annealing repair pathways [38]. Women with germline BRCA1/2 mutations are enriched for the HRD phenotype [39]. The underlying HRD phenotype explains why some HGSC patients are sensitive to platinum-based chemotherapy (carboplatin, paclitaxel, or docetaxel) or poly-(ADP-ribose)-polymerase 1 (PARP1) inhibitors (such as olaparib and niraparib). Platinum-based chemotherapy induces synthetic lethality by covalent binding with DNA, forming DNA-platinum adducts that eventually trigger double strand break. PARP1 inhibitors impede the PARP1-mediated repair of DNA single strand breaks, a component of the HRR pathway. In HGSC with underlying HRD, double strand breaks cannot be repaired efficiently and their accumulation in the genome result in cell death [38].

HGSC is diagnosed using the MD Anderson histologic 2-tier system [40,41]. Corroborating with the molecular event of p53 mutation, the diagnosis of HGSC can be further supported by performing immunohistochemical staining for p53. HGSC is staged using the current American Joint Committee on Cancer/College of American Pathologists Cancer Staging Form and the FIGO Staging System. The molecular diagnosis of ovarian cancer subtypes that correlate with prognosis may also be adopted as standard procedure in the future. Verhaak et al. analyzed the TCGA database and revealed four ovarian tumor subtypes, each associated with a different prognosis [42].

4. Molecular Studies Available for Diagnostic or Therapeutic Decision Support and Emerging Translational Research

We perform extensive molecular testing, including whole exome sequencing, transcriptomic sequencing, copy number information, mismatch repair (MMR) deficiency, microsatellite instability (MSI) status, tumor mutation burden (TMB), HRD, and PD-L1 protein expression levels, using paired formalin-fixed paraffin-embedded tumor tissue and patient saliva or peripheral blood. This comprehensive approach allows us to detect somatic and germline mutations, clinically actionable mutations, potential therapeutic targets, and markers to help guide checkpoint inhibitor therapy. The genomic analysis makes tailored therapy possible and informs clinical trial options that best match with patient tumor genotype.

Germline and somatic BRCA1 and BRCA2 mutations are assessed in specific clinical contexts to inform genetic counseling and therapy selection. Younger age at presentation and family history of tubo-ovarian and breast cancer malignancies are risk factors suggestive of the presence of germline cancer predisposition syndrome. Referral to a genetic counselor and establishing germline mutation information is crucial for informing patients about BRCA-related cancer risks for themselves and their family members. Most importantly, this allows patients the opportunity to access BRCA-related cancer risk reduction surgeries (e.g., risk-reducing salpingo-ophorectomy, mastectomy), where the timing of surgery can be crucial to successful risk reduction.

Germline and somatic BRCA1/2 mutation information is also important for informing PARP inhibitor eligibility in Stage II, III, and IV HGSC patients post primary treatment. The NCCN guidelines recommend screening for BRCA mutations early in the treatment course to avoid the possibility of delay in instituting PARP inhibitor therapy [43].

HRD positivity is determined by BRCA mutation status (deleterious or suspected deleterious) or HRD/genomic instability score (mathematically derived from genomic assessment of loss of heterozygosity, telomeric allelic imbalance, and large-scale state transitions). Due to the inherent biocomputational complexity with HRD score derivation and inter-laboratory analytic variability, most large medical centers perform HRD testing on a research basis and not for routine clinical diagnostic use.

Circulating miRNAs in blood and urine are being explored as potential early detection markers. However, the evidence on this approach is currently limited, and no consistent miRNA signatures have emerged [44–46]. The lack of reproducibility may be attributable, in part, to technical issues, such as different statistical modeling and approaches, the utilization of different miRNA detection platforms, and patient and tumor heterogeneity [46]. Besides early detection, liquid biopsy-based circulating tumor cells have been leveraged in a recent small pilot preclinical study to provide chemosensitivity information and therapy response prediction in patients presenting with recurrent ovarian cancer [47]. The quest for providing precision oncology to patients using minimally invasive liquid biopsies is expanding, and hopefully it will become a reality in the not so distant future.

With numerous genomic alterations present in HGSC, an integrative analytical approach is necessary to characterize the dominant biologic drivers of carcinogenesis, cancer progression, and prognosis. The TCGA (Cancer Genome Atlas Research Network) and CPTAC (Clinical Proteomic Tumor Analysis Consortium) investigators have paved the way for combining multiple omics in ovarian HGSC—including genomics, proteomics, and phosphoproteomics. Using transcriptomic data, TCGA has built a HGSC molecular taxonomy comprised of four subtypes: differentiated, mesenchymal, immunoreactive, and proliferative [35]. This framework was recapitulated using the proteomic data [36]. However, this molecular taxonomy does not correlate with patient survival [36]. Instead, proteomic signatures (cytoskeleton involved in invasion and migration, apoptosis, and epithelial junction/adhesion) showed more robust correlation with survival [36]. However, this proteomic signature is currently research-based only, awaiting further validation in larger independent cohorts, and is not currently used in clinical setting.

5. Adjuvant Chemotherapy

With the exception of patients with early-stage disease and low-grade cancers with a high cure rate, such as stage 1A and 1B grade 1 endometrioid ovarian cancer, mucinous carcinoma, and low grade serous carcinoma [48–50], patients with EOC who have undergone surgical debulking usually require adjuvant platinum- and taxane-based chemotherapy to reduce the risk of recurrence or prolong disease-free survival. Optimal time from surgery to initiate adjuvant chemotherapy has been shown to be 4–6 weeks [49,51]. Table 1 summarizes the main clinical studies of frontline treatment and maintenance of EOC. The standard adjuvant chemotherapy regimen includes: IV paclitaxel 175 mg/m^2 and carboplatin AUC 5–6 every 3 weeks. Alternatively, dose dense weekly paclitaxel 80 mg/m^2 and carboplatin AUC 5–6 every 3 weeks may be applied [52–55]—although this regimen has shown differing outcomes in different studies—the JGOG3016 study [52,56] showed a favorable outcome over every 3-week standard regimen, while the ICON-8 [55], and GOG-262 studies [53] failed to showed a significant improvement. The MITO-7 study used weekly paclitaxel 60 mg/m^2 and carboplatin AUC 2 for up to 18 weeks—this regimen has a high tolerance and is effective for elderly patients or those with poor performance status [54]. Single agent carboplatin is also acceptable if patients cannot tolerate the combination treatment. Docetaxel is an acceptable taxane alternative to paclitaxel with equivalent efficacy [57]. Carboplatin plus liposomal doxorubicin is also an acceptable combination for adjuvant chemotherapy when patients cannot tolerate taxanes [58,59]. Recently, bevacizumab was incorporated into the adjuvant chemotherapeutic regimen, showing improved progression-free survival and also overall survival in the high risk of progression subgroup, including those with stage IV disease and inoperable or sub-optimally debulked stage III disease (ICON-7, GOG-218) [60,61], especially in patients with ascites [60,62,63].

In patients with EOC, the peritoneal cavity is usually the primary site of recurrence. Thus, the administration of adjuvant IV/IP chemotherapy to treat residual cancer cells with highly concentrated chemotherapeutics is an attractive approach. The GOG-172 study showed that IV paclitaxel 135 mg/m^2 on day 1 plus IP cisplatin 75–100 mg/m^2 on day 2 and IP paclitaxel 60 mg/m^2 on day 8, every 3 weeks for up to six cycles, improved survival by 16 months in patients with optimally debulked stage III EOC compared with IV delivery of paclitaxel and cisplatin [27]; IP carboplatin is a suitable substitute for IP cisplatin in the GOG-252 study, as the median progression-free survival and overall survival were similar in the IP carboplatin and IP cisplatin arms [28]. However, the IV/IP chemotherapy regimen resulted in more side effects [64], including abdominal pain, catheter-related infection and blockage, and myelosuppression, all of which may delay treatment and compromise efficacy. We routinely use IV/IP adjuvant chemotherapy based on the favorable survival outcomes [27,65]. A recent publication showed that, when bevacizumab was added to IV/IV carboplatin and paclitaxel, IV/IP carboplatin and paclitaxel, or IV/IP cisplatin and paclitaxel, there was no significant difference in progression-free survival in all of these groups of patients [28]. Therefore, there is debate as to whether or not IP chemotherapy is still an acceptable option in primary adjuvant chemotherapy for patients with advanced EOC, given its higher toxicity, inconvenience, catheter complications, and uncertain long-term benefits [29]. At City of Hope, we have been treating patients with the IV/IP protocol. Due to recent advances in maintenance therapy, we are reconsidering if it is still necessary to perform the IP delivery of chemotherapeutics.

6. Maintenance Therapy

EOC patients who undergo surgical debulking and adjuvant chemotherapy still experience a high rate of disease recurrence. Thus, there is a need for effective maintenance therapy after adjuvant chemotherapy for patients with EOC to help prevent recurrence or prolong disease-free survival. In the past, patients who completed adjuvant chemotherapy usually underwent active surveillance with regular follow-up, labs, and imaging as needed. However, this practice was changed after the ICON-7 and GOG-218 studies showed clinical benefit by adding bevacizumab to the adjuvant chemotherapy regimen [59–62]. The ICON-7 study added bevacizumab (7.5 mg/kg) to IV paclitaxel and carboplatin on day 1, repeated every 3 weeks for 5–6 cycles, continuing bevacizumab for up to 12 additional cycles and showed a modest prolongation of progression-free survival by 2.4 months. Overall, survival was also increased in patients with a poor prognosis [61,66]. The GOG-218 study added bevacizumab to IV paclitaxel and carboplatin on day 1 of cycle 2 (15 mg/kg), every 3 weeks for up to 22 cycles. This regimen showed a significant benefit to progression-free survival (14.1 months vs. 10.3 months, $p < 0.001$). Patients with ascites who received bevacizumab in addition to paclitaxel and carboplatin had significantly improved progression-free survival and overall survival compared to those who received paclitaxel and carboplatin alone [63]. However, maintenance with PARP inhibitors may be favored over bevacizumab due to improved survival.

Following success in treating recurrent EOC, PARP inhibitors have also recently become an attractive choice for maintenance after adjuvant chemotherapy in newly diagnosed EOC patients. Olaparib was FDA-approved (2018) for the maintenance treatment of adult patients with deleterious or suspected deleterious germline or somatic BRCA-mutated advanced EOC who are experiencing a complete or partial response to first-line platinum-based chemotherapy. This is based on the SOLO-1 study [67], a randomized, double-blind, placebo-controlled, multi-center trial that compared the efficacy of olaparib with placebo in patients with BRCA-mutated advanced ovarian, fallopian tube, or primary peritoneal cancer following first-line platinum-based chemotherapy. After a median follow-up of 41 months, the risk of disease progression or death was 70% lower with olaparib than with placebo. In May 2020, the FDA expanded the indication of olaparib to include its combination with bevacizumab for first-line maintenance treatment of adult patients with advanced EOC who have complete or partial response to first-line platinum-based chemotherapy and whose cancers are HRD-positive, defined by either a deleterious or suspected deleterious BRCA mutation and/or genomic instability score. This recommendation was based on the study by Ray-Coquard et al. [68], which showed that, in patients with advanced EOC receiving first-line standard therapy bevacizumab, the addition of maintenance olaparib provided a significant progression-free survival benefit, which was substantial in patients with HRD-positive tumors (37.2 vs. 17.7 months). Patients with HRD-positivity but without a BRCA mutation also had significantly improved progression-free survival (28.1 vs. 16.6 months).

Niraparib, another PARP inhibitor, was granted approval by the FDA in April 2020 as a first-line maintenance treatment of adult patients with advanced EOC who experienced a complete or partial response to first-line platinum-based chemotherapy, regardless of biomarker status. This recommendation is based on the PRIMA study [69] (Table 1) which showed that patients with newly diagnosed advanced EOC who had a response to platinum-based chemotherapy and received niraparib had significantly longer progression-free survival than those who received placebo (13.8 vs. 8.2 months), regardless of the presence or absence of HRD. We use niraparib for patients without BRCA mutation or HRD, or patients with unknown BCRA/HRD status.

Additional maintenance options are being studied in clinical trials, including new PARP inhibitors, anti-angiogenesis agents, immune checkpoint inhibitors, agents targeting other signal transduction pathways, and new rational combinations. We expect to have improved maintenance options in the future to further reduce recurrence and prolong disease-free survival. Choosing the right maintenance therapy for each patient is highly complex and benefits from multi-disciplinary discussion. At COH, the community oncologists have access to the COH Gynecologic Cancer Tumor Board (discussed further below) to present their challenging cases for in-depth discussion.

Table 1. Major clinical trials on frontline treatment of epithelial ovarian cancer.

Study	Patients	Experimental	Control	Progression Free Survival	Overall Survival
JGOG 3016 [52,56]	Stage II-IV EOC	three-weekly carboplatin (AUC 6) and weekly paclitaxel (80 mg/m^2) for six cycles	three-weekly carboplatin (AUC 6) and paclitaxel (180 mg/m^2) for six cycles	28.0 vs. 17.2 months; HR 0.71, 95% CI 0.58-0.88; $p = 0.0015$	100.5 vs. 62.2 months (HR 0.79, 95% CI 0.63-0.99; $p = 0.039$
MITO-7 [54]	FIGO stage IC-IV EOC	Weekly carboplatin (AUC 2) and paclitaxel (60 mg/m^2) for 18 weeks	three-weekly carboplatin (AUC 6) and paclitaxel (175 mg/m^2) for six cycles	18.3 vs. 17.3 months; HR 0.96, 95% CI 0.80-1.16; $p = 0.66$	-
ICON-8 [55]	FIGO stage IC-IV EOC	Group 2: three-weekly carboplatin (AUC 5/6) and weekly paclitaxel (80 mg/m^2) for six cycles. Group 3: Weekly carboplatin (AUC 6) and paclitaxel (60 mg/m^2) for six cycles	Group 1: three-weekly carboplatin (AUC 5/6) and paclitaxel (175 mg/m^2) for six cycles	Group 1 vs. Group 2 vs. Group 3: 17.7 vs. 20.8 vs. 21.0 Group 2 vs. Group 1: $p = 0.35$ Group 3 vs. Group 1: $p = 0.51$	-
GOG-172 [57,58]	FIGO stage III with optimal debulking	paclitaxel 135 mg/m^2 continuous iv infusion over 24 h on day 1, cisplatin 100 mg/m^2 IP on day 2, paclitaxel 60 mg/m^2 IP on day 8 for six cycles	paclitaxel 135 mg/m^2 continuous IV infusion over 24 h on day 1, cisplatin 75 mg/m^2 IV on day 2 for six cycles	23.8 vs. 18.3 months; HR 0.80, 95% CI 0.64-1.00; $p = 0.05$	65.6 vs. 49.7 months; HR 0.75, 95% CI, 0.58-0.97; $p = 0.03$ 61.8 vs. 51.4 months; Adjusted HR 0.77; 95% CI, 0.65-0.90; $p = 0.002$
GOG-252 [58]	FIGO stage II-IV EOC	paclitaxel 80 mg/m^2 IV on days 1, 8, and 15 plus carboplatin AUC 6 IP on day 1 every 21 days for cycles 1–6 plus bevacizumab 15 mg/kg IV every 21 days for cycles 2–22 paclitaxel 135 mg/m^2 IV on day 1 plus cisplatin 75 mg/m^2 IP on day 2 plus paclitaxel 60 mg/m^2 IV on day 8 every 21 days for cycles 1–6 plus bevacizumab 15 mg/kg IV every 21 days for cycles 2–22	paclitaxel 80 mg/m^2 IV on days 1, 8, and 15 plus carboplatin AUC 6 IV on day 1 every 21 days for cycles 1–6 plus bevacizumab 15 mg/kg IV every 21 days for cycles 2–22	IV vs. IP-carboplatin vs. IP-cisplatin: 24.9 vs. 27.4 vs. 26.2 months IP-carboplatin: HR 0.93, 95% CI 0.80-1.07 IP-cisplatin: HR 0.98, 95% CI 0.84-1.13	IV vs. IP-carboplatin: IP-cisplatin: 75.5 vs. 78.9 vs. 72.9 months IP-carboplatin: HR 0.95, 95% CI 0.80-1.13 IP-cisplatin: HR 1.05, 95% CI; 0.88-1.24;
GOG-262 [59]	FIGO stage III-IV EOC	three-weekly carboplatin (AUC 6) and weekly paclitaxel (80 mg/m^2), plus/minus three-weekly bevacizumab 15 mg/kg for six cycles	three-weekly carboplatin (AUC 6) and paclitaxel (175 mg/m^2), plus/minus three-weekly bevacizumab 15 mg/kg for six cycles	With bevacizumab: 14.9 vs. 14.7 months; HR 0.99, 95% CI 0.83–1.20; $p = 0.60$ Without bevacizumab: 14.2 vs. 10.3 months; HR 0.62, 95% CI 0.40-0.95; $p = 0.03$	With and without bevacizumab: 40.2 vs. 39.0 months; HR 0.94; 95% CI, 0.72-1.2
SOLO-1 [67]	FIGO stage III or IV high-grade serous or endometrioid EOC patients with a deleterious or suspected deleterious germline or somatic BRCA1/2 mutation, completed frontline platinum-based chemotherapy	olaparib	placebo	Not reached vs. 13.8 months; HR 0.30, 95% CI 0.23–0.41); $p < 0.0001$ 3-year: 60% vs. 27% 4-year: 53% vs. 11%	-
PAOLA [68]	FIGO stage III or IV high-grade EOC patients after first-line treatment with platinum–taxane chemotherapy plus bevacizumab	olaparib plus bevacizumab	placebo plus bevacizumab	22.1 vs. 16.6 months; HR 0.59; 95% CI 0.49–0.72; $p < 0.001$ HRD plus BRCA mutation: 37.2 vs. 17.7 months; HR 0.33, 95% CI 0.25–0.45 HRD minus BRCA mutation: 28.1 vs. 16.6 months; HR 0.43, 95% CI 0.28–0.66	-
PRIMA [69]	FIGO stage III or IV high-grade serous or endometrioid EOC patients after first-line treatment with platinum-based chemotherapy	niraparib	placebo	Overall: 13.8 vs. 8.2 months; HR .62, 95% CI 0.50-0.76; $p < 0.001$ HRD-positive: 21.9 vs. 10.4 months; HR 0.43, 95% CI 0.31-0.59; $p < 0.001$	-

7. Genetic Counseling

HGSC is a single case indicator for germline genetic testing [70]. Germline genetic testing should be considered both due to the relatively high percentage of hereditary ovarian cancer with some studies estimating that more than 20% is hereditary in etiology [71–73], and due to the potential for treatment implications [74]. Generally, it is preferable for an individual to undergo germline testing as soon as diagnosis occurs [75,76]. This allows ample time to obtain and disclose results, especially in the setting of a patient who may have a guarded prognosis. Urgent testing of BRCA1/2 and other breast cancer genes with high or moderate penetrance by multi-gene panel can currently be performed. While this strategy is often used for women with breast cancer undergoing surgical decision-making, it can also be employed in the gynecologic oncology setting to provide results that may affect eligibility for PARP inhibitors or other therapies in a timely manner.

Germline testing in an affected individual is the most informative strategy and can help clarify risk for relatives. Close female relatives may have increased empiric risk to develop EOC, although older studies may include some families with risk alleles that would be identified by current technology [77,78]. The ascertainment of a multi-generational pedigree allows both for appropriate test selection as well as for proper assessment of family structure and identification of at-risk relatives [79]. Pedigree assessment in the setting of genetic counseling can also facilitate understanding of social relationships between relatives to help develop appropriate strategies to encourage familial communication about risk.

Germline testing for women with EOC at our center typically includes evaluation via a multi-gene panel to include EOC risk genes beyond BRCA1/2, such as the mismatch repair (Lynch syndrome) genes, BRIP1, RAD51C, and RAD51D [71,80]. Beyond informing therapeutic strategy, germline testing in the setting of appropriate counseling can have significant implications for patients and family members. Germline testing can help stratify the risk of developing other cancers and guide the development of appropriate management strategies, especially as the prognosis for EOC improves with better treatment options. For example, patients with Lynch syndrome are at significantly elevated risk to develop colorectal cancer [81] and patients with pathogenic alterations in the BRCA genes are at significantly elevated risk to develop breast cancer [82]. Understanding a patient's risk may help prevent a second primary cancer, especially in the setting of well-controlled ovarian disease or in the setting where the development of a new cancer may interfere with the patient's current treatment.

Germline testing may be even more impactful in terms of implications for relatives. Identifying an ovarian cancer risk allele can allow relatives with the same allele to undergo preventative measures, such as risk-reducing salpingo-oopherectomy, which is especially relevant when screening is not effective. Moreover, in some cases, over-treatment may be avoided in relatives who do not carry the risk allele but who may have otherwise chosen to move forward with preventative measures or screening due to concerns over risk, based on family history. Many genes implicated in EOC in the setting of a monoallelic pathogenic variant also have implications for typically childhood-onset syndromes in the setting of biallelic pathogenic variants. For example, biallelic variants in BRCA1/2, BRIP1, and RAD51C [83–86] are associated with Fanconi anemia and biallelic variants in the mismatch repair genes are associated with Constitutional Mismatch Repair Deficiency syndrome [81]. Thus, individuals contemplating childbearing may also wish to learn their germline status to inform reproductive decisions.

Importantly, negative somatic testing does not obviate the need for germline testing. Reasons for this can include the loss of a germline mutation in the tumor, limited analysis of the tumor genome, and differences in variant calling between somatic and germline laboratories. Conversely, somatic testing may identify variants that are germline in origin [87,88]. Therefore, patients should be counseled about this possibility, and if somatic results are available, they should be reviewed to help inform germline test selection. Other genes may also be included based on clinical suspicion and the evaluation of additional personal and family history. Reevaluation should be considered over time as changes to the family history, as well as advances in the field of cancer genetics, occur [79].

8. Team Medicine: Optimizing Partnerships and Clinical Research

We have a number of initiatives to ensure the inclusion of our community partners in research, education, and the integration of research-based advances into novel therapeutics by clinical trials. We aim to personalize therapy for patients so our community physicians can recommend improved therapy considerations, including clinical trials beyond the standard of care. One way we achieve this is via comprehensive molecular testing. All EOC patients at COH undergo GEM ExTra® testing (facilitated by TGen, a COH affiliate). This test reports clinically actionable mutations, copy number alterations, transcript variants, and fusions, detected in any gene in patient DNA or RNA. The goal is to uncover true tumor-specific (somatic) alterations by comparing the sequence of the tumor against the paired normal DNA from each patient. The test also includes whole-transcriptome RNA profiling, interrogating the patient's tumor transcriptome for fusions and transcriptional variants known to be relevant to cancer (e.g., EGFR vIII). Each tumor's cancer-specific alterations are then queried against a proprietary knowledge base algorithm to identify potential therapeutic associations. The final report provides the physician with a list of FDA-approved agents that are associated with tumor-specific DNA alterations, as well as biomarker summaries on the variants found and tumor-specific evidence for drug matches, including matches with investigational agents, as available on clinicaltrials.gov. The results are reviewed by our multidisciplinary gynecologic cancer research team to aid in treatment decision-making, highlight on-going studies and identify study candidates.

Our current clinical research portfolio in the frontline management of EOC focuses on developing superior treatment options for patients that reduce recurrence and prolong disease-free survival. We are exploring the use of HIPEC and PIPAC in the clinical trial setting as well as novel drug combinations that help to tailor and personalize treatment for superior results. Our HIPEC trial includes studying the molecular changes triggered by HIPEC to identify molecular signatures of response. Our PIPAC trial is the first in the United States to study aerosolized, pressurized chemotherapy for patients with peritoneal carcinomatosis, including ovarian cancer. Our community oncologists play an important role in these studies by referring patients, thereby allowing us to complete accrual expeditiously.

9. Summary

Management of EOC requires a multi-disciplinary approach, drawing on clinical expertise and collaboration combined with community practice and cutting edge clinical and translational research. Our goal is to understand the biology of this disease, advance therapy and connect our patients with the optimal treatment that offers the best possible outcomes.

Author Contributions: Conceptualization, E.W.W., C.H.W., S.L., S.J.-J.L., S.S. (Susan Shehayeb), S.G., R.L., S.S. (Siamak Saadat), J.S.; validation, E.W.W., M.C. and L.R.-R.; writing—original draft preparation, E.W.W., C.H.W., S.L., S.J.-J.L., S.S. (Susan Shehayeb), S.G., R.L., S.S. (Siamak Saadat), J.S.; writing—review and editing, E.W.W., C.H.W., S.L., S.J.-J.L., S.S. (Susan Shehayeb), T.D., E.S.H., D.S., S.W., M.C. and L.R.-R.; supervision, E.W.W. and L.R.-R.; project administration, E.W.W.; funding acquisition, E.W.W. All authors have read and agreed to the published version of the manuscript.

Funding: This research received no external funding.

Acknowledgments: The authors thank Nicola Welch, CMPP for assistance with writing and editing the manuscript. This work was supported by the National Cancer Institute of the National Institutes of Health under award number K12CA001727. The content is solely the responsibility of the authors and does not necessarily represent the official views of the National Institutes of Health.

Conflicts of Interest: The authors declare no conflict of interest.

References

1. Board PDQATE. *Ovarian Epithelial, Fallopian Tube, and Primary Peritoneal Cancer Treatment (PDQ(R)): Health Professional Version*; PDQ Cancer Information Summaries; National Cancer Institute: Bethesda, MD, USA, 2002.
2. Siegel, R.L.; Miller, K.D.; Jemal, A. Cancer statistics, 2020. *CA A Cancer J. Clin.* **2020**, *70*, 145–164. [CrossRef]

3. Nebgen, D.R.; Lu, K.H.; Bast, R.C., Jr. Novel Approaches to Ovarian Cancer Screening. *Curr. Oncol. Rep.* **2019**, *21*, 75. [CrossRef]
4. Howlader, N.N.A.; Krapcho, M.; Miller, D.; Brest, A.; Yu, M.; Ruhl, J.; Tatalovich, Z.; Mariotto, A.; Lewis, D.R.; Chen, H.S.; et al. *SEER Cancer Statistics Review, 1975–2017*; National Cancer Institute: Bethesda, MD, USA; Available online: https://seer.cancer.gov/csr/1975_2017/ (accessed on 25 August 2020).
5. Cliby, W.A.; Powell, M.A.; Al-Hammadi, N.; Chen, L.; Miller, J.P.; Roland, P.Y.; Mutch, D.G.; Bristow, R.E. Ovarian cancer in the United States: Contemporary patterns of care associated with improved survival. *Gynecol. Oncol.* **2015**, *136*, 11–17. [CrossRef] [PubMed]
6. Hoskins, W.J.; McGuire, W.P.; Brady, M.; Homesley, H.D.; Creasman, W.T.; Berman, M.; Ball, H.; Berek, J.S. The effect of diameter of largest residual disease on survival after primary cytoreductive surgery in patients with suboptimal residual epithelial ovarian carcinoma. *Am. J. Obs. Gynecol.* **1994**, *170*, 974–979. [CrossRef]
7. Eisenkop, S.M.; Friedman, R.L.; Wang, H.J. Complete cytoreductive surgery is feasible and maximizes survival in patients with advanced epithelial ovarian cancer: A prospective study. *Gynecol. Oncol.* **1998**, *69*, 103–108. [CrossRef] [PubMed]
8. Allen, D.G.; Heintz, A.P.; Touw, F.W. A meta-analysis of residual disease and survival in stage III and IV carcinoma of the ovary. *Eur. J. Gynaecol. Oncol.* **1995**, *16*, 349–356. [PubMed]
9. Chi, D.S.; Eisenhauer, E.L.; Lang, J.; Huh, J.; Haddad, L.; Abu-Rustum, N.R.; Sonoda, Y.; Levine, D.; Hensley, M.; Barakat, R. What is the optimal goal of primary cytoreductive surgery for bulky stage IIIC epithelial ovarian carcinoma (EOC)? *Gynecol. Oncol.* **2006**, *103*, 559–564. [CrossRef]
10. Winter, W.E., 3rd; Maxwell, G.L.; Tian, C.; Carlson, J.W.; Ozols, R.F.; Rose, P.G.; Markman, M.; Armstrong, D.K.; Muggia, F.; McGuire, W.P. Prognostic factors for stage III epithelial ovarian cancer: A Gynecologic Oncology Group Study. *J. Clin. Oncol. Off. J. Am. Soc. Clin. Oncol.* **2007**, *25*, 3621–3627. [CrossRef]
11. Wimberger, P.; Lehmann, N.; Kimmig, R.; Burges, A.; Meier, W.; Du Bois, A. Prognostic factors for complete debulking in advanced ovarian cancer and its impact on survival. An exploratory analysis of a prospectively randomized phase III study of the Arbeitsgemeinschaft Gynaekologische Onkologie Ovarian Cancer Study Group (AGO-OVAR). *Gynecol. Oncol.* **2007**, *106*, 69–74.
12. Bristow, R.E.; Tomacruz, R.S.; Armstrong, D.K.; Trimble, E.L.; Montz, F.J. Survival effect of maximal cytoreductive surgery for advanced ovarian carcinoma during the platinum era: A meta-analysis. *J. Clin. Oncol. Off. J. Am. Soc. Clin. Oncol.* **2002**, *20*, 1248–1259. [CrossRef]
13. Teramukai, S.; Ochiai, K.; Tada, H.; Fukushima, M. Japan Multinational Trial Organization OC. PIEPOC: A new prognostic index for advanced epithelial ovarian cancer–Japan Multinational Trial Organization OC01-01. *J. Clin. Oncol. Off. J. Am. Soc. Clin. Oncol.* **2007**, *25*, 3302–3306. [CrossRef] [PubMed]
14. Chang, S.J.; Hodeib, M.; Chang, J.; Bristow, R.E. Survival impact of complete cytoreduction to no gross residual disease for advanced-stage ovarian cancer: A meta-analysis. *Gynecol. Oncol.* **2013**, *130*, 493–498. [CrossRef] [PubMed]
15. Eisenkop, S.M.; Spirtos, N.M.; Lin, W.C. "Optimal" cytoreduction for advanced epithelial ovarian cancer: A commentary. *Gynecol. Oncol.* **2006**, *103*, 329–335. [CrossRef] [PubMed]
16. Winter, W.E., 3rd; Maxwell, G.L.; Tian, C.; Sundborg, M.J.; Rose, G.S.; Rose, P.G.; Rubin, S.C.; Muggia, F.; McGuire, W.P. Tumor residual after surgical cytoreduction in prediction of clinical outcome in stage IV epithelial ovarian cancer: A Gynecologic Oncology Group Study. *J. Clin. Oncol. Off. J. Am. Soc. Clin. Oncol.* **2008**, *26*, 83–89. [CrossRef] [PubMed]
17. Eisenhauer, E.L.; Abu-Rustum, N.R.; Sonoda, Y.; Aghajanian, C.; Barakat, R.R.; Chi, D.S. The effect of maximal surgical cytoreduction on sensitivity to platinum-taxane chemotherapy and subsequent survival in patients with advanced ovarian cancer. *Gynecol. Oncol.* **2008**, *108*, 276–281. [CrossRef] [PubMed]
18. Hoskins, W.J. Epithelial ovarian carcinoma: Principles of primary surgery. *Gynecologic Oncol.* **1994**, *55* (3 Pt 2), S91–S96. [CrossRef]
19. Elattar, A.; Bryant, A.; Winter-Roach, B.A.; Hatem, M.; Naik, R. Optimal primary surgical treatment for advanced epithelial ovarian cancer. *Cochrane Database Syst. Rev.* **2011**, *2011*, Cd007565. [CrossRef]
20. Wright, J.D.; Chen, L.; Hou, J.Y.; Burke, W.M.; Tergas, A.I.; Ananth, C.V.; Neugut, A.I.; Hershman, D.L. Association of Hospital Volume and Quality of Care With Survival for Ovarian Cancer. *Obstet. Gynecol.* **2017**, *130*, 545–553. [CrossRef]

21. Rutten, M.J.; Gaarenstroom, K.N.; Van Gorp, T.; van Meurs, H.S.; Arts, H.J.; Bossuyt, P.M.; Ter Brugge, H.G.; Hermans, R.H.; Opmeer, B.C.; Pijnenborg, J.M.; et al. Laparoscopy to predict the result of primary cytoreductive surgery in advanced ovarian cancer patients (LapOvCa-trial): A multicentre randomized controlled study. *BMC Cancer* **2012**, *12*, 31. [CrossRef]
22. Rutten, M.J.; van Meurs, H.S.; van de Vrie, R.; Gaarenstroom, K.N.; Naaktgeboren, C.A.; van Gorp, T.; Ter Brugge, H.G.; Hofhuis, W.; Schreuder, H.W.; Arts, H.J.; et al. Laparoscopy to Predict the Result of Primary Cytoreductive Surgery in Patients With Advanced Ovarian Cancer: A Randomized Controlled Trial. *J. Clin. Oncol. Off. J. Am. Soc. Clin. Oncol.* **2017**, *35*, 613–621. [CrossRef]
23. Fagotti, A.; Ferrandina, G.; Fanfani, F.; Ercoli, A.; Lorusso, D.; Rossi, M.; Scambia, G. A laparoscopy-based score to predict surgical outcome in patients with advanced ovarian carcinoma: A pilot study. *Ann. Surg. Oncol.* **2006**, *13*, 1156–1161. [CrossRef] [PubMed]
24. Wright, A.A.; Bohlke, K.; Armstrong, D.K.; Bookman, M.A.; Cliby, W.A.; Coleman, R.L.; Dizon, D.S.; Kash, J.J.; Meyer, L.A.; Moore, K.N.; et al. Neoadjuvant Chemotherapy for Newly Diagnosed, Advanced Ovarian Cancer: Society of Gynecologic Oncology and American Society of Clinical Oncology Clinical Practice Guideline. *J. Clin. Oncol. Off. J. Am. Soc. Clin. Oncol.* **2016**, *34*, 3460–3473. [CrossRef] [PubMed]
25. Harter, P.; Sehouli, J.; Lorusso, D.; Reuss, A.; Vergote, I.; Marth, C.; Kim, J.-W.; Raspagliesi, F.; Lampe, B.; Aletti, G.; et al. A Randomized Trial of Lymphadenectomy in Patients with Advanced Ovarian Neoplasms. *N. Engl. J. Med.* **2019**, *380*, 822–832. [CrossRef] [PubMed]
26. Walker, J.L.; Armstrong, D.K.; Huang, H.Q.; Fowler, J.; Webster, K.; Burger, R.A.; Clarke-Pearson, D. Intraperitoneal catheter outcomes in a phase III trial of intravenous versus intraperitoneal chemotherapy in optimal stage III ovarian and primary peritoneal cancer: A Gynecologic Oncology Group Study. *Gynecol. Oncol.* **2006**, *100*, 27–32. [CrossRef] [PubMed]
27. Armstrong, D.K.; Bundy, B.; Wenzel, L.; Huang, H.Q.; Baergen, R.; Lele, S.; Copeland, L.J.; Walker, J.; Burger, R.A. Intraperitoneal cisplatin and paclitaxel in ovarian cancer. *N. Engl. J. Med.* **2006**, *354*, 34–43. [CrossRef] [PubMed]
28. Walker, J.L.; Brady, M.F.; Wenzel, L.; Fleming, G.F.; Huang, H.Q.; DiSilvestro, P.A.; Fujiwara, K.; Alberts, D.S.; Zheng, W.; Tewari, K.S.; et al. Randomized Trial of Intravenous Versus Intraperitoneal Chemotherapy Plus Bevacizumab in Advanced Ovarian Carcinoma: An NRG Oncology/Gynecologic Oncology Group Study. *J. Clin. Oncol. Off. J. Am. Soc. Clin. Oncol.* **2019**, *37*, 1380–1390. [CrossRef] [PubMed]
29. Monk, B.J.; Chan, J.K. Is intraperitoneal chemotherapy still an acceptable option in primary adjuvant chemotherapy for advanced ovarian cancer? *Ann. Oncol. Off. J. Eur. Soc. Med. Oncol.* **2017**, *28* (Suppl. 8), viii40–viii45. [CrossRef]
30. van Driel, W.J.; Koole, S.N.; Sikorska, K.; Schagen van Leeuwen, J.H.; Schreuder, H.W.R.; Hermans, R.H.M.; De Hingh, I.H.; Van Der Velden, J.; Arts, H.J.; Massuger, L.F.; et al. Hyperthermic Intraperitoneal Chemotherapy in Ovarian Cancer. *N. Engl. J. Med.* **2018**, *378*, 230–240. [CrossRef]
31. Bouchard-Fortier, G.; Cusimano, M.C.; Fazelzad, R.; Sajewycz, K.; Lu, L.; Espin-Garcia, O.; May, T.; Bouchard-Fortier, A.; Ferguson, S.E. Oncologic outcomes and morbidity following heated intraperitoneal chemotherapy at cytoreductive surgery for primary epithelial ovarian cancer: A systematic review and meta-analysis. *Gynecol. Oncol.* **2020**, *158*, 218–228. [CrossRef]
32. Pletcher, E.; Gleeson, E.; Labow, D. Peritoneal Cancers and Hyperthermic Intraperitoneal Chemotherapy. *Surg. Clin. N. Am.* **2020**, *100*, 589–613. [CrossRef]
33. Nadiradze, G.; Horvath, P.; Sautkin, Y.; Archid, R.; Weinreich, F.J.; Königsrainer, A.; Reymond, M.A. Overcoming Drug Resistance by Taking Advantage of Physical Principles: Pressurized Intraperitoneal Aerosol Chemotherapy (PIPAC). *Cancers* **2019**, *12*, 34. [CrossRef]
34. Tate, S.J.; Torkington, J. Pressurized intraperitoneal aerosol chemotherapy: A review of the introduction of a new surgical technology using the IDEAL framework. *BJS Open* **2020**, *4*, 206–215. [CrossRef] [PubMed]
35. Cancer Genome Atlas Research Network. Integrated genomic analyses of ovarian carcinoma. *Nature* **2011**, *474*, 609–615. [CrossRef] [PubMed]
36. Zhang, H.; Liu, T.; Zhang, Z.; Payne, S.H.; Zhang, B.; McDermott, J.E.; Zhou, J.-Y.; Petyuk, V.A.; Chen, L.; Ray, D.; et al. Integrated Proteogenomic Characterization of Human High-Grade Serous Ovarian Cancer. *Cell* **2016**, *166*, 755–765. [CrossRef] [PubMed]
37. Gee, M.E.; Faraahi, Z.; McCormick, A.; Edmondson, R.J. DNA damage repair in ovarian cancer: Unlocking the heterogeneity. *J. Ovarian Res.* **2018**, *11*, 50. [CrossRef] [PubMed]

38. Milanesio, M.C.; Giordano, S.; Valabrega, G. Clinical Implications of DNA Repair Defects in High-Grade Serous Ovarian Carcinomas. *Cancers* **2020**, *12*, 1315. [CrossRef]
39. Takaya, H.; Nakai, H.; Takamatsu, S.; Mandai, M.; Matsumura, N. Homologous recombination deficiency status-based classification of high-grade serous ovarian carcinoma. *Sci. Rep.* **2020**, *10*, 2757. [CrossRef]
40. Bodurka, D.C.; Deavers, M.T.; Tian, C.; Sun, C.C.; Malpica, A.; Coleman, R.L.; Lu, K.H.; Sood, A.K.; Birrer, M.J.; Ozols, R.; et al. Reclassification of serous ovarian carcinoma by a 2-tier system: A Gynecologic Oncology Group Study. *Cancer* **2012**, *118*, 3087–3094. [CrossRef]
41. Malpica, A.; Deavers, M.T.; Lu, K.; Bodurka, D.C.; Atkinson, E.N.; Gershenson, D.M.; Silva, E.G. Grading ovarian serous carcinoma using a two-tier system. *Am. J. Surg. Pathol.* **2004**, *28*, 496–504. [CrossRef]
42. Verhaak, R.G.; Tamayo, P.; Yang, J.Y.; Hubbard, D.; Zhang, H.; Creighton, C.J.; Fereday, S.; Lawrence, M.; Carter, S.L.; Mermel, C.; et al. Prognostically relevant gene signatures of high-grade serous ovarian carcinoma. *J. Clin. Investig.* **2013**, *123*, 517–525. [CrossRef]
43. Armstrong, D.K.; Alvarez, R.D.; Bakkum-Gamez, J.N.; Barroilhet, L.; Behbakht, K.; Berchuck, A.; Berek, J.S.; Chen, L.-M.; Cristea, M.; DeRosa, M.; et al. NCCN Guidelines Insights: Ovarian Cancer, Version 1.2019. *J. Natl. Compr. Cancer Netw.* **2019**, *17*, 896–909. [CrossRef] [PubMed]
44. Yokoi, A.; Yoshioka, Y.; Hirakawa, A.; Yamamoto, Y.; Ishikawa, M.; Ikeda, S.I.; Kato, T.; Niimi, K.; Kajiyama, H.; Kikkawa, F.; et al. A combination of circulating miRNAs for the early detection of ovarian cancer. *Oncotarget* **2017**, *8*, 89811–89823. [CrossRef] [PubMed]
45. Otsuka, I.; Matsuura, T. Screening and Prevention for High-Grade Serous Carcinoma of the Ovary Based on Carcinogenesis-Fallopian Tube- and Ovarian-Derived Tumors and Incessant Retrograde Bleeding. *Diagnostics* **2020**, *10*, 120. [CrossRef] [PubMed]
46. Elias, K.M.; Fendler, W.; Stawiski, K.; Fiascone, S.J.; Vitonis, A.F.; Berkowitz, R.S.; Frendl, G.; Konstantinopoulos, P.A.; Crum, C.P.; Kedzierska, M.; et al. Diagnostic potential for a serum miRNA neural network for detection of ovarian cancer. *eLife* **2017**, *6*, e28932. [CrossRef] [PubMed]
47. Guadagni, S.; Clementi, M.; Masedu, F.; Fiorentini, G.; Sarti, D.; Deraco, M.; Kusamura, S.; Papasotiriou, I.; Apostolou, P.; Aigner, K.R.; et al. A Pilot Study of the Predictive Potential of Chemosensitivity and Gene Expression Assays Using Circulating Tumour Cells from Patients with Recurrent Ovarian Cancer. *Int. J. Mol. Sci.* **2020**, *21*, 4813. [CrossRef]
48. Young, R.C.; Walton, L.A.; Ellenberg, S.S.; Homesley, H.D.; Wilbanks, G.D.; Decker, D.G.; Miller, A.; Park, R.; Major, F. Adjuvant therapy in stage I and stage II epithelial ovarian cancer. Results of two prospective randomized trials. *N. Eng. J. Med.* **1990**, *322*, 1021–1027. [CrossRef]
49. Winter-Roach, B.A.; Kitchener, H.C.; Lawrie, T.A. Adjuvant (post-surgery) chemotherapy for early stage epithelial ovarian cancer. *Cochrane Database Syst. Rev.* **2012**, *3*, Cd004706.
50. Hogberg, T.; Glimelius, B.; Nygren, P. A systematic overview of chemotherapy effects in ovarian cancer. *Acta Oncolog.* **2001**, *40*, 340–360. [CrossRef]
51. Chan, J.K.; Java, J.J.; Fuh, K.; Monk, B.J.; Kapp, D.S.; Herzog, T.; Bell, J.; Young, R. The association between timing of initiation of adjuvant therapy and the survival of early stage ovarian cancer patients—An analysis of NRG Oncology/Gynecologic Oncology Group trials. *Gynecol. Oncol.* **2016**, *143*, 490–495. [CrossRef]
52. Harano, K.; Terauchi, F.; Katsumata, N.; Takahashi, F.; Yasuda, M.; Takakura, S.; Takano, M.; Yamamoto, Y.; Sugiyama, T. Quality-of-life outcomes from a randomized phase III trial of dose-dense weekly paclitaxel and carboplatin compared with conventional paclitaxel and carboplatin as a first-line treatment for stage II-IV ovarian cancer: Japanese Gynecologic Oncology Group Trial (JGOG3016). *Ann. Oncol. Off. J. Eur. Soc. Med.Oncol.* **2014**, *25*, 251–257.
53. Chan, J.K.; Brady, M.F.; Penson, R.T.; Huang, H.; Birrer, M.J.; Walker, J.L.; DiSilvestro, P.A.; Rubin, S.C.; Martin, L.P.; Davidson, S.A.; et al. Weekly vs. Every-3-Week Paclitaxel and Carboplatin for Ovarian Cancer. *N. Eng. J. Med.* **2016**, *374*, 738–748. [CrossRef] [PubMed]
54. Pignata, S.; Scambia, G.; Katsaros, D.; Gallo, C.; Pujade-Lauraine, E.; De Placido, S.; Bologna, A.; Weber, B.; Raspagliesi, F.; Panici, P.B.; et al. Carboplatin plus paclitaxel once a week versus every 3 weeks in patients with advanced ovarian cancer (MITO-7): A randomised, multicentre, open-label, phase 3 trial. *Lancet Oncol.* **2014**, *15*, 396–405. [CrossRef]

55. Clamp, A.R.; James, E.C.; McNeish, I.A.; Dean, A.; Kim, J.W.; O'Donnell, D.M.; Hook, J.; Coyle, C.; Blagden, S.; Brenton, J.D.; et al. Weekly dose-dense chemotherapy in first-line epithelial ovarian, fallopian tube, or primary peritoneal carcinoma treatment (ICON8): Primary progression free survival analysis results from a GCIG phase 3 randomised controlled trial. *Lancet* **2019**, *394*, 2084–2095. [CrossRef]
56. Katsumata, N.; Yasuda, M.; Isonishi, S.; Takahashi, F.; Michimae, H.; Kimura, E.; Aoki, D.; Jobo, T.; Kodama, S.; Terauchi, F.; et al. Long-term results of dose-dense paclitaxel and carboplatin versus conventional paclitaxel and carboplatin for treatment of advanced epithelial ovarian, fallopian tube, or primary peritoneal cancer (JGOG 3016): A randomised, controlled, open-label trial. *Lancet Oncol.* **2013**, *14*, 1020–1026. [CrossRef]
57. Hsu, Y.; Sood, A.K.; Sorosky, J.I. Docetaxel versus paclitaxel for adjuvant treatment of ovarian cancer: Case-control analysis of toxicity. *Am. J. Clin. Oncol.* **2004**, *27*, 14–18. [CrossRef]
58. Nguyen, J.; Solimando, D.A., Jr.; Waddell, J.A. Carboplatin and Liposomal Doxorubicin for Ovarian Cancer. *Hosp. Pharm.* **2016**, *51*, 442–449. [CrossRef]
59. Pignata, S.; Scambia, G.; Ferrandina, G.; Savarese, A.; Sorio, R.; Breda, E.; Gebbia, V.; Musso, P.; Frigerio, L.; Del Medico, P.; et al. Carboplatin plus paclitaxel versus carboplatin plus pegylated liposomal doxorubicin as first-line treatment for patients with ovarian cancer: The MITO-2 randomized phase III trial. *J. Clin. Oncol. Off. J. Am. Soc. Clin. Oncol.* **2011**, *29*, 3628–3635. [CrossRef]
60. Burger, R.A.; Brady, M.F.; Rhee, J.; Sovak, M.A.; Kong, G.; Nguyen, H.P.; Bookman, M.A. Independent radiologic review of the Gynecologic Oncology Group Study 0218, a phase III trial of bevacizumab in the primary treatment of advanced epithelial ovarian, primary peritoneal, or fallopian tube cancer. *Gynecol. Oncol.* **2013**, *131*, 21–26. [CrossRef]
61. Perren, T.J.; Swart, A.M.; Pfisterer, J.; Ledermann, J.A.; Pujade-Lauraine, E.; Kristensen, G.; Carey, M.S.; Beale, P.; Cervantes, A.; Kurzeder, C.; et al. A phase 3 trial of bevacizumab in ovarian cancer. *N. Eng. J. Med.* **2011**, *365*, 2484–2496. [CrossRef]
62. Burger, R.A.; Brady, M.; Bookman, M.A.; Fleming, G.F.; Monk, B.J.; Huang, H.; Mannel, R.S.; Homesley, H.D.; Fowler, J.; Greer, B.E.; et al. Incorporation of bevacizumab in the primary treatment of ovarian cancer. *N. Eng. J. Med.* **2011**, *365*, 2473–2483. [CrossRef]
63. Ferriss, J.S.; Java, J.J.; Bookman, M.A.; Fleming, G.F.; Monk, B.J.; Walker, J.L.; Homesley, H.D.; Fowler, J.; Greer, B.E.; Boente, M.P.; et al. Ascites predicts treatment benefit of bevacizumab in front-line therapy of advanced epithelial ovarian, fallopian tube and peritoneal cancers: An NRG Oncology/GOG study. *Gynecol. Oncol.* **2015**, *139*, 17–22. [CrossRef]
64. Wenzel, L.B.; Huang, H.Q.; Armstrong, D.K.; Walker, J.L.; Cella, D. Health-related quality of life during and after intraperitoneal versus intravenous chemotherapy for optimally debulked ovarian cancer: A Gynecologic Oncology Group Study. *J. Clin. Oncol. Off. J. Am. Soc. Clin. Oncol.* **2007**, *25*, 437–443. [CrossRef] [PubMed]
65. Tewari, D.; Java, J.J.; Salani, R.; Armstrong, D.K.; Markman, M.; Herzog, T.; Monk, B.J.; Chan, J.K. Long-term survival advantage and prognostic factors associated with intraperitoneal chemotherapy treatment in advanced ovarian cancer: A gynecologic oncology group study. *J. Clin. Oncol. Off. J. Am. Soc. Clin. Oncol.* **2015**, *33*, 1460–1466. [CrossRef]
66. Oza, A.M.; Cook, A.D.; Pfisterer, J.; Embleton, A.; Ledermann, J.A.; Pujade-Lauraine, E.; Kristensen, G.; Carey, M.S.; Beale, P.; Cervantes, A.; et al. Standard chemotherapy with or without bevacizumab for women with newly diagnosed ovarian cancer (ICON7): Overall survival results of a phase 3 randomised trial. *Lancet Oncol.* **2015**, *16*, 928–936. [CrossRef]
67. Moore, K.N.; Colombo, N.; Scambia, G.; Kim, B.-G.; Oaknin, A.; Friedlander, M.; Lisyanskaya, A.; Floquet, A.; Leary, A.; Sonke, G.S.; et al. Maintenance Olaparib in Patients with Newly Diagnosed Advanced Ovarian Cancer. *N. Eng. J. Med.* **2018**, *379*, 2495–2505. [CrossRef] [PubMed]
68. Ray-Coquard, I.; Pautier, P.; Pignata, S.; Pérol, D.; González-Martín, A.; Berger, R.; Fujiwara, K.; Vergote, I.; Colombo, N.; Mäenpää, J.; et al. Olaparib plus Bevacizumab as First-Line Maintenance in Ovarian Cancer. *N. Eng. J. Med.* **2019**, *381*, 2416–2428. [CrossRef] [PubMed]
69. González-Martín, A.; Pothuri, B.; Vergote, I.; Christensen, R.D.; Graybill, W.; Mirza, M.R.; McCormick, C.; Lorusso, D.; Hoskins, P.; Freyer, G.; et al. Niraparib in Patients with Newly Diagnosed Advanced Ovarian Cancer. *N. Engl. J. Med.* **2019**, *381*, 2391–2402. [CrossRef]
70. Daly, M.B.; Pilarski, R.; Yurgelun, M.B.; Berry, M.P.; Buys, S.S.; Dickson, P.; Domchek, S.M.; Elkhanany, A.; Friedman, S.; Garber, J.E.; et al. NCCN Guidelines Insights: Genetic/Familial High-Risk Assessment: Breast, Ovarian, and Pancreatic, Version 1.2020. *J. Natl. Compr. Cancer Netw.* **2020**, *18*, 380–391. [CrossRef]

71. Walsh, T.; Casadei, S.; Lee, M.K.; Pennil, C.C.; Nord, A.S.; Thornton, A.M.; Roeb, W.; Agnew, K.J.; Stray, S.M.; Wickramanayake, A.; et al. Mutations in 12 genes for inherited ovarian, fallopian tube, and peritoneal carcinoma identified by massively parallel sequencing. *Proc. Natl. Acad. Sci. USA* **2011**, *108*, 18032–18037. [CrossRef]
72. Zhang, S.; Royer, R.; Li, S.; McLaughlin, J.R.; Rosen, B.; Risch, H.A.; Fan, I.; Bradley, L.; Shaw, P.A.; Narod, S.A. Frequencies of BRCA1 and BRCA2 mutations among 1,342 unselected patients with invasive ovarian cancer. *Gynecol. Oncol.* **2011**, *121*, 353–357. [CrossRef]
73. Pal, T.; Permuth-Wey, J.; Betts, J.A.; Krischer, J.P.; Fiorica, J.; Arango, H.; Lapolla, J.; Hoffman, M.; Martino, M.A.; Wakeley, K.; et al. BRCA1 and BRCA2 mutations account for a large proportion of ovarian carcinoma cases. *Cancer* **2005**, *104*, 2807–2816. [CrossRef] [PubMed]
74. Fong, P.C.; Boss, D.S.; Yap, T.A.; Tutt, A.; Wu, P.; Mergui-Roelvink, M.; Mortimer, P.; Swaisland, H.; Lau, A.; O'Connor, M.J.; et al. Inhibition of poly(ADP-ribose) polymerase in tumors from BRCA mutation carriers. *N. Engl. J. Med.* **2009**, *361*, 123–134. [CrossRef] [PubMed]
75. Novetsky, A.; Smith, K.; Babb, S.A.; Jeffe, N.B.; Hagemann, A.R.; Thaker, P.H.; Powell, M.A.; Mutch, D.G.; Massad, L.S.; Zighelboim, I. Timing of referral for genetic counseling and genetic testing in patients with ovarian, fallopian tube, or primary peritoneal carcinoma. *Int. J. Gynecol. Cancer* **2013**, *23*, 1016–1021. [CrossRef] [PubMed]
76. Neviere, Z.; De La Motte Rouge, T.; Floquet, A.; Johnson, A.; Berthet, P.; Joly, F. How and when to refer patients for oncogenetic counseling in the era of PARP inhibitors. *Adv. Med. Oncol.* **2020**, *12*, 1758835919897530. [CrossRef]
77. Stratton, J.F.; Pharoah, P.; Smith, S.K.; Easton, D.; Ponder, B.A. A systematic review and meta-analysis of family history and risk of ovarian cancer. *Br. J. Obstet. Gynaecol.* **1998**, *105*, 493–499. [CrossRef] [PubMed]
78. Jervis, S.; Song, H.; Lee, A.; Dicks, E.; Harrington, P.; Baynes, C.; Manchanda, R.; Easton, U.F.; Jacobs, I.; Pharoah, P.P.D.; et al. A risk prediction algorithm for ovarian cancer incorporating BRCA1, BRCA2, common alleles and other familial effects. *J. Med. Genet.* **2015**, *52*, 465–475. [CrossRef]
79. Lu, K.H.; Wood, M.E.; Daniels, M.S.; Burke, C.; Ford, J.; Kauff, N.D.; Kohlmann, W.; Lindor, N.M.; Mulvey, T.M.; Robinson, L.; et al. American Society of Clinical Oncology Expert Statement: Collection and use of a cancer family history for oncology providers. *J. Clin. Oncol. Off. J. Am. Soc. Clin. Oncol.* **2014**, *32*, 833–840. [CrossRef]
80. Desmond, A.; Kurian, A.W.; Gabree, M.; Mills, M.A.; Anderson, M.J.; Kobayashi, Y.; Horick, N.; Yang, S.; Shannon, K.M.; Tung, N.; et al. Clinical Actionability of Multigene Panel Testing for Hereditary Breast and Ovarian Cancer Risk Assessment. *JAMA Oncol.* **2015**, *1*, 943–951. [CrossRef]
81. Wimmer, K.; Kratz, C.P. Constitutional mismatch repair-deficiency syndrome. *Haematologica* **2010**, *95*, 699–701. [CrossRef]
82. Ford, D.; Easton, D.; Stratton, M.; Narod, S.; Goldgar, D.; Devilee, P.; Bishop, D.T.; Weber, B.; Lenoir, G.; Chang-Claude, J.; et al. Genetic heterogeneity and penetrance analysis of the BRCA1 and BRCA2 genes in breast cancer families. The Breast Cancer Linkage Consortium. *Am. J. Hum. Genet.* **1998**, *62*, 676–689. [CrossRef]
83. Rafnar, T.; Gudbjartsson, D.F.; Sulem, P.; Jonasdottir, A.; Sigurdsson, A.; Jonasdottir, A.; Besenbacher, S.; Lundin, P.; Stacey, S.N.; Gudmundsson, J.; et al. Mutations in BRIP1 confer high risk of ovarian cancer. *Nat. Genet.* **2011**, *43*, 1104–1107. [CrossRef] [PubMed]
84. Vaz, F.; Hanenberg, H.; Schuster, B.; Barker, K.; Wiek, C.; Erven, V.; Neveling, K.; Endt, D.; Kesterton, I.; Autore, F.; et al. Mutation of the RAD51C gene in a Fanconi anemia-like disorder. *Nat. Genet.* **2010**, *42*, 406–409. [CrossRef] [PubMed]
85. Sawyer, S.L.; Tian, L.; Kähkönen, M.; Schwartzentruber, J.; Kircher, M.; Majewski, J.; Dyment, D.A.; Innes, A.M.; Boycott, K.M.; Moreau, L.A.; et al. Biallelic mutations in BRCA1 cause a new Fanconi anemia subtype. *Cancer Discov.* **2015**, *5*, 135–142. [CrossRef] [PubMed]
86. Wagner, J.E.; Tolar, J.; Levran, O.; Scholl, T.; Deffenbaugh, A.; Satagopan, J.; Ben-Porat, L.; Mah, K.; Batish, S.D.; Kutler, D.I.; et al. Germline mutations in BRCA2: Shared genetic susceptibility to breast cancer, early onset leukemia, and Fanconi anemia. *Blood* **2004**, *103*, 3226–3229. [CrossRef] [PubMed]

87. Ngeow, J.; Eng, C. Precision medicine in heritable cancer: When somatic tumour testing and germline mutations meet. *NPJ Genomic Med.* **2016**, *1*, 15006. [CrossRef]
88. Slavin, T.P.; Banks, K.C.; Chudova, D.; Oxnard, G.R.; Odegaard, J.I.; Nagy, R.J.; Tsang, K.W.; Neuhausen, S.L.; Gray, S.W.; Cristofanilli, M.; et al. Identification of Incidental Germline Mutations in Patients With Advanced Solid Tumors Who Underwent Cell-Free Circulating Tumor DNA Sequencing. *J. Clin. Oncol. Off. J. Am. Soc. Clin. Oncol.* **2018**, *36*, JCO1800328.

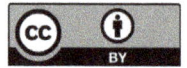

© 2020 by the authors. Licensee MDPI, Basel, Switzerland. This article is an open access article distributed under the terms and conditions of the Creative Commons Attribution (CC BY) license (http://creativecommons.org/licenses/by/4.0/).

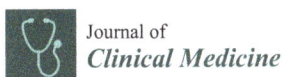

Review

Small Cell Lung Cancer from Traditional to Innovative Therapeutics: Building a Comprehensive Network to Optimize Clinical and Translational Research

Shanmuga Subbiah, Arin Nam, Natasha Garg, Amita Behal, Prakash Kulkarni and Ravi Salgia *

Department of Medical Oncology and Therapeutics Research, City of Hope National Medical Center, Duarte, CA 91010, USA; ssubbiah@coh.org (S.S.); anam@coh.org (A.N.); ngarg@coh.org (N.G.); abehal@coh.org (A.B.); pkulkarni@coh.org (P.K.)
* Correspondence: rsalgia@coh.org

Received: 21 June 2020; Accepted: 28 July 2020; Published: 30 July 2020

Abstract: Small cell lung cancer (SCLC) is an aggressive, complex disease with a distinct biology that contributes to its poor prognosis. Management of SCLC is still widely limited to chemotherapy and radiation therapy, and research recruitment still poses a considerable challenge. Here, we review the current standard of care for SCLC and advances made in utilizing immunotherapy. We also highlight research in the development of targeted therapies and emphasize the importance of a team-based approach to make clinical advances. Building an integrative network between an academic site and community practice sites optimizes biomarker and drug target discovery for managing and treating a difficult disease like SCLC.

Keywords: small cell lung cancer; translational research; immunotherapy; clinical trials; team medicine; community practice

1. Introduction

Lung cancer is the leading cause of cancer deaths in both men and women in the United States [1]. Small cell lung cancer (SCLC) is a subtype of lung cancer that has an incidence of 13% and is strongly associated with smoking [2,3]. A distinct biology, aggressive clinical course with distant metastasis, and poor survival outcomes characterize SCLC. The disease is classified into extensive stage and limited stage. While limited stage SCLC (LS-SCLC) is disease confined to one hemithorax that can be enclosed within a radiation field, extensive stage SCLC (ES-SCLC) is more prevalent (66%) and includes malignant pleural or pericardial effusions along with distant metastasis [4]. Despite the bleak prognosis, standard chemotherapies for patients with SCLC have not changed significantly in the last 30 years. However, recently, immunotherapy with checkpoint inhibitors have shown promising efficacy in advanced disease [5,6]. The lack of advances in SCLC therapies are partly due to disease complexity, research recruitment, and resource utilization. Thus, collaborative efforts between academic and community practices that combine knowledge, skills, experiences, and expertise of academicians, clinicians, and researchers, can accelerate advances in treatment and patient care. Academic centers are critical in the advancement of cancer treatment, but community hospital care plays an equally important and complementary role. Indeed, academic–community collaboration, or 'team medicine', has become an emerging culture to advance and shape clinical care.

In this article, we first highlight the current standard treatments in SCLC as well as recent advances in immunotherapies. We also review potential targeted therapies and underscore the importance of a team-based approach toward SCLC based on our experience at the City of Hope (COH).

2. Current Standard Therapies

2.1. Radiation Therapy

For LS-SCLC the standard of care is chemotherapy with concurrent radiation therapy [7]. Two meta-analyses established that concurrent cisplatin and etoposide treatment combined with radiation therapy improves survival compared to chemotherapy alone [8,9], although the dosage (once daily vs. twice daily) of radiation with chemotherapy remains equivocal. One study showed a significant survival advantage of patients who received 1.5 Gy in 30 fractions twice daily compared to 1.8 Gy in 25 fractions after a median follow-up of 8 years [10]. However, a more recent trial that randomized patients to receiving 1.5 Gy twice daily fractions (45 Gy dose) or 2 Gy once daily fractions (66 Gy dose) concurrently with platinum based chemotherapy showed that survival outcomes did not differ between the regimens, although the trial was not powered for equivalence [11]. The ongoing trial of CALGB 30,610 comparing 45 Gy twice daily to 70 Gy once daily (NCT00632853) is likely to shed more light on this issue.

2.2. Chemotherapy

Regardless of the stage, platinum with etoposide (EP) is the standard of care for patients with SCLC in the United States. Outside the United States, some patients are given platinum with irinotecan as an alternative treatment [12–14]. The overall response rates (ORR) range from 40–70% with up to 10% of the patients achieving complete radiographic response, and the median overall survival (OS) spans 7–12 months, with a two-year survival rate of less than 5% [15]. Eventually, however, most SCLC tumors become resistant to chemotherapy resulting in disease progression. For patients with disease relapse, topotecan as a single agent is the only approved second-line drug that has demonstrated increased survival compared to supportive care [16,17]. Nonetheless, the ORR of patients treated with topotecan is only about 5% [18] and even worse, in SCLC patients who develop disease recurrence within 3 months of the first-line platinum doublet chemotherapy, in which case topotecan is ineffective. Other chemotherapeutic agents such as gemcitabine, docetaxel, paclitaxel, temozolomide, irinotecan, and vinorelbine, may be used in certain cases based on limited clinical evidence [19–24]. Amrubicin is an anthracycline agent that has been developed more recently and approved only in Japan for second-line therapy [25]. Unfortunately, beyond second-line therapy, currently there are no standard guidelines of care although, newer immunotherapies appear promising in some patients.

2.3. Surgery

Compared to non-small cell lung cancer (NSCLC), SCLC is rarely treated surgically. However, over the years the fraction of SCLC patients treated surgically has increased considerably from 14.9% in 2004 to 28.5% in 2013. This is at least in part due to availability of better diagnostic tools in the form of positron emission tomography (PET) scans and increasing usage of low-dose computed tomography (CT) screening. Randomized trials reported in the late 1960s and early 1970s showed no survival advantage for surgery alone or in combination with radiation therapy compared with radiation therapy alone [26,27]. Subsequently, it was reported that chemotherapy given sequentially with radiation and then randomized to surgery vs. non-surgical group did not show any benefit to surgery [28]. However, recently there have been increasing numbers of retrospective studies showing survival benefit of surgery compared to non-surgical therapy [29–32]. For example, a meta-analysis published by Liu et al. [33], which included two randomized control trials described above and thirteen retrospective studies for a total of 41,483 patients, concluded that surgical resection significantly improved overall survival when compared to non-surgical treatment (hazard ratio (HR) = 0.56, $p < 0.001$) for retrospective studies, and in the two randomized trials there was no survival advantage to the surgical arm. This meta-analysis also showed that lobectomy was associated with superior OS compared with sub lobar resection (HR = 0.64, $p < 0.001$). Based on these data, the National Comprehensive Cancer Network (NCCN) also recommends surgery for T1-2N0M0 SCLC provided preoperative evaluation of mediastinal lymph nodes are done. Unfortunately, there are no ongoing randomized trials evaluating surgery in SCLC, since less than 5% of patients present with stage I SCLC. However, a collaborative engagement with community clinic sites where majority of cancer patients are seen and academic institutes similar to COH should help accrue enough patients to conduct a prospective trial.

3. Novel Therapies

Immunotherapy for SCLC was considered viable due to frequent somatic mutations as a result of smoking and the presence of paraneoplastic disorders [34–36]. Furthermore, in light of the remarkable success seen in NSCLC, parallel studies undertaken in SCLC have also shown considerable promise for immunotherapies that include antibodies against programmed cell death protein 1 (PD-1), programmed death-ligand 1 (PD-L1), and cytotoxic T-lymphocyte antigen 4 (CTLA4; Figure 1) [37,38] discussed below.

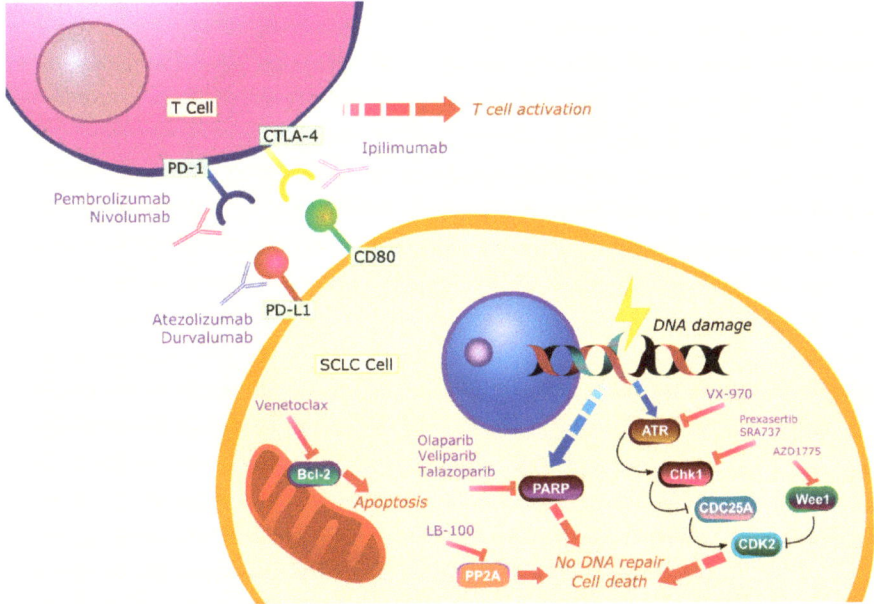

Figure 1. Current investigational immunotherapies and targeted therapies for small cell lung cancer SCLC.

3.1. Atezolizumab

In treatment-naïve ES-SCLC patients, a recently published a phase III trial involving 403 patients, IMpower-133, combining atezolizumab with carboplatin and etoposide (EP) demonstrated an improved progression-free survival (PFS) as well as overall survival (OS) [39]. More specifically, the patients who did not progress after 4 cycles of induction therapy, received atezolizumab or placebo as maintenance every 3 weeks until disease progression or intolerable toxicity. Median OS for those treated with atezolizumab was 12.3 months compared to 10.3 months for the placebo group, with a hazard ratio for death of 0.70. Median PFS was also improved in the atezolizumab group, which was 5.2 months vs. 4.3 months, with a hazard ratio for disease progression at 0.77, resulting in the approval of atezolizumab with EP for ES-SCLC in the first-line setting. However, blood-based tumor mutational burden (TMB) was not associated with clinical benefit in this study.

3.2. Durvalumab

Another phase III trial, the CASPIAN trial, which used durvalumab as the immunotherapy in combination with platinum with etoposide to treat treatment-naïve ES-SCLC patients, also showed improvement in OS compared to platinum-etoposide alone (13 months vs. 10.3 months, with a hazard ratio of 0.73) [40]. Based on these results, the Food and Drug Administration (FDA) also approved durvalumab for ES-SCLC.

3.3. Ipilimumab and Nivolumab

In contrast to atezolizumab or durvalumab, ipilimumab (an anti-cytotoxic T-lymphocyte-associated protein 4 (CTLA4) antibody) in combination with chemotherapy prolongs PFS, but does not improve OS in treatment-naïve ES-SCLC [41]. However, maintenance therapy in such patients with nivolumab/ipilimumab combination or nivolumab alone did not show improvement in OS, according to results from the phase III CheckMate 451 study presented at the recent European Lung Cancer Congress 2019 [42]. Another trial CheckMate 032 assessed nivolumab as a single agent or in combination with ipilimumab in previously treated SCLC and found that ORR with single agent nivolumab was 11% compared to 22% in the cohort with combination of nivolumab with ipilimumab. The median OS for nivolumab alone was 4.1 months, and for nivolumab with ipilimumab, it was 6 months to 7.8 months based on the doses received [43]. Because the long-term survival benefits with nivolumab alone demonstrated better outcomes compared to previous agents used in the third-line setting, nivolumab received FDA approval for third-line treatment of SCLC.

3.4. Pembrolizumab

Pembrolizumab was studied in relapsed SCLC patients in the KEYNOTE-028 and KEYNOTE-158 trials. In KEYNOTE-028, the study included only patients with PD-L1 combined positive score (CPS) ≥1%. Among 24 patients with relapsed SCLC, 12.5% were treated with pembrolizumab in the second-line setting and 50% in the third-line. ORR was 33%, median PFS was 1.9 months, one-year PFS was 23.8%, median OS was 9.7 months, and the one-year OS was 37.7% [44]. In the KEYNOTE-158 trial, 79% of 107 patients with relapsed SCLC were treated with pembrolizumab in the second-line or third-line setting. A total of 47% of patients were PD-L1-negative, with an ORR of 18.7% (35.7% in the PD-L1-positive subgroup and 6.0% PD-L1-negative subgroup). The median PFS was 2 months, and median OS was 9.1 months [45]. This led to the approval of pembrolizumab in metastatic SCLC patients whose disease progresses on or after platinum-based chemotherapy and at least one other line of treatment. Considered together, although immunotherapy appears promising for SCLC patients, its benefits are modest, and there is significant room for further improvement.

4. Targeted Therapy

Unlike in the case of NSCLC, there are currently no targeted therapies available for SCLC. The lack of knowledge of the key genetic mutations and molecular targets that drive SCLC initiation and progress to a more aggressive disease has been a major impediment in developing targeted therapies. However, recent genome-wide studies have identified the universal loss of tumor suppressor genes such as tumor protein 53 (TP53) in 75–90% of patients and retinoblastoma 1 (RB1) and by frequent 3P deletion [46–51]. Consistent with these observations, studies using genetically engineered mouse models have confirmed that the introduction of these two events in pulmonary cells can give rise to high frequency of SCLC development [52]. Nonetheless, more than 120 clinical trials are ongoing that are evaluating new drugs in SCLC targeting various/multiple pathways. Below, we review a few key studies and are depicted in Figure 1.

Aberrant signaling driven by epidermal growth factor receptor (EGFR), stem cell factor receptor tyrosine kinase (c-KIT), PI3K/AKT/mTOR, insulin-like growth factor receptor (IGFR1), and hedgehog signaling pathways have been identified in SCLC. However, inhibitors targeting these pathways have shown minimal efficacy in first-line, maintenance and relapsed SCLC [34,53–70]. Additionally, overexpression and amplification of MET and fibroblast growth factor receptor (FGFR) that are associated with regulating cell proliferation, survival, motility, ability of invasion, and chemoresistance were also observed in SCLC. However, therapies targeting these pathways have not fared well and next generation inhibitors need to be evaluated in combination with either chemotherapy or immunotherapy [71–76].

The apoptotic pathway and the cell cycle checkpoint are some of the other pathways that have been targeted in SCLC. In the former case, B-cell lymphoma 2 (BCL-2) is the favorite therapeutic target. However, BCL-2 antisense oligonucleotide oblimersen and other agents, including obatoclax and navitoclax, have not shown significant activity against SCLC in both phase I and phase II trials [77,78]. Another BCL-2-specific inhibitor venetoclax, demonstrated efficacy in SCLC cell lines expressing high levels of BCL-2 [79] and a phase I trial of venetoclax together with ABBV-075, a bromodomain and extra-terminal domain (BET) inhibitor, is currently under way (NCT02391480). As far as the cell cycle checkpoint is concerned, ataxia telangiectasia and Rad3-related protein (ATR), checkpoint kinase-1 (CHK1), WEE1, and aurora kinase (AURKA), have been the preferred targets among others [80].

In addition to the pathways discussed above, transcription and DNA repair pathways have also been investigated in SCLC. Of these, the MYC pathway stands out since MYC is amplified in a significant (~20%) fraction of SCLC patients and appears to have higher sensitivity to certain newer targeted therapies, such as AURKA and BET inhibitors [81–84]. Other agents that are currently being evaluated are: chiauranib, an aurora B kinase inhibitor for relapsed SCLC (NCT03216343), GSK525762, a BET inhibitor as monotherapy for patients harboring MYC amplification (NCT01587703), and in combination with trametinib for patients carrying RAS mutations (NCT03266159).

Wee-like protein kinase 1 (WEE1) is a key tyrosine kinase involved in halting the G2-to-M phase transition of the cell cycle upon DNA damage [85] that is overexpressed in SCLC [86]. In a preclinical study, the combination of Poly(ADP-Ribose) Polymerase (PARP) inhibitors and WEE1 inhibitors demonstrated a synergistic effect [87]. A phase II, multi-arm trial (BALTIC) is currently evaluating the efficacy of novel therapies in patients with ES-SCLC refractory to platinum-based agents. These novel therapies include PD-L1 inhibitor durvalumab, PARP inhibitor olaparib, and WEE1 kinase inhibitor AZD1775.

Poly (ADP-ribose) polymerase 1 (PARP1) another key player in DNA repair is overexpressed in SCLC [88]. PARP inhibitors prevent cancer cells from repairing DNA damage caused by cytotoxic drugs. Several PARP inhibitors have demonstrated antitumor efficacy in preclinical SCLC models and are currently being studied in several clinical trials. A phase II study investigating veliparib in combination with cisplatin and etoposide in untreated ES-SCLC patients showed improvement in the primary endpoint PFS (6.1 months vs. 5.5 months) although no significant differences in OS were observed [89]. However, Schlafen-11 (SLFN11), which is involved in regulating response to DNA damage and is overexpressed in about 48% of SCLC, has been identified as a potential biomarker for veliparib benefit [90]. Recently, another PARP inhibitor talazoparib also caused higher sensitization to radiotherapy in SCLC cell lines and patient-derived xenografts. Thus, PARP inhibitors have great potential to emerge as a promising therapy for SCLC [91].

Activation of the Notch pathway is oncogenic in some cancer types, but in SCLC, the inhibition of Notch pathway is involved in tumorigenic signaling, progression, and chemoresistance [92]. Consistently, the inhibitory Notch ligand Delta-like protein 3 (DLL3) is upregulated in 85% of SCLCs compared to normal lung [93]. Rovalpituzumab tesirine (Rova-T), a first-in-class DLL3 antibody-drug conjugate, initially exhibited promising results of 18% ORR in heavily pretreated SCLC [94]. Unfortunately, high toxicity rates in the phase II TRINITY trial (NCT02674568) precluded the study from meeting its primary endpoint. In addition, the phase III MERU trial (NCT03033511) evaluating Rova-T in the maintenance setting following first-line chemotherapy, was also terminated early as a result of lack of survival benefit at an interim analysis. Likewise, another phase III (TAHOE) study that assessed Rova-T as a second-line therapy for advanced SCLC compared to topotecan, stopped enrollment due to shorter OS in the Rova-T group compared with the topotecan control group [95,96]. A phase I/II study evaluating the safety of Rova-T administered in combination with nivolumab or nivolumab and ipilimumab for adults with ES-SCLC has been recently completed and could decide the future of Rova-T (NCT03026166).

5. Protein Phosphatase 2A (PP2A)

Protein phosphatase 2A (PP2A), a serine/threonine phosphatase that functions as a tumor suppressor in many cancers [97], is also involved in various cellular processes, such as protein synthesis, cellular signaling, cell cycle, apoptosis, metabolism, and stress responses [98]. Several small-molecule activators of PP2A (SMAPs) have emerged as first-in-class agents for this target [99–102]. Further, a recent study has shown that PP2A suppression leads to resistance to kinase inhibitors in KRAS-driven lung cancer cell lines. In KRAS-driven xenograft mouse models, combination treatment of SMAP and selumetinib (a MEK inhibitor used in clinical trials) led to significant tumor regression compared to either agent alone [103,104]. Although PP2A is generally held to have tumor suppressor function, several lines of evidence suggest that it could also function as an oncogene. Thus, small molecule inhibitors of PP2A such as LB-100 [105], are emerging as novel strategies for SCLC. Furthermore, since PP2A is also associated with immune response by downregulating cytotoxic T-lymphocyte function [106,107], PP2A inhibition combined with immunotherapy appears to be effective in mediating an antitumor response. Indeed, in colon cancer and melanoma cells, a combination of LB-100 and an immune checkpoint inhibitor led to greater T-cell-dependent anti-tumor response, with more effector T-cell and reduced regulatory T-cell infiltration [106]. Carbonic anhydrase IX (CAIX), an enzyme involved in hypoxia inducible factor 1 alpha (HIF-1α) hypoxic signaling, is a promising target for chimeric antigen receptor-T (CAR-T) cells in an intracranial mouse model for glioblastoma [108]. In this mouse model, LB-100 was shown to augment the cytotoxic response of anti-carbonic anhydrase (CAIX) CAR-T cells, underscoring the therapeutic potential of synergistic LB-100 and CAR-T cell therapy in SCLC and other solid tumors [109].

6. Mitochondria

Mitochondria play an essential role in cell survival, apoptosis, adenosine triphosphate (ATP) production, as well as tumorigenesis [110]. Multiple therapeutic strategies have been developed to target mitochondrial functions, such as oxidative phosphorylation, glycolysis, tricarboxylic acid (TCA) cycle, apoptosis, reactive oxygen species (ROS) regulation, permeability transition pore complex, mitochondrial DNA, and dihydroorotate de-hydrogenase (DHODH)-linked pyrimidine synthesis [111]. Drugs that target mitochondrial metabolism through inhibition of pyruvate dehydrogenase (CPI-613, dichloroacetate), isocitrate dehydrogenase (AG-22, AG-120, AG-881) and targeting apoptotic pathways (birinapant, Minnelide, ME-334, Debio 1143, ONC201, LCL161) have been studied in early phase clinical trials [112–117]. These drugs have modest clinical activity as single agents in various tumors including SCLC and are currently being explored as combination therapies with chemotherapy, immunotherapy, and other targeted therapies [118].

7. Stem Cell Therapy

Cancer stem cells (CSCs) are defined as a small population of cells within a heterogeneous tumor that exhibit similar traits of normal stem cells. CSCs can originate from either somatic stem cells or differentiated progenitor cells. They prompt tumorigenic activity by undergoing self-renewal and differentiation, leading to tumor relapse, resistance to therapy, and metastasis [119–121]. Hence, targeting CSCs has become a novel therapeutic strategy for cancer treatment. CSCs often have upregulated signaling involved in development and tissue homeostasis, such as Notch, Hedgehog and wingless type 1 (WNT) pathways, all of which can be found in SCLC [122,123]. Unfortunately, Notch signaling inhibition with Rova-T and tarextumab have failed, but combination therapies studies are ongoing that could potentially yield positive results. Lysine demethylase 1 (LSD1) is implicated in maintaining stemness properties and hence, has emerged as a potential target for inhibiting lung CSCs [124]. A phase II trial (CLEPSIDRA) investigating the LSD1 inhibitor iadademstat in combination with standard-of-care in relapsing SCLC patients showed remarkable response rates (up to 75%). Preclinical studies with another LSD1 inhibitor GSK2879552 using 150 cancer cell lines, showed that SCLC and acute myeloid leukemia (AML) cell lines were sensitive to growth inhibition by the LSD1 inhibitor [125–127]. Furthermore, dual inhibition of LSD1 and PD-1 appear to be more effective than either therapy alone [128]. Another route to target stem cells is through CD47 inhibition by RRx-001, which targets tumor-associated macrophages and CSCs via downregulation of the antiphagocytic CD47/SIRPα checkpoint axis. A phase II trial (QUADRUPLE THREAT) involving 26 previously platinum-treated third-line SCLC patients showed that the OS and PFS for patients treated with RRx-001 and a reintroduced platinum doublet were 8.6 months and 7.5 months, respectively, which is much higher for a third-line treatment reported in literature [129]. Interestingly, biopsies taken from patients have correlated response to CD47 inhibition with a high density of infiltrated tumor-associated macrophages that are abundant in SCLC. Based on these observations, a phase III (REPLATINUM) randomized study of RRx-001 with platinum doublet vs. only platinum doublet in third-line SCLC is currently ongoing (NCT03699956).

8. Improving Outcomes

8.1. Biomarker-Based Therapy

Although immunotherapy has improved median survival for treatment-naïve ES-SCLC patients, the benefits have been limited with improvement in both PFS and OS approximately 1 and 2 months, respectively, with only 12.6% of patients remaining progression-free after one-year [39]. To improve the outcomes, better selection of patients based on predictive biomarkers, given the high mutational load and rapid resistance in SCLC, and therapies targeting multiple pathways with combination strategies need to be developed.

PD-L1 remains the most common immune-based biomarker for several malignancies. PD-L1 staining in SCLC is less intense and infrequent compared to NSCLC [130]. In KEYNOTE-158, a combined score >1 for PD-L1 expression by the Dako 22C3 assay appeared to predict increased response to pembrolizumab and improved survival when compared with patients negative for PD-L1 [44]; however, the PD-L1 positivity based on Dako 28-8 assay as in the CheckMate 032 did not replicate those results [131]. The assays differ in that KEYNOTE-158 used a PD-L1 score based on staining of tumor cells, lymphocytes and macrophages, whereas CheckMate 032 used staining of only tumor cells to determine positivity. The ongoing phase II REACTION (NCT02580994) and the phase III KEYNOTE-604 (NCT03066778) trials will require measurement of PD-L1 at baseline to provide insight into the predictive role of PD-L1 expression. Higher tumor mutation burden (TMB) has been recognized as a likely predictor of response to immunotherapy across disease types [132]. In an exome-sequencing analysis of CheckMate 032, patients with high TMB appeared to have a greater improvement in OS when treated with nivolumab. Patients with high-, medium-, and low-TMB had a median OS of 5.4 months, 3.9 months, and 3.1 months, respectively; the one-year OS rates were 35.2%, 26.0%, and 22.1%, respectively [133]. However, in the IMpower-133, a blood-based TMB failed to predict benefit for atezolizumab, thus requiring further prospective randomized validation TMB studies. Circulating tumor cells (CTCs) can be detected in 85% of SCLC patients and can potentially serve as a biomarker [134]. CTCs have been explored in multiple studies as a biomarker to predict response and resistance to therapy; however, additional studies looking into the genomic, epigenetic, and transcriptomic heterogeneity of CTCs at diagnosis and during relapse need to be done before it can be applied in clinics [135,136]. Cell-free DNA (cfDNA) widely used in NSCLC has also been examined in SCLC. A study with 27 patients showed cfDNA was able to mirror treatment response and even identified disease recurrence before radiological progression [137]. Future work based on tumor or blood-based biomarkers will help a long way in understanding treatment resistance in SCLC.

8.2. Combination Therapy

To overcome treatment resistance, novel combination approaches targeting multiple pathways are being explored in combination with chemotherapy and immunotherapies. Lurbinectedin, a novel cytotoxic drug, is a transcriptional inhibitor that inhibits RNA polymerase II. In a phase II trial for both sensitive and resistant disease, lurbinectedin was active as a single agent in second-line SCLC with an ORR of 35.2% [138]. Based on this study, the FDA has approved lurbinectedin for the treatment of ES-SCLC patients with disease progression after platinum-based chemotherapy. A phase III study (ATLANTIS trial, NCT02566993) of lurbinectedin in combination with doxorubicin vs. chemotherapy has completed recruitment and results are pending. Current trials investigating targeted therapies with or without chemotherapy include WEE1 inhibitor AZD1775 in combination with carboplatin (NCT02937818) and olaparib (NCT02511795), checkpoint kinase 1 (CHK1) inhibitor SRA737 in combination with cisplatin/gemcitabine (NCT027979770), ataxia–telangiectasia and Rad3 related (ATR) inhibitor AZD6738 in combination with olaparib (NCT02937818), another ATR inhibitor VX-970 in combination with topotecan (NCT02487095), Bcl-2 inhibitor navitoclax and mTOR inhibitor vistusertib (NCT03366103), Bcl-2 inhibitor venetoclax and ABBV-075 (NCT02391480), and Aurora B kinase inhibitor (NCT02579226) are all ongoing, which should shed some light on the future of targeted therapy in SCLC. There are numerous early phase trials investigating the combination of immunotherapy and targeted drugs as well. Durvalumab with olaparib (NCT02734004, MENDIOLA), avelumab with utomilumab, which is a humanized monoclonal antibody (mAb) that stimulates signaling through CD137 (NCT02554812), nivolumab plus ipilimumab with dendritic cell-based p53 vaccine 9 (NCT03406715) in relapsed SCLC, atezolizumab with chemotherapy and a CDK 4/6 inhibitor trilaciclib (NCT03041311) in first-line ES-SCLC are some of the novel combinations of immunotherapy with targeted agents.

8.3. Other Modalities

Other modalities of therapies targeting cell surface antigens expressed on tumor cells by monoclonal antibodies or surface-targeting immunotherapies, such as CAR-T cells and bispecific T-cell engagers (BiTEs), are in early stages of development. CD56 is expressed in almost all SCLC tumors, and thus, presents to be an attractive target for treating SCLC [139]. In a preclinical study, promiximab-duocarmycin (DUBA), a CD56 antibody conjugated to a potent DNA alkylating agent with a novel linker, showed promising results. This antibody drug conjugate (ADC) demonstrated high efficacy in SCLC xenograft models [140], suggesting that further clinical evaluation of this compound may be beneficial. Another ADC sacituzumab govitecan is comprised of a humanized mAb targeting Trop-2 (trophoblastic antigen-2), which is highly expressed in several epithelial cancers [141], fused to SN-38 (the active metabolite of irinotecan), which induces double- and single-strand DNA breaks by inhibiting topoisomerase I [142]. Sacituzumab govitecan is currently being investigated in several trials, including a phase I/II trial where it is being evaluated as a single agent in patients with previously treated, advanced SCLC (NCT01631552). CAR-T cells targeting DLL3 have entered a phase I clinical trial (NCT03392064). AMG 757, a BiTE, is also being evaluated in a phase I trial that includes ES-SCLC patients requiring first-line maintenance therapy and those with SCLC recurrence (NCT03319940). In patients with metastatic solid tumors including relapsed SCLC, targeting other immune checkpoints, such as PD-1 and CTLA-4, with immunotherapies, including TIM3 and LAG3, are being evaluated in clinical trials in combination with anti-PD-1 or anti-PD-L1 antibodies (NCT03708328, NCT03365791). Finally, radiation therapy is assumed to modulate immune response, as it can increase tumor antigen production and presentation and also enhance cytotoxic T-lymphocyte activity [143]. Potential synergy of radiotherapy in combination with immunotherapy in patients with ES-SCLC is being evaluated in innovative ongoing trials, and results are expected in the near future. Altogether, advancement in biomarkers, targeting multiple critical pathways, and enhancing immunotherapy efficacy in SCLC will hopefully improve the survival outcomes for SCLC patients, which has been elusive for many years.

9. Community Network-City of Hope Experience

City of Hope is a National Cancer Institute (NCI)-designated Comprehensive Cancer Center and a member of the National Comprehensive Cancer Network (NCCN). In addition, all clinical sites accept the Via Oncology Pathways (modified by City of Hope) for evaluation, antitumor treatment and surveillance after treatments have concluded. City of Hope is composed of a central academic site in Duarte and several satellite sites within Southern California. At the academic center, preclinical work is performed, and clinical trials on that translational research can be rapidly deployed across the entire enterprise, making bench-to-bedside research feasible and fascicle. The collaboration between basic research done on the main campus and clinical research done at both the main and satellite campuses, furthers the discovery of disease biomarkers and novel drug targets. This results in more rational drug design, improved therapeutic efficacy, and quicker optimization of high priority drugs for clinical use (Figure 2).

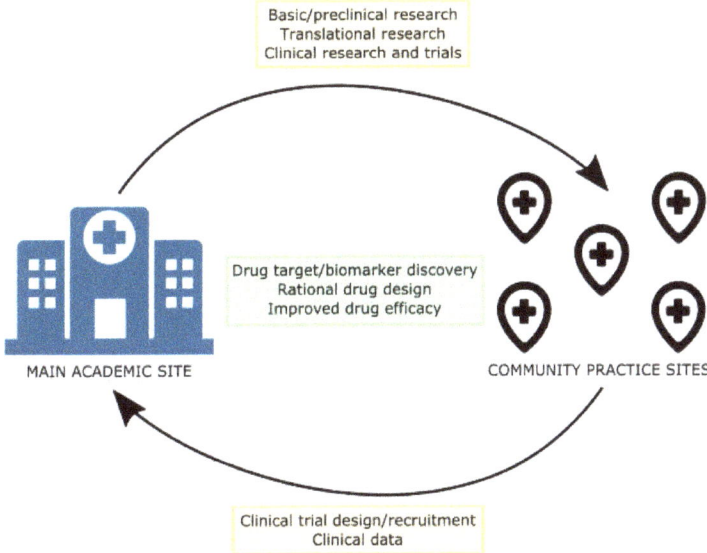

Figure 2. Collaboration between main academic site and community sites for clinical research.

Clinical trials are initiated at the academic campus in Duarte and at one or more of our 27 affiliated network community cancer center offices that are staffed with 43 medical oncologists, 40 radiation oncologists, seven advanced practice providers (APPs) and a clinical trials coordinator. As directed by the Recalcitrant Cancer Research Congressional Act of 2012 (H.R.733), the National Cancer Institute (NCI) allocates resources for research and treatment of recalcitrant cancers having five-year relative survival rates of <20% and estimated to cause at least 30,000 deaths in the US per year. SCLC is considered a recalcitrant cancer having a dismal five-year survival rate of less than 7%. One of the major limitations to ongoing research in SCLC is tumor tissue availability, as the disease is rarely treated surgically. Another issue is many clinical trials in SCLC cannot be completed due to lack of accrual. Using the academic collaboration model with the academic center along with 27 community sites, enrollment becomes more feasible. The rapid progression of disease in SCLC relapse also places research on an urgent timeline to test new agents with a small window to observe treatment efficacy. Given single Institutional Review Board (IRB) approval in our institution, clinical trials can be opened at multiple sites in a rapid fashion. At the academic site, preclinical investigations are done, and clinical trials based on translational research data can be rapidly designed and disseminated across the entire enterprise, facilitating bench-to-bedside SCLC research in a more feasible manner. The collective knowledge gained from the interaction between the academic and community sites will provide insight into how to overcome challenges that continuously hinder therapeutic advancements in SCLC.

10. Future Directions

Traditionally, SCLC has been regarded as a homogenous disease, which led to most SCLC patients being treated with essentially one standard regimen. Recent studies from molecular analysis of patient tissues and genetically defined models indicate that there is notable heterogeneity among SCLCs in terms of histology, growth characteristics, expression of neuroendocrine cell differentiation markers, MYC activation, Notch pathway inactivation, and role of neuronal lineage-specific transcription factors in this disease (ASCL1, achaete-scute homologue 1; NeuroD1, neurogenic differentiation factor 1; POU2F3, POU class 2 homeobox 3; YAP1, yes-associated protein 1) [144–148]. Currently, SCLC is classified into four subtypes based on increased expression of different markers: ASCL1 high (SCLC-A), NEUROD1 high (SCLC-N), POU2F3 high (SCLC-P), and YAP1 high (SCLC-Y) [79]. SCLC-A and SCLC-N are neuroendocrine subtypes, whereas SCLC-P and SCLC-Y are non-neuroendocrine subtypes. These subtypes can be associated with specific biomarkers that are either drug-specific targets or predictors of drug response (e.g., DLL3 in SCLC-A, AURKA in SCLC-N, CDK4/6 in SCLC-Y and IGF1R in SCLC-P). These distinct gene expression profiles will guide us in designing new clinical trials. Recent advances in using patient-derived xenograft (PDX) models based on biopsy/resected tumors, CTCs, genetically engineered mouse models (GEMM), as well as omics profiling will drastically enhance our capacity to identify and test novel drugs and discover biomarkers for treatment and prognostication [93,149].

In conclusion, we recommend: (i) setting up a centralized biobank and repository leading to creation of a database incorporating full genomic, proteomic, and microRNA information; (ii) enrolling a higher proportion of SCLC patients into clinical trials with obligatory biomarker analysis; (iii) creating a master protocol which will help reduce duplicative effort and thus ease the eligibility requirements for clinical trials; (iv) create and incentivize academic and community research partnership centers of excellence, since most SCLC patients are treated in community sites; (v) collaborate with bioengineers, cancer biologists, and biophysicists to gather the genetic aberrations discovered and harness the power of computational modeling of genetic information, which will be a powerful tool in understanding SCLC and developing future therapies. Given the academic and community partnership we have established at City of Hope, this should be achievable and pave way for success in treating this challenging disease.

Author Contributions: Conceptualization, S.S., A.N., and R.S.; methodology, S.S., A.N., and N.G.; writing—original draft preparation, S.S. and A.N.; writing—review and editing, S.S., A.N., N.G., A.B., P.K., and R.S.; supervision, R.S.; project administration, P.K.; funding acquisition, R.S. All authors have read and agreed to the published version of the manuscript.

Funding: This research received no external funding.

Conflicts of Interest: The authors declare no conflict of interest.

References

1. Centers for Disease Control and Prevention. National Center for Health Statistics. CDC On-Line Database, Compiled from Compressed Mortality File 1999–2016 Series 20 No. 2V, 2017. Available online: https://www.cdc.gov/nchs/data_access/cmf.htm (accessed on 28 July 2020).
2. Gazdar, A.F.; Bunn, P.A.; Minna, J.D. Small-cell lung cancer: What we know, what we need to know and the path forward. *Nat. Rev. Cancer* **2017**, *17*, 765. [CrossRef] [PubMed]
3. Herbst, R.S.; Morgensztern, D.; Boshoff, C. The biology and management of non-small cell lung cancer. *Nature* **2018**, *553*, 446–454. [CrossRef] [PubMed]
4. Kalemkerian, G.P. Staging and imaging of small cell Lung cancer. *Cancer Imaging* **2012**, *11*, 253–258. [CrossRef] [PubMed]

5. Navarro, A.; Felip, E. Pembrolizumab in advanced pretreated small cell lung cancer patients with PD-L1 expression: Data from the KEYNOTE-028 trial: A reason for hope? *Transl. Lung Cancer Res.* **2017**, *6* (Suppl. S1), S78–S83. [CrossRef]
6. U.S. Food & Drug Administration. FDA Grants Nivolumab Accelerated Approval for Third-Line Treatment of Metastatic Small Cell Lung Cancer. Available online: https://www.fda.gov/drugs/resources-information-approved-drugs/fda-grants-nivolumab-accelerated-approval-third-line-treatment-metastatic-small-cell-lung-cancer (accessed on 28 July 2020).
7. NCCN. *NCCN Clinical Practice Guidelines in Oncology: Small Cell Lung Cancer*; The National Comprehensive Cancer Network (NCCN): Whitemarsh, PA, USA, 2019.
8. Warde, P.; Payne, D. Does thoracic irradiation improve survival and local control in limited-stage small-cell carcinoma of the lung? A meta-analysis. *J. Clin. Oncol.* **1992**, *10*, 890–895. [CrossRef]
9. Pignon, J.P.; Arriagada, R.; Ihde, D.C.; Johnsosn, D.H.; Perry, M.C.; Souhami, R.L.; Brodin, O.; Joss, R.A.; Kies, M.S.; Lebeau, B.; et al. A meta-analysis of thoracic radiotherapy for small-cell lung cancer. *N. Engl. J. Med.* **1992**, *327*, 1618–1624. [CrossRef]
10. Turrisi, A.T., III; Kim, K.; Blum, R.; Sause, W.T.; Livingston, R.B.; Komaki, R.; Wagner, H.; Aisner, S.; Johnson, D.H. Twice-daily compared with once-daily thoracic radiotherapy in limited small-cell lung cancer treated concurrently with cisplatin and etoposide. *N. Engl. J. Med.* **1999**, *340*, 265–271. [CrossRef]
11. Faivre-Finn, C.; Snee, M.; Ashcroft, L.; Appel, W.; Barlesi, F.; Bhatnagar, A.; Bezjak, A.; Cardenal, F.; Fournel, P.; Harden, S.; et al. Concurrent once-daily versus twice-daily chemoradiotherapy in patients with limited-stage small-cell lung cancer (CONVERT): An open-label, phase 3, randomised, superiority trial. *Lancet Oncol.* **2017**, *18*, 1116–1125. [CrossRef]
12. Fukuoka, M.; Furuse, K.; Saijo, N.; Nishiwaki, Y.; Ikegami, H.; Tamura, T.; Shimoyama, M.; Suemasu, K. Randomized trial of cyclophosphamide, doxorubicin, and vincristine versus cisplatin and etoposide versus alternation of these regimens in small-cell lung cancer. *J. Natl. Cancer Inst.* **1991**, *83*, 855–861. [CrossRef]
13. Roth, B.J.; Johnson, D.H.; Einhorn, L.H.; Schacter, L.P.; Cherng, N.C.; Cohen, H.J.; Crawford, J.; Randolph, J.A.; Goodlow, J.L.; Broun, G.O.; et al. Randomized study of cyclophosphamide, doxorubicin, and vincristine versus etoposide and cisplatin versus alternation of these two regimens in extensive small-cell lung cancer: A phase III trial of the Southeastern cancer study group. *J. Clin. Oncol.* **1992**, *10*, 282–291. [CrossRef]
14. Noda, K.; Nishiwaki, Y.; Kawahara, M.; Negoro, S.; Sugiura, T.; Yokoyama, A.; Fukuoka, M.; Mori, K.; Watanabe, K.; Tamura, T.; et al. Irinotecan plus cisplatin compared with etoposide plus cisplatin for extensive small-cell lung cancer. *N. Engl. J. Med.* **2002**, *346*, 85–91. [CrossRef] [PubMed]
15. Jackman, D.M.; Johnson, B.E. Small-cell lung cancer. *Lancet* **2005**, *366*, 1385–1396. [CrossRef]
16. O'Brien, M.E.R.; Ciuleanu, T.E.; Tsekov, H.; Shparyk, Y.; Cuceviá, B.; Juhasz, G.; Thatcher, N.; Ross, G.A.; Dane, G.C.; Crofts, T. Phase III trial comparing supportive care alone with supportive care with oral topotecan in patients with relapsed small-cell lung cancer. *J. Clin. Oncol.* **2006**, *24*, 5441–5447. [CrossRef] [PubMed]
17. Von Pawel, J.; Schiller, J.H.; Shepherd, F.A.; Fields, S.Z.; Kleisbauer, J.P.; Chrysson, N.G.; Stewart, D.J.; Clark, P.I.; Palmer, M.C.; Depierre, A.; et al. Topotecan versus cyclophosphamide, doxorubicin, and vincristine for the treatment of recurrent small-cell lung cancer. *J. Clin. Oncol.* **1999**, *17*, 658–667. [CrossRef]
18. Horita, N.; Yamamoto, M.; Sato, T.; Tsukahara, T.; Nagakura, H.; Tashiro, K.; Shinata, Y.; Watanabe, H.; Nagai, K.; Inoue, M.; et al. Topotecan for relapsed small-cell lung cancer: Systematic review and meta-analysis of 1347 patients. *Sci. Rep.* **2015**, *5*, 15437. [CrossRef]
19. Masters, G.A.; Declerck, L.; Blanke, C.; Sandler, A.; DeVore, R.; Miller, K.; Johnson, D.; Eastern Cooperative Oncology Group. Phase II trial of gemcitabine in refractory or relapsed small-cell lung cancer: Eastern Cooperative Oncology Group Trial 1597. *J. Clin. Oncol.* **2003**, *21*, 1550–1555. [CrossRef]
20. Smyth, J.F.; Smith, I.E.; Sessa, C.; Schoffski, P.; Wanders, J.; Franklin, H.; Kaye, S.B. Activity of docetaxel (Taxotere) in small cell lung cancer: The Early Clinical Trials Group of the EORTC. *Eur. J. Cancer* **1994**, *30A*, 1058–1060. [CrossRef]
21. Yamamoto, N.; Tsurutani, J.; Yoshimura, N.; Asai, G.; Moriyama, A.; Nakagawa, K.; Kudoh, S.; Takada, M.; Minato, Y.; Fukuoka, M. Phase II study of weekly paclitaxel for relapsed and refractory small cell lung cancer. *Anticancer Res.* **2006**, *26*, 777–781.

22. Pietanza, M.C.; Kadota, K.; Huberman, K.; Sima, C.S.; Fiore, J.J.; Sumner, D.K.; Travis, W.D.; Heguy, A.; Ginsberg, M.S.; Holodny, A.I.; et al. Phase II trial of temozolomide in patients with relapsed sensitive or refractory small cell lung cancer, with assessment of methylguanine-DNA methyltransferase as a potential biomarker. *Clin. Cancer Res.* **2012**, *18*, 1138–1145. [CrossRef]
23. Masuda, N.; Fukuoka, M.; Kusunoki, Y.; Matsui, K.; Takifuji, N.; Kudoh, S.; Negoro, S.; Nishioka, M.; Nakagawa, K.; Takada, M. CPT-11: A new derivative of camptothecin for the treatment of refractory or relapsed small-cell lung cancer. *J. Clin. Oncol.* **1992**, *10*, 1225–1229. [CrossRef]
24. Jassem, J.; Karnicka-Mlodkowska, H.; van Pottelsberghe, C.; van Glabbeke, M.; Noseda, M.A.; Ardizzoni, A.; Gozzelino, F.; Planting, A.; van Zandwijk, N. Phase II study of vinorelbine (Navelbine) in previously treated small cell lung cancer patients: EORTC Lung Cancer Cooperative Group. *Eur. J. Cancer* **1993**, *29A*, 1720–1722. [CrossRef]
25. Ding, Q.; Zhan, J. Amrubicin: Potential in combination with cisplatin or carboplatin to treat small-cell lung cancer. *Drug Des. Dev. Ther.* **2013**, *7*, 681–689.
26. Miller, A.B.; Fox, W.; Tall, R. Five-year follow-up of the Medical Research Council comparative trial of surgery and radiotherapy for the primary treatment of small-celled or oat-celled carcinoma of the bronchus. *Lancet* **1969**, *2*, 501–505. [CrossRef]
27. Fox, W.; Scadding, J.G. Treatment of oat-celled carcinoma of the bronchus. *Lancet* **1973**, *2*, 616–617. [CrossRef]
28. Lad, T.; Piantadosi, S.; Thomas, P.; Payne, D.; Ruckdeschel, J.; Giaccone, G. A prospective randomized trial to determine the benefit of surgical resection of residual disease following response of small cell lung cancer to combination chemotherapy. *Chest* **1994**, *106* (Suppl. S6), 320S–323S. [CrossRef]
29. Rostad, H.; Naalsund, A.; Jacobsen, R.; Strand, T.E.; Scott, H.; Strøm, E.H.; Norstein, J. Small cell lung cancer in Norway. Should more patients have been offered surgical therapy? *Eur. J. Cardiothorac. Surg.* **2004**, *26*, 782–786. [CrossRef]
30. Brock, M.V.; Hooker, C.M.; Syphard, J.E.; Westra, W.; Xu, L.; Alberg, A.J.; Mason, D.; Baylin, S.B.; Herman, J.G.; Yung, R.C.; et al. Surgical resection of limited disease small cell lung cancer in the new era of platinum chemotherapy: Its time has come. *J. Thorac. Cardiovasc. Surg.* **2005**, *129*, 64–72. [CrossRef]
31. Lim, E.; Belcher, E.; Yap, Y.K.; Nicholson, A.G.; Goldstraw, P. The role of surgery in the treatment of limited disease small cell lung cancer: Time to reevaluate. *J. Thorac. Oncol.* **2008**, *3*, 1267–1271. [CrossRef]
32. Schreiber, D.; Rineer, J.; Weedon, J.; Vongtama, D.; Wortham, A.; Kim, A.; Han, P.; Choi, K.; Rotman, M. Survival outcomes with the use of surgery in limited-stage small cell lung cancer: Should its role be re-evaluated? *Cancer* **2010**, *116*, 1350–1357. [CrossRef]
33. Liu, T.; Chen, Z.; Dang, J.; Li, G. The role of surgery in stage I to III small cell lung cancer: A systematic review and meta-analysis. *PLoS ONE* **2018**, *13*, e0210001. [CrossRef]
34. Peifer, M.; Fernández-Cuesta, L.; Sos, M.L.; George, J.; Seidel, D.; Kasper, L.H.; Plenker, D.; Leenders, F.; Sun, R.; Zander, T.; et al. Integrative genome analyses identify key somatic driver mutations of small-cell lung cancer. *Nat. Genet.* **2012**, *44*, 1104–1110. [CrossRef] [PubMed]
35. Alexandrov, L.B.; Nik-Zainal, S.; Wedge, D.C.; Aparicio, S.A.; Behjati, S.; Biankin, A.V.; Bignell, G.R.; Bolli, N.; Borg, A.; Børrensen-Dale, A.L.; et al. Signatures of mutational processes in human cancer. *Nature* **2013**, *500*, 415–421. [CrossRef] [PubMed]
36. Horn, L.; Reck, M.; Spigel, D.R. The future of immunotherapy in the treatment of small cell lung cancer. *Oncologist* **2016**, *21*, 910–921. [CrossRef] [PubMed]
37. Reck, M.; Heigener, D.; Reinmuth, N. Immunotherapy for small-cell lung cancer: Emerging evidence. *Future Oncol.* **2016**, *12*, 931–943. [CrossRef] [PubMed]
38. Horn, L.; Mansfield, A.S.; Szczęsna, A.; Havel, L.; Krzakowski, M.; Hochmair, M.J.; Huemer, F.; Losonczy, G.; Johnson, M.L.; IMpower133 Study Group; et al. First-line atezolizumab plus chemotherapy in extensive-stage small-cell lung cancer. *N. Engl. J. Med.* **2018**, *379*, 2220–2229. [CrossRef]
39. Paz-Ares, L.; Dvorkin, M.; Chen, Y.; Reinmuth, N.; Hotta, K.; Trukhin, D.; Statsenko, G.; Hochmair, M.J.; Özgüroğlu, M.; Ji, J.H.; et al. Durvalumab plus platinum–etoposide versus platinum–etoposide in first-line treatment of extensive-stage small-cell lung cancer (CASPIAN): A randomised, controlled, open-label, phase 3 trial. *Lancet* **2019**, *394*, 1929–1939. [CrossRef]

40. Reck, M.; Luft, A.; Szczesna, A.; Havel, L.; Kim, S.-W.; Akerley, W.; Pietanza, M.C.; Wu, Y.-L.; Zielinski, C.; Thomas, M.; et al. Phase III randomized trial of ipilimumab plus etoposide and platinum versus placebo plus etoposide and platinum in extensive-stage small-cell lung cancer. *J. Clin. Oncol.* **2016**, *34*, 3740–3748. [CrossRef]
41. Owonikoko, T.K.; Kim, H.R.; Govindan, R.; Ready, N.; Reck, M.; Peters, S.; Dakhil, S.R.; Navarro, A.; Rodriguez-Cid, J.; Schenker, M.; et al. Nivolumab (nivo) plus ipilimumab (ipi), nivo, or placebo (pbo) as maintenance therapy in patients (pts) with extensive disease small cell lung cancer (ED-SCLC) after first-line (1L) platinum-based chemotherapy (chemo): Results from the double-blind, randomized phase III CheckMate 451 study. *Ann. Oncol.* **2019**, *30* (Suppl. S2), ii77–ii80.
42. Ready, N.E.; Ott, P.A.; Hellmann, M.D.; Zugazagoitia, J.; Hann, C.L.; de Braud, F.; Antonia, S.J.; Ascierto, P.A.; Moreno, V.; Atmaca, A.; et al. Nivolumab Monotherapy and Nivolumab Plus Ipilimumab in Recurrent Small Cell Lung Cancer: Results from the CheckMate 032 Randomized Cohort. *J. Thorac. Oncol.* **2020**, *15*, 426–435. [CrossRef]
43. Ott, P.A.; Elez, E.; Hiret, S.; Kim, D.-W.; Morosky, A.; Saraf, S.; Piperdi, B.; Mehnert, J.M. Pembrolizumab in patients with extensive-stage small-cell lung cancer: Results from the phase Ib KEYNOTE-028 study. *J. Clin. Oncol.* **2017**, *35*, 3823–3829. [CrossRef]
44. Chung, H.C.; Lopez-Martin, J.A.; Kao, S.C.-H.; Miller, W.H.; Ros, W.; Gao, B.; Marabelle, A.; Gottfried, M.; Zer, A.; Delord, J.-P.; et al. Phase 2 study of pembrolizumab in advanced small-cell lung cancer (SCLC): KEYNOTE-158. *J. Clin. Oncol.* **2018**, *15*, 8506. [CrossRef]
45. Rudin, C.M.; Poirier, J.T. Small-cell lung cancer in 2016: Shining light on novel targets and therapies. *Nat. Rev. Clin. Oncol.* **2017**, *14*, 75–76. [CrossRef] [PubMed]
46. Miller, C.W.; Simon, K.; Aslo, A.; Kok, Y.; Yokota, J.; Buys, C.H.; Terada, M.; Koeffler, H.P. p53 mutations in human lung tumors. *Cancer Res.* **1992**, *52*, 1695–1698. [PubMed]
47. Takahashi, T.; Takahashi, T.; Suzuki, H.; Hida, T.; Sekido, Y.; Ariyoshi, Y.; Ueda, R. The p53 gene is very frequently mutated in small-cell lung cancer with a distinct nucleotide substitution pattern. *Oncogene* **1991**, *6*, 1775–1778. [PubMed]
48. Helin, K.; Holm, K.; Niebuhr, A.; Eiberg, H.; Tommerup, N.; Hougaard, S.; Poulsen, H.S.; Spang-Thomsen, M.; Norgaard, P. Loss of the retinoblastoma protein-related p130 protein in small cell lung carcinoma. *Proc. Natl. Acad. Sci. USA* **1997**, *94*, 6933–6938. [CrossRef] [PubMed]
49. Kaye, F.J. RB and cyclin dependent kinase pathways: Defining a distinction between RB and p16 loss in lung cancer. *Oncogene* **2002**, *21*, 6908–6914. [CrossRef]
50. Wistuba, I.I.; Behrens, C.; Virmani, A.K.; Mele, G.; Milchgrub, S.; Girard, L.; Fondon, J.W., 3rd; Garner, H.R.; McKay, B.; Latif, F.; et al. High resolution chromosome 3p allelotyping of human lung cancer and preneoplastic/preinvasive bronchial epithelium reveals multiple, discontinuous sites of 3p allele loss and 3 regions of frequent breakpoints. *Cancer Res.* **2000**, *60*, 1949–1960.
51. Wistuba, I.I.; Berry, J.; Behrens, C.; Maitra, A.; Shivapurkar, N.; Milchgrub, S.; Mackay, B.; Minna, J.D.; Gazdar, A.F. Molecular changes in the bronchial epithelium of patients with small cell lung cancer. *Clin. Cancer Res.* **2000**, *6*, 2604–2610.
52. Bordi, P.; Tiseo, M.; Barbieri, F.; Bavieri, M.; Sartori, G.; Marchetti, A.; Buttitta, F.; Bortesi, B.; Ambrosini-Spaltro, A.; Gnetti, L.; et al. Gene mutations in small-cell lung cancer (SCLC): Results of a panel of 6 genes in a cohort of Italian patients. *Lung Cancer* **2014**, *86*, 324–328. [CrossRef]
53. Ross, J.S.; Wang, K.; Elkadi, O.R.; Tarasen, A.; Foulke, L.; Sheehan, C.E.; Otto, G.A.; Palmer, G.; Yelensky, R.; Lipson, D.; et al. Next-generation sequencing reveals frequent consistent genomic alterations in small cell undifferentiated lung cancer. *J. Clin. Pathol.* **2014**, *67*, 772–776. [CrossRef]
54. Wakuda, K.; Kenmotsu, H.; Serizawa, M.; Koh, Y.; Isaka, M.; Takahashi, S.; Ono, A.; Taira, T.; Naito, T.; Murakami, H.; et al. Molecular profiling of small cell lung cancer in a Japanese cohort. *Lung Cancer* **2014**, *84*, 139–144. [CrossRef] [PubMed]
55. Metro, G.; Duranti, S.; Fischer, M.J.; Cappuzzo, F.; Crinò, L. Emerging drugs for small cell lung cancer—An update. *Expert Opin. Emerg. Drugs* **2012**, *17*, 31–36. [CrossRef] [PubMed]
56. Rudin, C.M.; Durinck, S.; Stawiski, E.W.; Poirier, J.T.; Modrusan, Z.; Shames, D.S.; Bergbower, E.A.; Guan, Y.; Shin, J.; Guillory, J.; et al. Comprehensive genomic analysis identifies SOX2 as a frequently amplified gene in small-cell lung cancer. *Nat. Genet.* **2012**, *44*, 1111–1116. [CrossRef]

57. Umemura, S.; Mimaki, S.; Makinoshima, H.; Tada, S.; Ishii, G.; Ohmatsu, H.; Niho, S.; Yoh, K.; Matsumoto, S.; Takahashi, A.; et al. Therapeutic priority of the PI3K/AKT/mTOR pathway in small cell lung cancers as revealed by a comprehensive genomic analysis. *J. Thorac. Oncol.* **2014**, *9*, 1324–1331. [CrossRef] [PubMed]
58. Umemura, S.; Tsuchihara, K.; Goto, K. Genomic profiling of small-cell lung cancer: The era of targeted therapies. *Jpn. J. Clin. Oncol.* **2015**, *45*, 513–519. [CrossRef] [PubMed]
59. Badzio, A.; Wynes, M.W.; Dziadziuszko, R.; Merrick, D.T.; Pardo, M.; Rzyman, W.; Kowalczyk, A.; Singh, S.; Ranger-Moore, J.; Manriquez, G.; et al. Increased insulin-like growth factor 1 receptor protein expression and gene copy number in small cell lung cancer. *J. Thorac. Oncol.* **2010**, *5*, 1905–1911. [CrossRef] [PubMed]
60. Potti, A.; Moazzam, N.; Ramar, K.; Hanekom, D.S.; Kargas, S.; Koch, M. CD117 (c-KIT) overexpression in patients with extensive-stage small-cell lung carcinoma. *Ann. Oncol.* **2003**, *14*, 894–897. [CrossRef]
61. Park, K.S.; Martelotto, L.G.; Peifer, M.; Sos, M.L.; Karnezis, A.N.; Mahjoub, M.R.; Bernard, K.; Conklin, J.F.; Szczepny, A.; Yuan, J.; et al. A crucial requirement for Hedgehog signaling in small cell lung cancer. *Nat. Med.* **2011**, *17*, 1504–1508. [CrossRef]
62. Belani, C.P.; Dahlberg, S.E.; Rudin, C.M.; Fleisher, M.; Chen, H.X.; Takebe, N.; Ramalingam, S.S.; Schiller, J.H. Three-arm randomized phase II study of cisplatin and etoposide (CE) versus CE with either vismodegib (V) or cixutumumab (Cx) for patients with extensive stage-small cell lung cancer (ES-SCLC) (ECOG 1508). *J. Clin. Oncol.* **2013**, *31*, 7508. [CrossRef]
63. Johnson, B.E.; Fischer, T.; Fischer, B.; Dunlop, D.; Rischin, D.; Silberman, S.; Kowalski, M.O.; Sayles, D.; Dimitrijevic, S.; Fletcher, C.; et al. Phase II study of imatinib in patients with small cell lung cancer. *Clin. Cancer Res.* **2003**, *9*, 5880–5887.
64. Pandya, K.J.; Dahlberg, S.; Hidalgo, M.; Cohen, R.B.; Lee, M.W.; Schiller, J.H.; Johnson, D.H.; Eastern Cooperative Oncology Group. A randomized, phase II trial of two dose levels of temsirolimus (CCI-779) in patients with extensive-stage small cell lung cancer who have responding or stable disease after induction chemotherapy: A trial of the Eastern Cooperative Oncology Group (E1500). *J. Thorac. Oncol.* **2007**, *2*, 1036–1041. [CrossRef] [PubMed]
65. Schneider, B.J.; Kalemkerian, G.P.; Ramnath, N.; Kraut, M.J.; Wozniak, A.J.; Worden, F.P.; Ruckdeschel, J.C.; Zhang, X.; Chen, W.; Gadgeel, S.M. Phase II trial of imatinib maintenance therapy after irinotecan and cisplatin in patients with c-Kit-positive, extensive-stage small-cell lung cancer. *Clin. Lung Cancer* **2010**, *11*, 223–227. [CrossRef] [PubMed]
66. Spigel, D.R.; Hainsworth, J.D.; Simons, L.; Meng, C.; Burris, H.A., 3rd; Yardley, D.A.; Grapski, R.; Schreeder, M.; Mallidi, P.V.; Greco, F.A.; et al. Irinotecan, carboplatin, and imatinib in untreated extensive-stage small-cell lung cancer: A phase II trial of the Minnie Pearl Cancer Research Network. *J. Thorac. Oncol.* **2007**, *2*, 854–861. [CrossRef]
67. Krug, L.M.; Crapanzano, J.P.; Azzoli, C.G.; Miller, V.A.; Rizvi, N.; Gomez, J.; Kris, M.G.; Pizzo, B.; Tyson, L.; Dunne, M.; et al. Imatinib mesylate lacks activity in small cell lung carcinoma expressing c-kit protein: A phase II clinical trial. *Cancer* **2005**, *103*, 2128–2131. [CrossRef]
68. Moore, A.M.; Einhorn, L.H.; Estes, D.; Govindan, R.; Axelson, J.; Vinson, J.; Breen, T.E.; Yu, M.; Hanna, N.H. Gefitinib in patients with chemo-sensitive and chemo-refractory relapsed small cell cancers: A Hoosier Oncology Group phase II trial. *Lung Cancer* **2006**, *52*, 93–97. [CrossRef]
69. Tarhini, A.; Kotsakis, A.; Gooding, W.; Shuai, Y.; Petro, D.; Friedland, D.; Belani, C.P.; Dacic, S.; Argiris, A. Phase II study of everolimus (RAD001) in previously treated small cell lung cancer. *Clin. Cancer Res.* **2010**, *16*, 5900–5907. [CrossRef]
70. Sattler, M.; Salgia, R. Molecular and cellular biology of small cell lung cancer. *Semin. Oncol.* **2003**, *30*, 57–71. [CrossRef]
71. Bikfalvi, A.; Klein, S.; Pintucci, G.; Rifkin, D.B. Biological roles of fibroblast growth factor-2. *Endocr. Rev.* **1997**, *18*, 26–45.
72. Ruotsalainen, T.; Joensuu, H.; Mattson, K.; Salven, P. High Pretreatment Serum Concentration of Basic Fibroblast Growth Factor Is a Predictor of Poor Prognosis in Small Cell Lung Cancer. *Cancer Epidemiol. Biomark. Prev.* **2002**, *11*, 1492–1495.
73. Dai, S.; Zhou, Z.; Chen, Z.; Xu, G.; Chen, Y. Fibroblast Growth Factor Receptors (FGFRs): Structures and Small Molecule Inhibitors. *Cells* **2019**, *8*, 614. [CrossRef] [PubMed]
74. Koch, J.P.; Aebersold, D.M.; Zimmer, Y.; Medová, M. MET targeting: Time for a rematch. *Oncogene* **2020**, *39*, 2845–2862. [CrossRef] [PubMed]

75. Desai, A.; Adjei, A.A. FGFR signaling as a target for lung cancer therapy. *J. Thorac. Oncol.* **2016**, *11*, 9–20. [CrossRef] [PubMed]
76. Rudin, C.M.; Salgia, R.; Wang, X.; Hodgson, L.D.; Masters, G.A.; Green, M.; Vokes, E.E. Randomized phase II study of carboplatin and etoposide with or without the bcl-2 antisense oligonucleotide oblimersen for extensive-stage small-cell lung cancer: CALGB 30103. *J. Clin. Oncol.* **2008**, *26*, 870–876. [CrossRef] [PubMed]
77. Rudin, C.M.; Hann, C.L.; Garon, E.B.; de Oliveira, M.R.; Bonomi, P.D.; Camidge, D.R.; Chu, Q.; Giaccone, G.; Khaira, D.; Ramalingam, S.S.; et al. Phase II study of single-agent navitoclax (ABT-263) and biomarker correlates in patients with relapsed small cell lung cancer. *Clin. Cancer Res.* **2012**, *18*, 3163–3169. [CrossRef] [PubMed]
78. Lochmann, T.L.; Floros, K.V.; Naseri, M.; Powell, K.M.; Cook, W.; March, R.J.; Stein, G.T.; Greninger, P.; Maves, Y.K.; Saunders, L.R.; et al. Venetoclax is effective in small-cell lung cancers with high BCL-2 expression. *Clin. Cancer Res.* **2018**, *24*, 360–369. [CrossRef]
79. Rudin, C.M.; Poirier, J.T.; Byers, L.A.; Dive, C.; Dowlati, A.; George, J.; Heymach, J.V.; Johnson, J.E.; Lehman, J.M.; MacPherson, D.; et al. Molecular subtypes of small cell lung cancer: A synthesis of human and mouse model data. *Nat. Rev. Cancer* **2019**, *19*, 289–297. [CrossRef]
80. Simos, D.; Sajjady, G.; Sergi, M.; Liew, M.S.; Califano, R.; Ho, C.; Leighl, N.; White, S.; Summers, Y.; Petrcich, W.; et al. Third-line chemotherapy in small-cell lung cancer: An international analysis. *Clin. Lung Cancer* **2014**, *15*, 110–118. [CrossRef]
81. Sos, M.L.; Dietlein, F.; Peifer, M.; Schöttle, J.; Balke-Want, H.; Müller, C.; Koker, M.; Richters, A.; Heynck, S.; Malchers, F.; et al. A framework for identification of actionable cancer genome dependencies in small cell lung cancer. *Proc. Natl. Acad. Sci. USA* **2012**, *109*, 17034–17039. [CrossRef]
82. Mertz, J.A.; Conery, A.R.; Bryant, B.M.; Sandy, P.; Balasubramanian, S.; Mele, D.A.; Bergeron, L.; Sims, R.J., 3rd. Targeting MYC dependence in cancer by inhibiting BET bromodomains. *Proc. Natl. Acad. Sci. USA* **2011**, *108*, 16669–16674. [CrossRef]
83. Owonikoko, T.; Nackaerts, K.; Csoszi, T.; Ostoros, G.; Baik, C.; Ullmann, C.D.; Zagadailov, E.; Sheldon-Waniga, E.; Huebner, D. OA05.05 randomized phase 2 study: Alisertib (MLN8237) or placebo + paclitaxel as second-line therapy for small-cell lung cancer (SCLC). *J. Thorac. Oncol.* **2017**, *12*, S261–S262. [CrossRef]
84. Mir, S.E.; De Witt Hamer, P.C.; Krawczyk, P.M.; Balaj, L.; Claes, A.; Niers, J.M.; Van Tilborg, A.A.G.; Zwinderman, A.H.; Geerts, D.; Kaspers, G.J.L.; et al. In silico analysis of kinase expression identifies WEE1 as a gatekeeper against mitotic catastrophe in glioblastoma. *Cancer Cell* **2010**, *18*, 244–257. [CrossRef] [PubMed]
85. Sen, T.; Tong, P.; Diao, L.; Li, L.; Fan, Y.; Hoff, J.; Heymach, J.V.; Wang, J.; Byers, L.A. Targeting AXL and mTOR pathway overcomes primary and acquired resistance to WEE1 inhibition in small-cell lung cancer. *Clin. Cancer Res.* **2017**, *23*, 6239–6253. [CrossRef] [PubMed]
86. Fang, Y.; McGrail, D.J.; Sun, C.; Labrie, M.; Chen, X.; Zhang, D.; Ju, Z.; Vellano, C.P.; Lu, Y.; Li, Y.; et al. Sequential therapy with PARP and WEE1 inhibitors minimizes toxicity while maintaining efficacy. *Cancer Cell* **2019**, *35*, 851.e7–867.e7. [CrossRef] [PubMed]
87. Cardnell, R.J.; Feng, Y.; Mukherjee, S.; Diao, L.; Tong, P.; Stewart, C.A.; Masrorpour, F.; Fan, Y.; Nilsson, M.; Shen, Y.; et al. Activation of the PI3K/mTOR pathway following PARP inhibition in small cell Lung cancer. *PLoS ONE* **2016**, *11*, e0152584. [CrossRef]
88. Owonikoko, T.K.; Dahlberg, S.E.; Sica, G.L.; Wagner, L.I.; Wade, J.L.; Srkalovic, G.; Lash, B.W.; Leach, J.W.; Leal, T.B.; Aggarwal, C.; et al. Randomized phase II trial of cisplatin and etoposide in combination with veliparib or placebo for extensive-stage small-cell lung cancer: ECOG-ACRIN 2511 study. *J. Clin. Oncol.* **2018**, *3*, 222–229. [CrossRef]
89. Inno, A.; Stagno, A.; Gori, S. Schlafen-11 (SLFN11): A step forward towards personalized medicine in small-cell lung cancer? *Transl. Lung Cancer Res.* **2018**, *7* (Suppl. S4), S341–S345. [CrossRef]
90. Laird, J.H.; Lok, B.H.; Ma, J.; Bell, A.; de Stanchina, E.; Poirier, J.T.; Rudin, C.M. Talazoparib is a potent radiosensitizer in small cell lung cancer cell lines and xenografts. *Clin. Cancer Res.* **2018**, *24*, 5143–5152. [CrossRef]
91. Kunnimalaiyaan, M.; Chen, H. Tumor suppressor role of Notch-1 signaling in neuroendocrine tumors. *Oncologist* **2007**, *12*, 535–542. [CrossRef]

92. Chapman, G.; Sparrow, D.B.; Kremmer, E.; Dunwoodie, S.L. Notch inhibition by the ligand DELTA-LIKE 3 defines the mechanism of abnormal vertebral segmentation in spondylocostal dysostosis. *Hum. Mol. Genet.* **2011**, *20*, 905–916. [CrossRef]
93. Saunders, L.R.; Bankovich, A.J.; Anderson, W.C.; Aujay, M.A.; Bheddah, S.; Black, K.; Desai, R.; Escarpe, P.A.; Hampl, J.; Laysang, A.; et al. A DLL3-targeted antibody-drug conjugate eradicates high-grade pulmonary neuroendocrine tumor initiating cells in vivo. *Sci. Transl. Med.* **2015**, *7*, 302ra136. [CrossRef]
94. Morgenszter, D.; Besse, B.; Greillier, L.; Santana-Davila, R.; Ready, N.; Hann, C.L.; Glisson, B.S.; Farago, A.F.; Dowlati, A.; Rudin, C.M.; et al. Efficacy and safety of rovalpituzumab tesirine in third-line and beyond patients with DLL3-Expressing, relapsed/refractory small-cell lung cancer: Results from the phase II trinity study. *Clin. Cancer Res.* **2019**, *25*, 6958–6966. [CrossRef] [PubMed]
95. Mullard, A. Cancer stem cell candidate Rova-T discontinued. *Nat. Rev. Drug Discov.* **2019**, *18*, 814. [CrossRef] [PubMed]
96. Mumby, M. PP2A: Unveiling a reluctant tumor suppressor. *Cell* **2007**, *130*, 21–24. [CrossRef] [PubMed]
97. Perrotti, D.; Neviani, P. Protein phosphatase 2A: A target for anticancer therapy. *Lancet Oncol.* **2013**, *14*, e229–e238. [CrossRef]
98. Neviani, P.; Perrotti, D. SETting OP449 into the PP2A-activating drug family. *Clin. Cancer Res.* **2014**, *20*, 2026–2028. [CrossRef] [PubMed]
99. Matsuoka, Y.; Nagahara, Y.; Ikekita, M.; Shinomiya, T. A novel immunosuppressive agent FTY720 induced Akt dephosphorylation in leukemia cells. *Br. J. Pharmacol.* **2003**, *138*, 1303–1312. [CrossRef]
100. Cristóbal, I.; Madoz-Gúrpide, J.; Manso, R.; González-Alonso, P.; Rojo, F.; García-Foncillas, J. Potential anti-tumor effects of FTY720 associated with PP2A activation: A brief review. *Curr. Med. Res. Opin.* **2016**, *32*, 1137–1141. [CrossRef]
101. Gutierrez, A.; Pan, L.; Groen, R.W.J.; Baleydier, F.; Kentsis, A.; Marineau, J.; Grebliunaite, R.; Kozakewich, E.; Reed, C.; Pflumio, F.; et al. Phenothiazines induce PP2A-mediated apoptosis in T cell acute lymphoblastic leukemia. *J. Clin. Investig.* **2014**, *124*, 644–655. [CrossRef]
102. Kauko, O.; O'Connor, C.M.; Kulesskiy, E.; Sangodkar, J.; Aakula, A.; Izadmehr, S.; Yetukuri, L.; Yadav, B.; Padzik, A.; Laajala, T.D.; et al. PP2A inhibition is a druggable MEK inhibitor resistance mechanism in KRAS-mutant lung cancer cells. *Sci. Transl. Med.* **2018**, *10*, eaaq1093. [CrossRef]
103. Shimizu, T.; Tolcher, A.W.; Papadopoulos, K.P.; Beeram, M.; Rasco, D.W.; Smith, L.S.; Gunn, S.; Smetzer, L.; Mays, T.A.; Kaiser, B.; et al. The clinical effect of the dual-targeting strategy involving PI3K/AKT/mTOR and RAS/MEK/ERK pathways in patients with advanced cancer. *Clin. Cancer Res.* **2012**, *18*, 2316–2325. [CrossRef]
104. Chung, V.; Mansfield, A.S.; Braiteh, F.; Richards, D.; Durivage, H.; Ungerleider, R.S.; Johnson, F.; Kovach, J.S. Safety, Tolerability, and Preliminary Activity of LB-100, an Inhibitor of Protein Phosphatase 2A, in Patients with Relapsed Solid Tumors: An Open-Label, Dose Escalation, First-in-Human, Phase I Trial. *Clin. Cancer Res.* **2017**, *23*, 3277–3284. [CrossRef] [PubMed]
105. Ho, W.S.; Wang, H.; Maggio, D.; Kovach, J.S.; Zhang, Q.; Song, Q.; Marincola, F.M.; Heiss, J.D.; Gilbert, M.R.; Lu, R.; et al. Pharmacologic inhibition of protein phosphatase-2A achieves durable immune-mediated antitumor activity when combined with PD-1 blockade. *Nat. Commun.* **2018**, *9*, 2126. [CrossRef] [PubMed]
106. Taffs, R.E.; Redegeld, F.A.; Sitkovsky, M.V. Modulation of cytolytic T lymphocyte functions by an inhibitor of serine/threonine phosphatase, okadaic acid. Enhancement of cytolytic T lymphocyte-mediated cytotoxicity. *J. Immunol.* **1991**, *147*, 722–728. [PubMed]
107. Cui, J.; Wang, H.; Medina, R.; Zhang, Q.; Xu, C.; Indig, I.H.; Zhou, J.; Song, Q.; Dmitriev, P.; Sun, M.Y.; et al. Inhibition of PP2A with LB-100 Enhances Efficacy of CAR-T Cell Therapy Against Glioblastoma. *Cancers* **2020**, *12*, 139. [CrossRef] [PubMed]
108. Hong, C.S.; Ho, W.; Zhang, C.; Yang, C.; Elder, J.B.; Zhuang, Z. LB100, a small molecule inhibitor of PP2A with potent chemo- and radio-sensitizing potential. *Cancer Biol. Ther.* **2015**, *16*, 821–833. [CrossRef]
109. Cui, Q.; Wen, S.; Huang, P. Targeting cancer cell mitochondria as a therapeutic approach: Recent updates. *Future Med. Chem.* **2017**, *9*, 929–949. [CrossRef]
110. Kalyanaraman, B.; Cheng, G.; Hardy, M.; Quari, M.; Lopez, M.; Joseph, J.; Zielonka, J.; Dwinell, M.B. A review of the basics of mitochondrial bioenergetics, metabolism, and related signaling pathways in cancer cells: Therapeutic targeting of tumor mitochondria with lipophilic cationic compounds. *Redox Biol.* **2018**, *14*, 316–327. [CrossRef]

111. Hamilton, E.P.; Birrer, M.J.; DiCarlo, B.A.; Gaillard, S.; Martin, L.P.; Nemunaitis, J.J.; Perez, R.P.; Schilder, R.J.; Annunziata, C.M.; Begley, C.G.; et al. A phase 1b, open-label, non-randomized multicenter study of birinapant in combination with conatumumab in subjects with relapsed epithelial ovarian cancer, primary peritoneal cancer, or fallopian tube cancer. *J. Clin. Oncol.* **2015**, *33*, 5571. [CrossRef]
112. Hurwitz, H.I.; Smith, D.C.; Pitot, H.C.; Brill, J.M.; Chugh, R.; Rouits, E.; Rubin, J.; Strickler, J.; Vuagniaux, G.; Sorensen, J.M.; et al. Safety, pharmacokinetics and pharmacodynamics properties of oral DEBIO1143 (AT-406) in patients with advanced cancer: Results of a first-in-man study. *Cancer Chemother. Pharmacol.* **2015**, *75*, 851–859. [CrossRef]
113. Bendell, J.C.; Patel, M.R.; Infante, J.R.; Kurkjian, C.D.; Jones, S.F.; Pant, S.; Burris, H.A., 3rd; Moreno, O.; Esquibel, V.; Levin, W.; et al. Phase 1, open-label, dose escalation, safety, and pharmacokinetics study of ME-344 as a single agent in patients with refractory solid tumors. *Cancer* **2015**, *121*, 1056–1063. [CrossRef]
114. Diamond, J.R.; Goff, B.; Forster, M.D.; Bendell, J.C.; Britten, C.D.; Gordon, M.S.; Gabra, H.; Waterhouse, D.M.; Poole, M.; Camidge, D.R.; et al. Phase Ib study of the mitochondrial inhibitor ME-344 plus topotecan in patients with previously treated, locally advanced or metastatic small cell lung, ovarian and cervical cancers. *Investig. New Drugs* **2017**, *35*, 627–633. [CrossRef] [PubMed]
115. Greeno, E.; Borazanci, E.H.; Gockerman, J.P.; Korn, R.L.; Saluja, A.; VonHoff, D.D. Phase I dose escalation and pharmokinetic study of a modified schedule of 14-ophosphonooxymethyltriptolide. *J. Clin. Oncol.* **2016**, *34*, TPS472. [CrossRef]
116. Stein, M.N.; Bertino, J.R.; Kaufman, H.L.; Mayer, T.; Moss, R.; Silk, A.; Chan, N.; Malhotra, J.; Rodriguez, L.; Aisner, J.; et al. First-in-human clinical trial of oral ONC201 in patients with refractory solid tumors. *Clin. Cancer Res.* **2017**, *23*, 4163–4169. [CrossRef] [PubMed]
117. Roth, K.G.; Mambetsariev, I.; Kulkarni, P.; Salgia, R. The mitochondrion as an emerging therapeutic target in cancer. *Trends Mol. Med.* **2020**, *26*, 119–134. [CrossRef] [PubMed]
118. Lobo, N.A.; Shimono, Y.; Qian, D.; Clarke, M.F. The biology of cancer stem cells. *Annu. Rev. Cell Dev. Biol.* **2007**, *23*, 675–699. [CrossRef]
119. Yang, Y.M.; Chang, J.W. Current status and issues in cancer stem cell study. *Cancer Investig.* **2008**, *26*, 741–755. [CrossRef]
120. Wicha, M.S.; Liu, S.; Dontu, G. Cancer stem cells: An old idea—A paradigm shift. *Cancer Res.* **2006**, *66*, 1883–1896. [CrossRef]
121. Takebe, N.; Miele, L.; Harris, P.J.; Jeong, W.; Bando, H.; Kahn, M.; Yang, S.X.; Ivy, S.P. Targeting Notch, Hedgehog, and Wnt pathways in cancer stem cells: Clinical update. *Nat. Rev. Clin. Oncol.* **2015**, *12*, 445–464. [CrossRef]
122. Codony-Servat, J.; Verlicchi, A.; Rosell, R. Cancer stem cells in small cell lung cancer. *Transl. Lung Cancer Res.* **2016**, *5*, 16–25.
123. Stewart, C.A.; Byers, L.A. Altering the course of small cell lung cancer: Targeting cancer stem cells via LSD1 inhibition. *Cancer Cell* **2015**, *28*, 4–6. [CrossRef]
124. Bauer, T.M.; Besse, B.; Martinez-Marti, A.; Trigo, J.M.; Moreno, V.; Garrido, P.; Ferron-Brady, G.; Wu, Y.; Park, J.; Collingwood, T.; et al. Phase I, Open-Label, Dose-Escalation Study of the Safety, Pharmacokinetics, Pharmacodynamics, and Efficacy of GSK2879552 in Relapsed/Refractory SCLC. *J. Thorac. Oncol.* **2019**, *14*, 1828–1838. [CrossRef] [PubMed]
125. Mohammad, H.P.; Kruger, R.G. Antitumor activity of LSD1 inhibitors in Lung cancer. *Mol. Cell Oncol.* **2016**, *3*, e1117700. [CrossRef] [PubMed]
126. Ropacki, M.; Navarro, A.; Maes, T.; Gutierrez, S.; Bullock, R.; Buesa, C. P2.12-04 CLEPSIDRA: A Phase II Trial Combining Iadademstat with Platinum-Etoposide in Platinum-Sensitive Relapsed SCLC Patients. *J. Thorac. Oncol.* **2019**, *14*, S813. [CrossRef]
127. Sheng, W.; LaFleur, M.W.; Nguyen, T.H.; Chen, S.; Chakravarthy, A.; Conway, J.R.; Li, Y.; Chen, H.; Yang, H.; Hsu, P.-H.; et al. LSD1 ablation stimulates anti-tumor immunity and enables checkpoint blockade. *Cell* **2018**, *174*, 549–563. [CrossRef]
128. Morgensztern, D.; Rose, M.; Waqar, S.N.; Morris, J.; Ma, P.C.; Reid, T.; Brzezniak, C.E.; Zeman, K.G.; Padmanabhan, A.; Hirth, J.; et al. RRx-001 followed by platinum plus etoposide in patients with previously treated small-cell lung cancer. *Br. J. Cancer* **2019**, *121*, 211–217. [CrossRef] [PubMed]

129. Weiskopf, K.; Jahchan, N.S.; Schnorr, P.J.; Cristea, S.; Ring, A.M.; Maute, R.L.; Volkmer, A.K.; Volkmer, J.-P.; Liu, J.; Lim, J.S.; et al. CD47-blocking immunotherapies stimulate macrophage-mediated destruction of small-cell lung cancer. *J. Clin. Investig.* **2016**, *126*, 2610–2620. [CrossRef]
130. Bonanno, L.; Pavan, A.; Dieci, M.V.; Di Liso, E.; Schiavon, M.; Comacchio, G.; Attili, I.; Pasello, G.; Calabrese, F.; Rea, F.; et al. The role of immune microenvironment in small-cell lung cancer: Distribution of PD-L1 expression and prognostic role of FOXP3-positive tumour infiltrating lymphocytes. *Eur. J. Cancer* **2018**, *101*, 191–200. [CrossRef]
131. Antonia, S.J.; López-Martin, J.A.; Bendell, J.; Ott, P.A.; Taylor, M.; Eder, J.P.; Jäger, D.; Pietanza, M.C.; Le, D.T.; de Braud, F.; et al. Nivolumab alone and nivolumab plus ipilimumab in recurrent small-cell lung cancer (CheckMate 032): A multicentre, open-label, phase 1/2 trial. *Lancet Oncol.* **2016**, *17*, 883–895. [CrossRef]
132. Goodman, A.M.; Kato, S.; Bazhenova, L.; Patel, S.P.; Frampton, G.M.; Miller, V.; Stephens, P.J.; Daniels, G.A.; Kurzrock, R. Tumor mutational burden as an independent predictor of response to immunotherapy in diverse cancers. *Mol. Cancer Ther.* **2017**, *16*, 2598–2608. [CrossRef]
133. Hellmann, M.D.; Callahan, M.K.; Awad, M.M.; Calvo, E.; Ascierto, P.A.; Atmaca, A.; Rizvi, N.A.; Hirsch, F.R.; Selvaggi, G.; Szustakowski, J.; et al. Tumor mutational burden and efficacy of Nivolumab monotherapy and in combination with ipilimumab in small-cell lung cancer. *Cancer Cell* **2018**, *33*, 853.e4–861.e4. [CrossRef]
134. Hou, J.M.; Krebs, M.G.; Lancashire, L.; Sloane, R.; Backen, A.; Swain, R.K.; Priest, L.J.; Greystoke, A.; Zhou, C.; Morris, K.; et al. Clinical significance and molecular characteristics of circulating tumor cells and circulating tumor microemboli in patients with small-cell lung cancer. *J. Clin. Oncol.* **2012**, *30*, 525–532. [CrossRef] [PubMed]
135. Belani, C.P.; Dahlberg, S.E.; Rudin, C.M.; Fleisher, M.; Chen, H.X.; Takebe, N.; Velasco, M.R., Jr.; Tester, W.J.; Sturtz, K.; Hann, C.L.; et al. Vismodegib or cixutumumab in combination with standard chemotherapy for patients with extensive-stage small cell lung cancer: A trial of the ECOG-ACRIN Cancer Research Group (E1508). *Cancer* **2016**, *122*, 2371–2378. [CrossRef] [PubMed]
136. Pietanza, M.C.; Litvak, A.M.; Varghese, A.M.; Krug, L.M.; Fleisher, M.; Teitcher, J.B.; Holodny, A.I.; Sima, C.S.; Woo, K.M.; Ng, K.K.; et al. A phase I trial of the Hedgehog inhibitor, sonidegib (LDE225), in combination with etoposide and cisplatin for the initial treatment of extensive stage small cell lung cancer. *Lung Cancer* **2016**, *99*, 23–30. [CrossRef] [PubMed]
137. Almodovar, K.; Iams, W.T.; Meador, C.B.; Zhao, Z.; York, S.; Horn, L.; Yan, Y.; Hernandez, J.; Chen, H.; Shyr, Y.; et al. Longitudinal cell-free DNA analysis in patients with small cell lung cancer reveals dynamic insights into treatment efficacy and disease relapse. *J. Thorac. Oncol.* **2018**, *13*, 112–123. [CrossRef]
138. Paz-Ares, L.G.; Trigo Perez, J.M.; Besse, B.; Moreno, V.; Lopez, R.; Sala, M.A.; Aix, S.P.; Fernandez, C.M.; Siguero, M.; Kahatt, C.M.; et al. Efficacy and safety profile of lurbinectedin in second-line SCLC patients: Results from a phase II single-agent trial. *J. Clin. Oncol.* **2019**, *37*, 8506. [CrossRef]
139. Kontogianni, K.; Nicholson, A.G.; Butcher, D.; Sheppard, M.N. CD56: A useful tool for the diagnosis of small cell lung carcinomas on biopsies with extensive crush artefact. *J. Clin. Pathol.* **2005**, *58*, 978–980. [CrossRef]
140. Yu, L.; Lu, Y.; Yao, Y.; Liu, Y.; Wang, Y.; Lai, Q.; Zhang, R.; Li, W.; Wang, R.; Fu, Y.; et al. Promiximab-duocarmycin, a new CD56 antibody-drug conjugates, is highly efficacious in small cell lung cancer xenograft models. *Oncotarget* **2017**, *9*, 5197–5207. [CrossRef]
141. Zaman, S.; Jadid, H.; Denson, A.C.; Gray, J.E. Targeting Trop-2 in solid tumors: Future prospects. *Onco Targets Ther.* **2019**, *12*, 1781–1790. [CrossRef]
142. Ocean, A.J.; Starodub, A.N.; Bardia, A.; Vahdat, L.T.; Isakoff, S.J.; Guarino, M.; Messersmith, W.A.; Picozzi, V.J.; Mayer, I.A.; Wegener, W.A.; et al. Sacituzumab govitecan (IMMU-132), an Anti-Trop-2-SN-38 antibody-drug conjugate for the treatment of diverse epithelial cancers: Safety and pharmacokinetics. *Cancer* **2017**, *123*, 3843–3854. [CrossRef]
143. Simone, C.B., 2nd; Berman, A.T.; Jabbour, S.K. Harnessing the potential synergy of combining radiation therapy and immunotherapy for thoracic malignancies. *Transl. Lung Cancer Res.* **2017**, *6*, 109–112. [CrossRef]
144. McColl, K.; Wildey, G.; Sakre, N.; Lipka, M.B.; Behtaj, M.; Kresak, A.; Chen, Y.; Yang, M.; Velcheti, V.; Fu, P.; et al. Reciprocal expression of INSM1 and YAP1 defines subgroups in small cell lung cancer. *Oncotarget* **2017**, *8*, 73745–73756. [CrossRef] [PubMed]
145. Huang, Y.H.; Klingbeil, O.; He, X.Y.; Wu, X.S.; Arun, G.; Lu, B.; Somerville, T.; Milazzo, J.P.; Wilkinson, J.E.; Demerdash, O.E.; et al. POU2F3 is a master regulator of a tuft cell-like variant of small cell lung cancer. *Genes Dev.* **2018**, *32*, 915–928. [CrossRef] [PubMed]

146. Polley, E.; Kunkel, M.; Evans, D.; Silvers, T.; Delosh, R.; Laudeman, J.; Ogle, C.; Reinhart, R.; Selby, M.; Connelly, J.; et al. Small cell lung cancer screen of oncology drugs, investigational agents, and gene and microRNA expression. *J. Natl. Cancer Inst.* **2016**, *108*, djw122. [CrossRef] [PubMed]
147. Barretina, J.; Caponigro, G.; Stransky, N.; Venkatesan, K.; Margolin, A.A.; Kim, S.; Wilson, C.J.; Lehár, J.; Kryukov, G.V.; Sonkin, D.; et al. The Cancer Cell Line Encyclopedia enables predictive modelling of anticancer drug sensitivity. *Nature* **2012**, *483*, 603–607. [CrossRef]
148. Mollaoglu, G.; Guthrie, M.R.; Böhm, S.; Brägelmann, J.; Can, I.; Ballieu, P.M.; Marx, A.; George, J.; Heinen, C.; Chalishazar, M.D.; et al. MYC drives progression of small cell lung cancer to a variant neuroendocrine subtype with vulnerability to aurora kinase inhibition. *Cancer Cell* **2017**, *31*, 270–285. [CrossRef]
149. Sonkin, D.; Vural, S.; Thomas, A.; Teicher, B.A. Neuroendocrine negative SCLC is mostly RB1 WT and may be sensitive to CDK4/6 inhibition: Supplemental Tables. *bioRxiv* **2019**. [CrossRef]

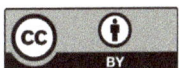

© 2020 by the authors. Licensee MDPI, Basel, Switzerland. This article is an open access article distributed under the terms and conditions of the Creative Commons Attribution (CC BY) license (http://creativecommons.org/licenses/by/4.0/).

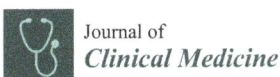

Review

The Community Oncology and Academic Medical Center Alliance in the Age of Precision Medicine: Cancer Genetics and Genomics Considerations

Marilena Melas [1], Shanmuga Subbiah [2], Siamak Saadat [3], Swapnil Rajurkar [4] and Kevin J. McDonnell [5,6,*

[1] The Steve and Cindy Rasmussen Institute for Genomic Medicine, Nationwide Children's Hospital, Columbus, OH 43205, USA; Marilena.Melas@nationwidechildrens.org
[2] Department of Medical Oncology and Therapeutics Research, City of Hope Comprehensive Cancer Center, Glendora, CA 91741, USA; ssubbiah@coh.org
[3] Department of Medical Oncology and Therapeutics Research, City of Hope Comprehensive Cancer Center, Colton, CA 92324, USA; ssaadat@coh.org
[4] Department of Medical Oncology and Therapeutics Research, City of Hope Comprehensive Cancer Center, Upland, CA 91786, USA; srajurkar@coh.org
[5] Department of Medical Oncology and Therapeutics Research, City of Hope Comprehensive Cancer Center and Beckman Research Institute, Duarte, CA 91010, USA
[6] Center for Precision Medicine, City of Hope Comprehensive Cancer Center, Duarte, CA 91010, USA
* Correspondence: kemcdonnell@coh.org

Received: 13 June 2020; Accepted: 2 July 2020; Published: 6 July 2020

Abstract: Recent public policy, governmental regulatory and economic trends have motivated the establishment and deepening of community health and academic medical center alliances. Accordingly, community oncology practices now deliver a significant portion of their oncology care in association with academic cancer centers. In the age of precision medicine, this alliance has acquired critical importance; novel advances in nucleic acid sequencing, the generation and analysis of immense data sets, the changing clinical landscape of hereditary cancer predisposition and ongoing discovery of novel, targeted therapies challenge community-based oncologists to deliver molecularly-informed health care. The active engagement of community oncology practices with academic partners helps with meeting these challenges; community/academic alliances result in improved cancer patient care and provider efficacy. Here, we review the community oncology and academic medical center alliance. We examine how practitioners may leverage academic center precision medicine-based cancer genetics and genomics programs to advance their patients' needs. We highlight a number of project initiatives at the City of Hope Comprehensive Cancer Center that seek to optimize community oncology and academic cancer center precision medicine interactions.

Keywords: community oncology; academic cancer center; precision medicine; cancer genetics; cancer genomics

1. Introduction

Historically, the practice and delivery of healthcare in the community contrasted significantly with medical care provided at the academic medical center [1,2]. These differences manifested across specialty practices, including oncology [3,4]. Rapid advances in molecular diagnostics, the advent of targeted therapies and the introduction of precision medicine amplified differences between community and academic oncology practices [5,6]. Reversing this historical divide, however, new financial realities, public policy initiatives and legislative mandateshave forced community oncologists and academic cancer centers to more closely align their healthcare efforts [7]. This forced alliance has lessened the separation between community and academic oncology practices and permitted broader access and utilization of precision medicine-based cancer genetics services and tumor genomic analyses. The alliance between community and academic oncology expands the capabilities and effectiveness of the community practitioner, reinforces the mission of the academic cancer center and, ultimately, secures better oncologic care for the cancer patient.

2. The Emergence and Evolution of the Community Health Care and Academic Medical Center Alliance

A number of key distinctions differentiate the medical care provided at community health centers (CHCs) versus academic health centers (AHCs); these differences result in complementary advantages. The overwhelming majority of patients receive their healthcare through CHCs; the CHC patient population typically exhibits great diversity across economic, racial, ethnic and social spectra [8]. CHCs offer their patients increased accessibility and enhanced client engagement [9]. In contrast, AHCs, characteristically, have focused on specialty medical care, biomedical research, the education and training of health care professionals and the stopgap provision of health care to uninsured and destitute populations [10]. These activities underlie the strengths of AHCs. These strengths include the presence of medical expertise, scientific innovation and clinical trial availability; additionally, AHCs possess unique physical resources such as libraries, computerized database management and informatics infrastructure, research laboratories and emergency room facilities [11,12]. Leveraging these strengths, AHCs have established their reputations and acquired leadership roles in shaping medical care and policy [10].

Until two decades ago, CHCs and AHCs functioned largely in parallel, without administrative or operational intersection. A variety of recent economic, social and regulatory circumstances, however, diminished the independence of AHCs. With the rise of community-based health care markets, particularly managed care plans, many of the operations traditionally carried out at AHCs shifted to CHCs; this shift often undercut the previously reliable revenue streams of AHCs. This situation forced reconsideration of the AHC financial model and provided impetus for the implementation of more efficient, cost-effective health care delivery strategies [13–18]. At the same time, governmental funding agencies, to ensure faithful representation of population diseases, placed a premium on the inclusion of community patients into research protocols. These agencies also issued directives to AHCs to provide comprehensive population care and mandated the formal reporting of AHC involvement with community patient populations [19–25]. Overall, these influences forced AHCs to redefine their core mission with a new emphasis on the integration of the CHC and their patient populations [26–28]. Given their previous work in shaping medical policy, their stewardship of medical education, and their diverse and extensive resources, AHCs readily assumed a leadership role in the restructuring of the CHC/AHC relationship and the creation of integrated partnerships [2,29–35].

The alliance between CHCs and AHCs provides advantages to both partners. CHCs and AHCs enjoy better positioning within the healthcare marketplace. The improved marketplace positioning results primarily from economy of scale pricing that accompanies the integration and expansion of patient services, procedures and therapeutics; the alliance secures for both partners more stable financial footings [36]. The alliance makes possible specific benefits for the CHC. This alliance permits the CHC more direct access to AHC-generated experimental therapeutics, clinical trials, translational research, medical devices and protocols [37]. Further, evidence suggests that affiliation with an AHC often enhances the prestige and attractiveness of the CHC, increases patient and clinical staff retention, fosters more opportunity for continuing professional development, frequently results in greater professional satisfaction and has the potential to enhance the quality and efficacy of the CHC [38–40]. For the AHC, partnerships with a CHC allow for enhanced opportunities to interact more tangibly with the community patient population and expand and diversify patient pools for translational research and clinical trial enrollment; partnerships also increase the ability of AHCs to mitigate outcomes and patient access disparities [41]. Multiple examples of successful CHC/AHC partnerships exist; they serve as models for the feasibility and potential future CHC/AHC partnerships [42–44].

3. Community Oncology and Academic Cancer Center Alliance

The integration of CHCs with AHCs most tangibly manifests as practice changes within specific departments, including, prominently, medical oncology [45–51]. During recent years cancer care has transitioned from primarily private, CHC-based oncology practices to AHC-affiliated and -integrated network cancer centers [51–55]. This transition has advantaged the community cancer patient as the services associated with the academic cancer center provide added value.

At the City of Hope Comprehensive Cancer Center (COHCCC), patients identify a number of key value elements associated with the academic cancer center including access to cancer disease specialists, the availability of clinical, translational and basic science researchers, potential for clinical trial participation and enhanced comprehensive care coordinated through multidisciplinary clinical teams [56].

Across a broad range of cancers, patients experience improved survival when receiving treatment at an academic cancer center or at a community hospital associated with an AHC [57–64]. Academic cancer centers provide additional value to community practices through the discovery and provision of novel drugs, experimental medical devices, treatment protocols and technological advancements [65–71]. Reciprocally, academic cancer centers benefit from their alliance with community oncology practices by expanding clinical trial portfolios [72–74], increasing patient diversity in cancer translational and basic research initiatives [75–79], enhancing cancer center core mission accomplishment through community cancer patient engagement [80] and reducing cancer care costs resulting from increased patient volumes [81].

The introduction of new technologies and scientific techniques underscores the importance and potential of the alliance between community oncology practices and academic cancer centers. Specifically, recent advances in genetics and tumor genomics have provided a foundation for the emergence of precision oncology; the community/academic oncology alliance promises to accelerate significantly the clinical utility of precision oncology for the cancer care of community patients [82–85].

4. The Age of Precision Oncology

Cancers exhibit highly complex genomic and epigenomic alterations; these alterations dictate their overall phenotypic behavior that includes growth characteristics, metastatic potential, interplay between cells and microenvironmental interactions and responses. Over the past several decades, scientific strategies to prevent, diagnose and treat cancer have radically shifted from histology-based to genomically- and immunologically-informed approaches [86].

Since completion of the Human Genome Project in 2003 [87], a series of convergent technological advances resulted from academic-based initiatives. These advances include the introduction and adoption of next generation nucleic acid sequencing (NGS), exponential improvements in computer hardware capabilities, optimization of data processing approaches, evolution of increasingly sophisticated computational biological methods and the discovery and utilization of targeted cancer therapies. Together these advances made possible precision medicine and, more exactly, precision oncology [82,88–90].

NGS arose from innovative DNA sequencing methodologies, most notably massively parallel signature sequencing [91,92]. NGS permits tractable high throughput sequencing of immensely large and complex DNA samples such as whole human exomes and genomes [93,94]. Geneticists first employed NGS to sequence accurately and rapidly the human germline genome [95], allowing insights into the cause of inherited disease [96,97]; investigators then extended the technology to sequence somatic cancer genomes [98]. Scientists further refined the applications of NGS technology. New applications permitted assessment of not only single nucleotide variation and nucleotide insertions and deletions, but also the transcriptome to assess gene expression [99–101], copy number variation [102], complex genomic structural variation [103], protein-DNA interactions [104], targetable epigenetic alterations [105] and epigenetic mechanisms regulating 3D genome structure [106].

In addition to examining tumor genomics, there arose an interest in understanding the immune profiles of the tumor and its microenvironment using NGS; in part, this interest developed from the recognition that tumor genomic changes frequently result in the production of unique, highly immunogenic neoantigens that render the tumor vulnerable to immune surveillance and destruction [107,108]. With the appreciation that the immune system plays an important role in cancer initiation and progression, there has also occurred new interest in targeted therapies aimed at activation of the immune axis [109,110].

NGS generates enormous caches of data; use of these immense data sets for precision oncology requires ever increasing levels of computer hardware performance. Employment of Dennard scaling [111] and multicore architectures [112] have sustained exponential increases in computer chip performance [113–115]. Data processing innovations have included parallel algorithm implementation [116] and parallel data computing [117]; such innovations have force multiplied the efficiency and speed of computation. These approaches allow data analysts to keep pace with the ever increasing information workloads of precision oncology [118].

The realization of precision oncology required adoption of computational biological approaches. The creation of computational biology as an independent academic discipline resulted from the complexity and size of biological data sets. In the case of NGS, the sheer number of nucleotides reads, the task of aligning these reads to reference sequences, predicting functional consequences of genomic variation and the translation of these findings into clinically actionable information necessitated computational biological expertise [119–122]. Computational biological analysis now constitutes an integral element of the data workflow in precision oncology [123–126]; effective clinical translation depends inextricably upon the availability of these computational resources [127–130].

In the early 1970's, Drs. Janet Rowley, Peter Nowell and Alfred Knudson, studying leukemia cell chromosomes under the microscope, suggested that a specific chromosomal translocation that resulted in the formation of the BCR-ABL fusion oncogene caused chronic myelogenous leukemia (CML); this observation established a foundation for clinical cancer genomics [131]. Oncogenic proteins consequently became a focus of therapeutic drug design; targeted therapies aimed to suppress the aberrant functions of these proteins in order to inhibit tumor progression [132,133].

The successful harnessing of precision therapeutics in oncology ultimately relies upon the availability and efficacy of targeted agents. The discovery that imatinib effectively treats CML harboring the BCR-ABL fusion protein [134] led to the drug's FDA approval in 2001 [135], demonstrated the utility of targeted cancer therapy [136,137], kindled enthusiasm for the identification of other genetically vulnerable cancers and their treatments [90,138] and underscored the clinical value and potential of precision oncology [98,139,140]. Since the success of imatinib, the FDA has approved a multitude of additional therapies to target molecularly-altered cancers [141,142].

The clinical provision of precision oncology requires multidisciplinary support [143]; the complexity of this support will become more intense as precision oncology continues to undergo accelerating change [144–146]. AHCs possess the resources and organization to create this support structure; their alliance with CHC oncology practitioners will make precision oncology available to the larger CHC cancer population.

5. The Community Oncology/Academic Cancer Center Alliance in Germline Cancer Genetics

NGS and precision oncology have had a profound effect upon the practice of cancer genetics, including the evaluation and care of community patients with hereditary predisposition to cancer [147–151]. Until recently, genetic testing involved clinical assessment followed by sequential, single gene Sanger sequencing of suspect genes [152–156]. The advent of NGS brought high throughput germline multigene panel [157–161], whole exome [162–167] and whole genome assessment [168–172] to clinical cancer genetics. These platforms provide tremendous benefit to cancer genetics patients both in community oncology practices and at academic cancer centers; these advantages include increased diagnostic yield, increased speed of testing, optimized testing workflows, decreased expense and the discovery of new cancer-causing genes [173–177]. However, together with advantages, challenges and limitations arise; AHCs have the specialized resources to address these issues.

In accordance with the American College of Medical Genetics and the Association for Molecular Pathology guidelines, variants from clinical genetic testing fall along a spectrum ranging from pathogenic/likely pathogenic to benign/likely benign [178]; variants of uncertain significance (VUS) occur when there exists insufficient information for variant assignment to either the pathogenic or benign categories [179,180]. For pathogenic/likely pathogenic and benign/likely benign variants, genetic providers typically have the ability to communicate clear interpretation of results and to provide consensus health recommendations. As their pathogenicity remains uncertain, VUS challenge health care specialists to formulate and relay unambiguous health care instructions [181–185]; furthermore, VUS frequently cause confusion and anxiety for the patient [186–190]. VUS impose a significant clinical burden. More than one third of NGS-based cancer gene panel tests result in identification of a VUS [191]; whole exome and genome testing generate even greater numbers of VUS [192–195]. Moreover, if a patient belongs to a minority group, for whom genome annotations remain less well confirmed, VUS additionally increase [196].

Geneticists classify genes according to their penetrance, that is, how likely will a pathogenic variant of a gene cause disease [197]. For pathogenic variants of high penetrance genes, clinicians more often have firmly established guidelines that inform recommendations for patient screening and surveillance. However, for pathological variants of low penetrance genes, less definitive clinical guidelines exist. NGS-based testing results in increasing detection of pathogenic variants of low penetrance genes; this increased detection adds complexity and uncertainty to patient management [198,199].

Clinicians face another challenge when selecting NGS gene panels for genetic evaluation: they must select the composition of the gene panel that they will employ. This selection requires specialized education and training [200,201]. The cancer genetics expertise required to address this challenge remains scarce [202–205]; the wider use of NGS platforms in clinical oncology and continued technological advances has made this expertise even more scarce [206–208].

AHCs possess the clinical expertise, facilities, support personnel, and administrative structures to meet the burgeoning demands of cancer genetics and to overcome the obstacles associated with the use of NGS in the clinic. Allied community oncology practices and their patients have access to these resources and services through their partnerships with AHCs. Four access models enable community oncology patient engagement with the AHC: (1) patient consultation visits to the academic cancer center, (2) cancer genetics specialist visits to community oncology sites, (3) telemedicine- and web-based remote visits and (4) AHC-sponsored genetic education initiatives that train community oncology practitioners to assess and manage cancer genetic risk and disease (Figure 1).

Conventionally, community oncology patients have received their cancer genetics care by consulting, in person, with a specialist at an AHC [155,209–211]. This model disadvantages community patients who live substantial distances from an AHC as it involves significant travel time and cost commitments [210,212,213]. Alternative cancer genetics delivery models have the potential to mitigate these problems.

In the community satellite clinic model, AHC cancer genetic specialists travel to the CHC clinic on an interval basis to meet the cancer genetic needs of community patients. This approach has proven successful in a variety of circumstances where logistical or economic challenges create barriers to effective cancer genetics care [214–217].

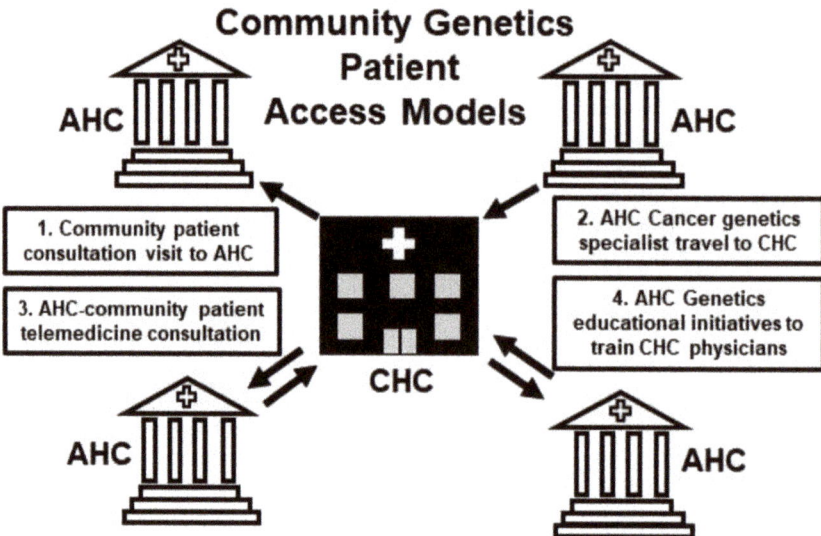

Figure 1. Community health center (CHC) patients requiring genetics care interface with specialists at academic health centers (AHC) through four modes of interaction. (1) The CHC patient may travel to the AHC for assessment. (2) The AHC genetics specialist may travel to a satellite CHC genetics clinic to evaluate the CHC patient. (3) CHC patients and AHC genetic specialists may interact via telemedicine consultation. (4) In order to provide genetics care to their patients, CHC physicians may undergo genetics specialty training sponsored by AHCs.

In our digital era, innovative cancer genetics delivery models have emerged; telemedicine platforms that involve both telephony and video communication platforms represent one such model [218–222]. The Division of Clinical Cancer Genetics (CCG) at COHCCC has assumed a national leadership position in the adoption of digital age technologies to provide academic center cancer genetic services to community oncology practices and their patients.

The CCG formed the Cancer Screening and Program Network (CSPPN), building a bridge to community oncology practices; the CSPPN utilizes innovative videoconferencing, telemedicine and wed-based applications to provide cancer genetics services [223]. Innovation continues at the CCG with the ongoing construction of new software and web-based platforms to permit effective communication between academic cancer genetics providers and community-based patients and practitioners [224]. Alongside the use of these digital platforms, the CCG has administered a landmark educational program to provide community oncology healthcare providers with the necessary training that allows them to function as competent cancer risk assessment specialists in their own communities [225]. This program, funded by the National Cancer Institute, has expanded the workforce of qualified germline genetics providers and has helped to alleviate the shortage of cancer genetics expertise in CHC practices.

Educational programs, such as that sponsored by the CCG, have acquired additional practical importance as many healthcare systems now require, prior to genetic testing, assessment by a healthcare provider trained in genetics. These requirements may hinder effective cancer genetics care, particularly in underserved communities [226]; the availability of training will help eliminate this hindrance.

6. The Community Oncology/Academic Cancer Center Alliance in Somatic Tumor Genomics

The use of clinical NGS in oncology has risen exponentially [227]. Hundreds of commercial and academic laboratories now offer NGS-based clinical sequencing of cancer specimens [119,228]. The NGS sequencing formats for somatic tumor sequencing include, among others, whole exome, whole genome, targeted panel, transcriptome and liquid biopsy assessments [229–235]. Various factors have driven the increased clinical application of NGS for somatic tumor assessment. The number of targetable genomic alterations increases substantially each year. Currently, there exist well over one hundred FDA-approved targeted therapies available for the treatment of both solid and hematological cancers [98]; over the past year alone, the FDA granted approval to nearly 20 new drugs or new indications for previously approved drugs [96]. With inclusion of therapy based upon molecular pathway considerations or off-label usage based on tissue-agnostic variant matching, the set of molecular targets and usage indications expands geometrically [236–244]. Purposing NGS-based somatic testing to determine clinical trial eligibility further increases the utility of NGS [245–248]; moreover, the demonstrated efficacy of testing to achieve improved outcomes has also motivated demand [248–252]. The decision by the Centers for Medicare and Medicaid Services to provide insurance coverage for NGS-based sequencing tests removed a financial barrier against the use of NGS, and contributed to the expanded use of this technology [253–255]. All told, currently over three quarters of oncologists use now NGS-base clinical testing to guide treatment decisions [256].

Significant challenges, however, temper enthusiasm for the clinical institution of somatic tumor NGS. A majority of oncologists report difficulty interpreting NGS somatic tumor testing, lack understanding of the clinical indications for testing and have inadequate opportunities to acquire the necessary training to properly use testing. One quarter of oncologists refer patients to other specialists to assist with NGS testing, and approximately 1 in 5 oncologists did not feel they had the proper knowledge to use properly NGS testing [256–258]. Additionally, oncologists report challenges with managing the large data volumes generated from NGS somatic testing. Oncologists also feel that they do not have the ability to distill from these reports actionable information; further, they lack the skill to manage germline variants detected as incidental findings in somatic NGS tumor testing [259–262]. These obstacles may be amplified for the CHC-based oncologist who lacks access to the necessary computational resources, logistical support and expertise in targeted therapeutics [263–266].

The CHC/AHC alliance provides solutions to alleviate these obstacles. Innovative AHC-based web applications make available to community oncologists an analytic framework and the computational tools to aid in the interpretation and clinical implementation of NGS sequencing results (Table 1). CIViC, an open access web resource, serves as a public central repository of NGS data "supporting clinical interpretations related to cancer" [267]. OncoKB, a precision oncology database, aids therapeutic decision-making based upon cancer gene variant status [268]; similarly, the web applications Personalized Cancer Therapy and My Cancer Genome assist both community and academic oncologists in selecting therapeutic options resulting from the somatic NGS of tumor specimens [269,270]. The SMART Cancer Navigator aggregates variant and clinical data from multiple data bases to assist community-based oncologists with the processing of NGS reports and the identification of effective targeted therapies [271]. At the COHCCC, investigators have configured an interactive web interface, HOPE-Genomics, that community patients and oncologists may use to better understand genomic sequencing results and treatment recommendations [224]. The COHCCC also provides to its community practice partners in-house NGS panel testing as part of its HOPESEQ molecular testing panel [272]; HOPESEQ includes genomic test reports designed to assist clinicians with interpreting the genetic testing results and clinical decision making. Furthermore, COHCCC physicians and community partners have access to Via Oncology; this tool provides a web-based clinical pathway system to help match patients with clinical trials and insurance reimbursement for NGS driven treatments [273].

Precision oncology tumor boards (POTBs) represent another solution to the problem of implementing NGS data in the CHC oncology clinic. POTBs arose from the need to assess, process and generate clinical treatment plans from the highly dense and complex data sets that arise from somatic NGS of tumor specimens [274]. POTBs serve two primary functions: targeted therapy drug matching and molecularly-informed clinical trial enrollment [275–280] (Figure 2).

Table 1. Web-based genomics resources available to community oncologists.

WEB-BASED RESOURCE	URL
CIViC	civicdb.org
OncoKB	oncokb.org
Personalized Cancer Therapy	pct.mdanderson.org
My Cancer Genome	mycancergenome.org
SMART Cancer Navigator	smart-cancer-navigator.github.io/home
ASCO Multidisciplinary Molecular Tumor Boards	elearning.asco.org/product-details/multidisciplinary-molecular-tumor/boards-mmtbs
Helio Learn Genomics	healio.com
Know Your Tumor	pancan.org

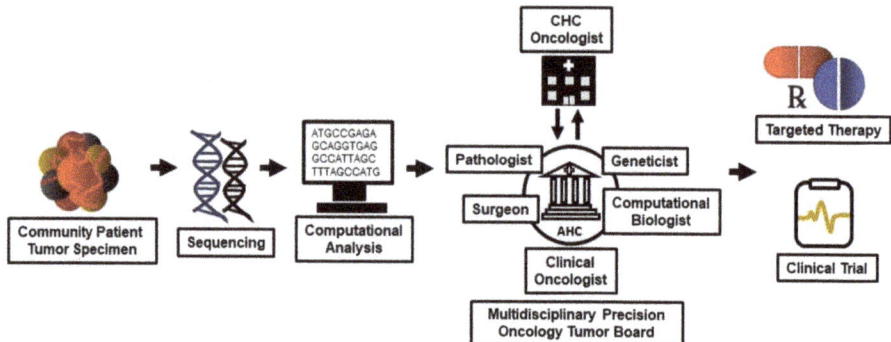

Figure 2. Multidisciplinary precision oncology tumor boards (POTBs) provide expert targeted drug matching and molecularly informed clinical trial enrollment for community oncology patients. Tumor specimens from community patients undergo nucleic acid sequencing with computational analysis to identify molecular alterations; this information provides a basis to discover candidate targeted therapies and determine clinical trial eligibility. An academic health center (AHC) POTB comprising, among others, clinical oncologists, pathologists, surgeons, geneticists and computational biologists, in consultation with community health center (CHC) oncologists, reviews patients' clinical cases and their sequencing results to select appropriate targeted therapies and clinical trials.

POTBs originated within AHCs as these centers possess the multidisciplinary expertise including, among others, clinical oncologists, pathologists, genomics specialists, computational biologists, pharmacologists and clinical geneticists to efficiently identify targeted therapies and clinical trials [281–290]. Targeted therapy drug matching requires comprehensive molecular mutational profiling and downstream pathway analyses of the tumor, combined with the identification of safe and effective therapeutic agents that redress these molecular alterations [291–293]; CHCs typically do not possess the analytic or pharmacologic capabilities to adequately perform these activities. Most clinical trials fail [294–296]; these failures result from a number of factors including deficient clinical trial design, poor proof of concept planning and insufficient administrative support and compliance [297–300]. Such failures have adverse consequences for both the clinical trial sponsors as well as the patients; failure has significant economic cost and results in lost therapeutic opportunity, in addition to potentially exposing the patient to harm from the investigational protocol and drugs [301–303]. These clinical trial-related matters may be more acute at CHCs given their more limited resources and the absence of experienced clinical trialists [304–307]. The POTB provides appropriate, molecularly-informed clinical trial assignment for patients, maximizing both the utility of clinical trial participation and potential patient benefit [308–320].

Given the resource limitations of the CHC oncology clinic, community POTB operation requires innovation and dedicated planning [83,321,322]. One innovation available to community oncologists, the web-based ASCO Multidisciplinary Molecular Tumor Boards, assists oncologists with understanding precision medicine-based tumor testing and the therapy recommendations resulting from these tests [323] (Table 1). Helio Learn Genomics, another web platform, offers a number of educational modules, including POTB cases, to help providers understand the molecular bases of carcinogenesis and precision therapeutics [324]. The Pancreatic Cancer Action Network administers a Know Your Tumor program, a turn-key precision medicine initiative, that allows community oncology practitioners to submit their patients' pancreatic cancer specimens for NGS molecular testing and to receive back a precision medicine-based treatment plan [325].

Another version of the POTB, the virtual POTB, permits the distance participation of community oncologists in an academic POTB. In this model an AHC hosts the POTB and reviews the clinical history and precision oncology testing results of the community oncology patient; subsequently, the POTB discusses with the community oncologist, using a live interactive video teleconferencing link, targeted treatment and clinical trial recommendations [263,311,326–330]. The Translational Genomics Research Institute (TGEN), an academic affiliate of the COHCCC, has successfully built a comprehensive, integrated, high-throughput sequencing and reporting framework that, when combined with remote teleconferencing, has proven tremendously successful in establishing efficient collaborative POTBs [331–335]. Together, these various models of providing clinical somatic NGS demonstrate the feasibility of leveraging precision oncology for the community-based cancer oncologist and their patients.

7. Conclusions

We have entered the age of precision oncology. Precision oncology offers the potential of molecularly informed medicine for the assessment of inherited cancer predisposition, as well as for the diagnosis and treatment of cancers. Realization of this potential depends upon access to specialized expertise and significant analytic and technological resources. While frequently available at AHCs, these resources have previously been limited for CHC oncology practices and their patients. In this paper, we have examined the CHC/AHC alliance and discussed examples illustrating how this alliance provides a structure that allows community cancer patients to benefit from germline and somatic precision oncology advances. Looking forward, multidisciplinary efforts, improved technology and continuing innovation promise to strengthen and facilitate the CHC/AHC alliance in oncology; this alliance offers community oncologists and their patients the prospect of unambiguous interpretation of genetic and genomic test results and optimized precision oncology care.

Author Contributions: Writing-Original Draft Preparation, M.M., S.S. (Shanmuga Subbiah), K.J.M.; Writing-Review and Editing, S.S. (Swapnil Rajurkar). All authors have read and agreed to the published version of the manuscript.

Funding: This research received no external funding.

Conflicts of Interest: The authors declare no conflict of interest.

References

1. Wartman, S.A. *The Transformation of Academic Health Centers: Meeting The Challenges Of Healthcare's Changing Landscape*; Academic Press: Fribourg, Switzerland, 2015.
2. Dzau, V.J.; Ackerly, D.C.; Sutton-Wallace, P.; Merson, M.H.; Williams, R.S.; Krishnan, K.R.; Taber, R.C.; Califf, R.M. The role of academic health science systems in the transformation of medicine. *Lancet* **2010**, *375*, 949–953. [CrossRef]
3. Desch, C.E.; Blayney, D.W. Making the choice between academic oncology and community practice: the big picture and details about each career. *J. Oncol. Pract.* **2006**, *2*, 132–136. [CrossRef]
4. Todd, R.F., III. A guide to planning careers in hematology and oncology. *Hematol. Am. Soc. Hemat.* **2001**, *2001*, 499–506. [CrossRef] [PubMed]

5. Levit, L.A.; Kim, E.S.; McAneny, B.L.; Nadauld, L.D.; Levit, K.; Schenkel, C.; Schilsky, R.L. Implementing precision medicine in community-based oncology programs: Three models. *J. Oncol. Pract.* **2019**, *15*, 325–329. [CrossRef] [PubMed]
6. Thompson, M.A.; Godden, J.J.; Weissman, S.M.; Wham, D.; Wilson, A.; Ruggeri, A.; Mullane, M.P.; Weese, J.L. Implementing an oncology precision medicine clinic in a large community health system. *Am. J. Manag. Care* **2017**, *23*, SP425–SP427.
7. Levine, D.M.; Becker, D.M.; Bone, L.R.; Hill, M.N.; Tuggle, M.B., II; Zeger, S.L. Community-academic health center partnerships for underserved minority populations. One solution to a national crisis. *J. Am. Med. Assoc.* **1994**, *272*, 309–311. [CrossRef]
8. Shin, P.; Sharac, J.; Rosenbaum, S. Community health centers and medicaid at 50: An. Enduring relationship essential for health system transformation. *Health Aff. (Millwood)* **2015**, *34*, 1096–1104. [CrossRef]
9. Sharma, A.E.; Huang, B.; Knox, M.; Willard-Grace, R.; Potter, M.B. Patient engagement in community health center leadership: How does it happen? *J. Community Health* **2018**, *43*, 1069–1074. [CrossRef] [PubMed]
10. Blumenthal, D.; Meyer, G.S. Academic health centers in a changing environment. *Health Aff. (Millwood)* **1996**, *15*, 200–215. [CrossRef]
11. Nash, D.B.; Veloski, J.J. Emerging opportunities for educational partnerships between managed care organizations and academic health centers. *West. J. Med.* **1998**, *168*, 319–327. [PubMed]
12. Roper, W.L.; Newton, W.P. The role of academic health centers in improving health. *Ann. Fam. Med.* **2006**, *4*, S55–S57. [CrossRef] [PubMed]
13. Blumenthal, D.; Meyer, G.S. The future of the academic medical center under health care reform. *N. Engl. J. Med.* **1993**, *329*, 1812–1814. [CrossRef]
14. Fox, P.D.; Wasserman, J. Academic medical centers and managed care: Uneasy partners. *Health Aff. (Millwood)* **1993**, *12*, 85–93. [CrossRef]
15. Epstein, A.M. US teaching hospitals in the evolving health care system. *J. Am. Med. Assoc.* **1995**, *273*, 1203–1207. [CrossRef]
16. Iglehart, J.K. Academic medical centers enter the market: The case of Philadelphia. *N. Engl. J. Med.* **1995**, *333*, 1019–1023. [CrossRef] [PubMed]
17. Lofgren, R.; Karpf, M.; Perman, J.; Higdon, C.M. The U.S. health care system is in crisis: Implications for academic medical centers and their missions. *Acad. Med.* **2006**, *81*, 713–720. [CrossRef]
18. Park, B.; Frank, B.; Likumahuwa-Ackman, S.; Brodt, E.; Gibbs, B.K.; Hofkamp, H.; DeVoe, J. Health equity and the tripartite mission: Moving from academic health centers to academic-community health systems. *Acad. Med.* **2019**, *94*, 1276–1282. [CrossRef]
19. Bartlett, S.J.; Barnes, T.; McIvor, R.A. Integrating patients into meaningful real-world research. *Ann. Am. Thorac. Soc.* **2014**, *11*, S112–S117. [CrossRef]
20. Gourevitch, M.N. Population health and the academic medical center: The time is right. *Acad. Med.* **2014**, *89*, 544–549. [CrossRef] [PubMed]
21. Vitale, K.; Newton, G.L.; Abraido-Lanza, A.F.; Aguirre, A.N.; Ahmed, S.; Esmond, S.L.; Evans, J.; Gelmon, S.B.; Hart, C.; Hendricks, D.; et al. Community engagement in academic health centers: A model for capturing and advancing our successes. *J. Commun. Engagem. Scholarsh.* **2018**, *10*, 81–90.
22. Zerhouni, E. Medicine: The NIH roadmap. *Science* **2003**, *302*, 63–72. [CrossRef] [PubMed]
23. Schwenk, T.L.; Green, L.A. The Michigan Clinical Research Collaboratory: Following the NIH Roadmap to the community. *Ann. Fam. Med.* **2006**, *4*, S49–S54. [CrossRef] [PubMed]
24. Zerhouni, E.A. Translational and clinical science—Time for a new vision. *N. Engl. J. Med.* **2005**, *353*, 1621–1623. [CrossRef] [PubMed]
25. Zerhouni, E.A. US biomedical research: Basic, translational, and clinical sciences. *J. Am. Med. Assoc.* **2005**, *294*, 1352–1358. [CrossRef]
26. Kassirer, J.P. Academic medical centers under siege. *N. Engl. J. Med.* **1994**, *331*, 1370–1371. [CrossRef]
27. Iglehart, J.K. Rapid changes for academic medical centers. 2. *N. Engl. J. Med.* **1995**, *332*, 407–411. [CrossRef]
28. Iglehart, J.K. Rapid changes for academic medical centers. 1. *N. Engl. J. Med.* **1994**, *331*, 1391–1395. [CrossRef]
29. Moses, H., III; Matheson, D.H.M.; Poste, G. Serving individuals and populations within integrated health systems: A bridge too far? *J. Am. Med. Assoc.* **2019**, *321*, 1975–1976. [CrossRef]
30. Cutler, D.M.; Morton, F.S. Hospitals, market share, and consolidation. *J. Am. Med. Assoc.* **2013**, *310*, 1964–1970. [CrossRef]

31. Moses, H., III; Matheson, D.H.; Dorsey, E.R.; George, B.P.; Sadoff, D.; Yoshimura, S. The anatomy of health care in the United States. *J. Am. Med. Assoc.* **2013**, *310*, 1947–1963. [CrossRef]
32. Cohen, M.D.; Jennings, G. Mergers involving academic medical institutions: Impact on academic radiology departments. *J. Am. Coll. Radiol.* **2005**, *2*, 174–182. [CrossRef] [PubMed]
33. Denham, A.C.; Hay, S.S.; Steiner, B.D.; Newton, W.P. Academic health centers and community health centers partnering to build a system of care for vulnerable patients: Lessons from Carolina Health Net. *Acad. Med.* **2013**, *88*, 638–643. [CrossRef] [PubMed]
34. Rieselbach, R.E.; Rieselbach, R.E.; Epperly, T.; Friedman, A.; Keahey, D.; McConnell, E.; Nichols, K.; Nycz, G.; Roberts, J.; Schmader, K.; et al. A new community health center/academic medicine partnership for medicaid cost control, powered by the Mega Teaching Health Center. *Acad. Med.* **2018**, *93*, 406–413. [CrossRef]
35. Blumenthal, D.; Campbell, E.G.; Weissman, J.S. The social missions of academic health centers. *N. Engl. J. Med.* **1997**, *337*, 1550–1553. [CrossRef]
36. Fleishon, H.B.; Itri, J.N.; Boland, G.W.; Duszak, R., Jr. Academic medical centers and community hospitals integration: Trends and strategies. *J. Am. Coll. Radiol.* **2017**, *14*, 45–51. [CrossRef]
37. Ellner, A.L.; Stout, S.; Sullivan, E.E.; Griffiths, E.P.; Mountjoy, A.; Phillips, R.S. Health systems innovation at academic health centers: Leading in a new era of health care delivery. *Acad. Med.* **2015**, *90*, 872–880. [CrossRef] [PubMed]
38. Moore, G.T.; Inui, T.S.; Ludden, J.M.; Schoenbaum, S.C. The "teaching HMO": A new academic partner. *Acad. Med.* **1994**, *69*, 595–600. [CrossRef] [PubMed]
39. Poncelet, A.N.; Mazotti, L.A.; Blumberg, B.; Wamsley, M.A.; Grennan, T.; Shore, W.B. Creating a longitudinal integrated clerkship with mutual benefits for an academic medical center and a community health system. *Perm. J.* **2014**, *18*, 50–56. [CrossRef]
40. Berkowitz, S.A.; Brown, P.; Brotman, D.J.; Deutschendorf, A.; Dunbar, L.; Everett, A.; Hickman, D.; Howell, E.; Purnell, L.; Sylvester, C.; et al. Case Study: Johns Hopkins Community Health Partnership: A model for transformation. *Healthc (Amst.)* **2016**, *4*, 264–270. [CrossRef]
41. Institute of Medicine (US) Committee on Understanding and Eliminating Racial and Ethnic Disparities in Health Care. *Unequal Treatment: Confronting Racial and Ethnic Disparities in Health Care*; Smedley, B.D., Stith, A.Y., Nelson, A.R., Eds.; National Academies Press: Washington, DC, USA, 2003.
42. Ahmed, S.M.; Maurana, C.; Nelson, D.; Meister, T.; Young, S.N.; Lucey, P. Opening the black box: Conceptualizing community engagement from 109 community-academic partnership programs. *Prog. Community Health Partnersh.* **2016**, *10*, 51–61. [CrossRef]
43. Croft, C.R.; Dial, R.; Doyle, G.; Schaadt, J.; Merchant, L. Integrating a community hospital-based radiology department with an academic medical center. *J. Am. Coll. Radiol.* **2016**, *13*, 300–302. [CrossRef]
44. Sussman, A.J.; Otten, J.R.; Goldszer, R.C.; Hanson, M.; Trull, D.J.; Paulus, K.; Brown, M.; Dzau, V.; Brennan, T.A. Integration of an academic medical center and a community hospital: The Brigham and Women's/Faulkner hospital experience. *Acad. Med.* **2005**, *80*, 253–260. [CrossRef] [PubMed]
45. Spalluto, L.B.; Thomas, D.; Beard, K.R.; Campbell, T.; Audet, C.M.; McBride Murry, V.; Shrubsole, M.J.; Barajas, C.P.; Joosten, Y.A.; Dittus, R.S.; et al. A community-academic partnership to reduce health care disparities in diagnostic imaging. *J. Am. Coll. Radiol.* **2019**, *16*, 649–656. [CrossRef] [PubMed]
46. Kelley-Quon, L.I.; Thomas, D.; Beard, K.R.; Campbell, T.; Audet, C.M.; McBride Murry, V.; Shrubsole, M.J.; Barajas, C.P.; Joosten, Y.A.; Dittus, R.S.; et al. Academic-community partnerships improve outcomes in pediatric trauma care. *J. Pediatr. Surg.* **2015**, *50*, 1032–1036. [CrossRef] [PubMed]
47. Phillip, C.R.; Mancera-Cuevas, K.; Leatherwood, C.; Chmiel, J.S.; Erickson, D.L.; Freeman, E.; Granville, G.; Dollear, M.; Walker, K.; McNeil, R.; et al. Implementation and dissemination of an African American popular opinion model to improve lupus awareness: An academic-community partnership. *Lupus* **2019**, *28*, 1441–1451. [CrossRef] [PubMed]
48. Rees, T. Academic medical center, community hospital partner to market center of excellence. *Profiles Healthc. Mark.* **1999**, *15*, 40–43.
49. Yaggy, S.D.; Michener, J.L.; Yaggy, D.; Champagne, M.T.; Silberberg, M.; Lyn, M.; Johnson, F.; Yarnall, K.S. Just for Us: An academic medical center-community partnership to maintain the health of a frail low-income senior population. *Gerontologist* **2006**, *46*, 271–276. [CrossRef]
50. Natesan, R.; Yang, W.T.; Tannir, H.; Parikh, J. Strategic expansion models in academic radiology. *J. Am. Coll. Radiol.* **2016**, *13*, 329–334. [CrossRef]

51. Kirkwood, M.K.; Hanley, A.; Bruinooge, S.S.; Garrett-Mayer, E.; Levit, L.A.; Schenkel, C.; Seid, J.E.; Polite, B.N.; Schilsky, R.L. The State of oncology practice in America, 2018: results of the ASCO practice census survey. *J. Oncol. Pract.* **2018**, *14*, e412–e420. [CrossRef]
52. OBR New Perspective Catalyst. *Most Cancer Patients Will Be Treated in Integrated Delivery Networks (IDN) and Cancer Institutions by 2016, Predicts New Report*; OBR New Perspective Catalyst: Sausalito, CA, USA, 2012; Volume 11.
53. Genetech. *The 2018 Genentech Oncology Trend Report*; Genetech: San Francisco, CA, USA, 2018.
54. Genetech. *The 2019 Genentech Oncology Trend Report*; Genetech: San Francisco, CA, USA, 2019.
55. Academic Cancer Centers (NCCC). *Trends Impacting Key Account. Management*; Academic Cancer Centers: Pipersville, PA, USA, 2016.
56. Nardi, E.A.; Wolfson, J.A.; Rosen, S.T.; Diasio, R.B.; Gerson, S.L.; Parker, B.A.; Alvarnas, J.C.; Levine, H.A.; Fong, Y.; Weisenburger, D.D.; et al. Value, access, and cost of cancer care delivery at academic cancer centers. *J. Natl. Compr. Cancer Netw.* **2016**, *14*, 837–847. [CrossRef]
57. Speicher, P.J.; Englum, B.R.; Ganapathi, A.M.; Wang, X.; Hartwig, M.G.; D'Amico, T.A.; Berry, M.F. Traveling to a high-volume center is associated with improved survival for patients with esophageal cancer. *Ann. Surg.* **2017**, *265*, 743–749. [CrossRef] [PubMed]
58. Lidsky, M.E.; Sun, Z.; Nussbaum, D.P.; Adam, M.A.; Speicher, P.J.; Blazer, D.G., III. Going the extra mile: Improved survival for pancreatic cancer patients traveling to high-volume centers. *Ann. Surg.* **2017**, *266*, 333–338. [CrossRef] [PubMed]
59. David, J.M.; Ho, A.S.; Luu, M.; Yoshida, E.J.; Kim, S.; Mita, A.C.; Scher, K.S.; Shiao, S.L.; Tighiouart, M.; Zumsteg, Z.S. Treatment at high-volume facilities and academic centers is independently associated with improved survival in patients with locally advanced head and neck cancer. *Cancer* **2017**, *123*, 3933–3942. [CrossRef]
60. Chen, A.Y.; Fedewa, S.; Pavluck, A.; Ward, E.M. Improved survival is associated with treatment at high-volume teaching facilities for patients with advanced stage laryngeal cancer. *Cancer* **2010**, *116*, 4744–4752. [CrossRef] [PubMed]
61. Pfister, D.G.; Rubin, D.M.; Elkin, E.B.; Neill, U.S.; Duck, E.; Radzyner, M.; Bach, P.B. Risk adjusting survival outcomes in hospitals that treat patients with cancer without information on cancer stage. *JAMA Oncol.* **2015**, *1*, 1303–1310. [CrossRef] [PubMed]
62. Schmitz, R.; Adam, M.A.; Blazer, D.G., III. Overcoming a travel burden to high-volume centers for treatment of retroperitoneal sarcomas is associated with improved survival. *World J. Surg. Oncol.* **2019**, *17*, 180. [CrossRef] [PubMed]
63. Dillman, R.O.; Chico, S.D. Cancer patient survival improvement is correlated with the opening of a community cancer center: Comparisons with intramural and extramural benchmarks. *J. Oncol. Pract.* **2005**, *1*, 84–92. [CrossRef] [PubMed]
64. Ramalingam, S.; Dinan, M.A.; Crawford, J. Survival comparison in patients with stage iv lung cancer in academic versus community centers in the United States. *J. Thorac. Oncol.* **2018**, *13*, 1842–1850. [CrossRef] [PubMed]
65. Carugo, A.; Draetta, G.F. Academic discovery of anticancer drugs: Historic and future perspectives. *Ann. Rev. Cancer Biol.* **2019**, *3*, 385–408. [CrossRef]
66. Everett, J.R. Academic drug discovery: Current status and prospects. *Expert Opin. Drug Discov.* **2015**, *10*, 937–944. [CrossRef] [PubMed]
67. Matter, A. Bridging academic science and clinical research in the search for novel targeted anti-cancer agents. *Cancer Biol. Med.* **2015**, *12*, 316–327. [PubMed]
68. Dorfman, G.S.; Lawrence, T.S.; Matrisian, L.M.; Translational Research Working Group. The Translational Research Working Group developmental pathway for interventive devices. *Clin. Cancer Res.* **2008**, *14*, 5700–5706. [CrossRef] [PubMed]
69. Barrios, C.H.; Reinert, T.; Werutsky, G. Global breast cancer research: Moving forward. *Am. Soc. Clin. Oncol. Educ. Book.* **2018**, *38*, 441–450. [CrossRef] [PubMed]
70. Huber, M.A.; Kraut, N. Key drivers of biomedical innovation in cancer drug discovery. *EMBO Mol. Med.* **2015**, *7*, 12–16. [CrossRef] [PubMed]

71. Grodzinski, P.; Liu, C.H.; Hartshorn, C.M.; Morris, S.A.; Russell, L.M. NCI Alliance for Nanotechnology in Cancer—From academic research to clinical interventions. *Biomed. Microdev.* **2019**, *21*, 32. [CrossRef] [PubMed]
72. Clauser, S.B.; Johnson, M.R.; O'Brien, D.M.; Beveridge, J.M.; Fennell, M.L.; Kaluzny, A.D. Improving clinical research and cancer care delivery in community settings: Evaluating the NCI community cancer centers program. *Implement. Sci.* **2009**, *4*, 63. [CrossRef]
73. Hirsch, B.R.; Locke, S.C.; Abernethy, A.P. Experience of the national cancer institute community cancer centers program on community-based cancer clinical trials activity. *J. Oncol. Pract.* **2016**, *12*, e350-8. [CrossRef]
74. Copur, M.S.; Ramaekers, R.; Gonen, M.; Gulzow, M.; Hadenfeldt, R.; Fuller, C.; Scott, J.; Einspahr, S.; Benzel, H.; Mickey, M.; et al. Impact of the national cancer institute community cancer centers program on clinical trial and related activities at a community cancer center in rural Nebraska. *J. Oncol. Pract.* **2016**, *12*, 67–68. [CrossRef]
75. DH, F. Clinical trials have the best medicine but do not enroll the patients who need it. *Sci. Am.* **2019**, *320*, 61–65.
76. Copur, M.S. Inadequate awareness of and participation in cancer clinical trials in the community oncology setting. *Oncology* **2019**, *33*, 54–57.
77. Green, M.A.; Michaels, M.; Blakeney, N.; Odulana, A.A.; Isler, M.R.; Richmond, A.; Long, D.G.; Robinson, W.S.; Taylor, Y.J.; Corbie-Smith, G. Evaluating a community-partnered cancer clinical trials pilot intervention with African American communities. *J. Cancer Educ.* **2015**, *30*, 158–166. [CrossRef] [PubMed]
78. Best, A.; Hiatt, R.A.; Cameron, R.; Rimer, B.K.; Abrams, D.B. The evolution of cancer control research: An international perspective from Canada and the United States. *Cancer Epidemiol Biomarkers Prev.* **2003**, *12*, 705–712. [PubMed]
79. Greenwald, P.; Cullen, J.W. The new emphasis in cancer control. *J. Natl. Cancer. Inst.* **1985**, *74*, 543–551. [CrossRef]
80. Noel, L.; Phillips, F.; Tossas-Milligan, K.; Spear, K.; Vanderford, N.L.; Winn, R.A.; Vanderpool, R.C.; Eckhardt, S.G. Community-academic partnerships: Approaches to engagement. *Am. Soc. Clin. Oncol. Educ. Book.* **2019**, *39*, 88–95. [CrossRef]
81. Harris, A.; Kumar, P.; Sutaria, S. *Unlocking the Potential of Acdemic and Community Health System Partnerships*; McKinsey and Company: New York, NY, USA, 2015.
82. Johnson, T.M. Perspective on precision medicine in oncology. *Pharmacotherapy* **2017**, *37*, 988–989. [CrossRef] [PubMed]
83. Ersek, J.L.; Black, L.J.; Thompson, M.A.; Kim, E.S. Implementing precision medicine programs and clinical trials in the community-based oncology practice: Barriers and best practices. *Am. Soc. Clin. Oncol. Educ. Book.* **2018**, *38*, 188–196. [CrossRef]
84. Nadauld, L.D.; Ford, J.M.; Pritchard, D.; Brown, T. Strategies for clinical implementation: Precision oncology at three distinct institutions. *Health Aff. (Millwood)* **2018**, *37*, 751–756. [CrossRef]
85. Thompson, M.A.; Godden, J.J.; Wham, D.; Ruggeri, A.; Mullane, M.P.; Wilson, A.; Virani, S.; Weissman, S.M.; Ramczyk, B.; Vanderwall, P.; et al. Coordinating an oncology precision medicine clinic within an integrated health system: lessons learned in year one. *J. Patient Cent. Res. Rev.* **2019**, *6*, 36–45. [CrossRef]
86. Carpten, J.C.; Mardis, E.R. The era of precision oncogenomics. *Cold Spring Harb. Mol. Case Stud.* **2018**, *4*. [CrossRef]
87. International Human Genome Sequencing Consortium. Finishing the euchromatic sequence of the human genome. *Nature* **2004**, *431*, 931–945. [CrossRef]
88. Ashley, E.A. Towards precision medicine. *Nat. Rev. Genet.* **2016**, *17*, 507–522. [CrossRef] [PubMed]
89. Sanchez, N.S.; Mills, G.B.; Mills Shaw, K.R. Precision oncology: Neither a silver bullet nor a dream. *Pharmacogenomics* **2017**, *18*, 1525–1539. [CrossRef] [PubMed]
90. Berger, M.F.; Mardis, E.R. The emerging clinical relevance of genomics in cancer medicine. *Nat. Rev. Clin. Oncol.* **2018**, *15*, 353–365. [CrossRef] [PubMed]
91. Mitra, R.D.; Church, G.M. In situ localized amplification and contact replication of many individual DNA molecules. *Nucleic Acids Res.* **1999**, *27*, e34. [CrossRef]
92. Brenner, S.; Johnson, M.; Bridgham, J.; Golda, G.; Lloyd, D.H.; Johnson, D.; Luo, S.; McCurdy, S.; Foy, M.; Ewan, M.; et al. Gene expression analysis by massively parallel signature sequencing (MPSS) on microbead arrays. *Nat. Biotechnol.* **2000**, *18*, 630–634. [CrossRef]

93. Mardis, E.R. Next-generation DNA sequencing methods. *Annu. Rev. Genomics Hum. Genet.* **2008**, *9*, 387–402. [CrossRef]
94. Shendure, J.; Ji, H. Next-generation DNA sequencing. *Nat. Biotechnol.* **2008**, *26*, 1135–1145. [CrossRef] [PubMed]
95. Bentley, D.R.; Balasubramanian, S.; Swerdlow, H.P.; Smith, G.P.; Milton, J.; Brown, C.G.; Hall, K.P.; Evers, D.J.; Barnes, C.L.; Bignell, H.R.; et al. Accurate whole human genome sequencing using reversible terminator chemistry. *Nature* **2008**, *456*, 53–59. [CrossRef] [PubMed]
96. Mardis, E.R. The impact of next-generation sequencing technology on genetics. *Trends Genet.* **2008**, *24*, 133–141. [CrossRef]
97. Tucker, T.; Marra, M.; Friedman, J.M. Massively parallel sequencing: The next big thing in genetic medicine. *Am. J. Hum. Genet.* **2009**, *85*, 142–154. [CrossRef]
98. Ley, T.J.; Mardis, E.R.; Ding, L.; Fulton, B.; McLellan, M.D.; Chen, K.; Dooling, D.; Dunford-Shore, B.H.; McGrath, S.; Hickenbotham, M.; et al. DNA sequencing of a cytogenetically normal acute myeloid leukaemia genome. *Nature* **2008**, *456*, 66–72. [CrossRef] [PubMed]
99. Reinartz, J.; Bruyns, E.; Lin, J.Z.; Burcham, T.; Brenner, S.; Bowen, B.; Kramer, M.; Woychik, R. Massively parallel signature sequencing (MPSS) as a tool for in-depth quantitative gene expression profiling in all organisms. *Brief. Funct. Genomic. Proteomic.* **2002**, *1*, 95–104. [CrossRef] [PubMed]
100. Torres, T.T.; Metta, M.; Ottenwalder, B.; Schlotterer, C. Gene expression profiling by massively parallel sequencing. *Genome Res.* **2008**, *18*, 172–177. [CrossRef] [PubMed]
101. Cancer Genome Atlas Research, N.; Weinstein, J.N.; Collisson, E.A.; Mills, G.B.; Shaw, K.R.; Ozenberger, B.A.; Ellrott, K.; Shmulevich, I.; Sander, C.; Stuart, J.M. The cancer genome atlas pan-cancer analysis project. *Nat. Genet.* **2013**, *45*, 1113–1120.
102. Wang, H.; Nettleton, D.; Ying, K. Copy number variation detection using next generation sequencing read counts. *BMC Bioinform.* **2014**, *15*, 109. [CrossRef] [PubMed]
103. Medvedev, P.; Stanciu, M.; Brudno, M. Computational methods for discovering structural variation with next-generation sequencing. *Nat. Methods* **2009**, *6*, S13–S20. [CrossRef]
104. Johnson, D.S.; Mortazavi, A.; Myers, R.M.; Wold, B. Genome-wide mapping of in vivo protein-DNA interactions. *Science* **2007**, *316*, 1497–1502. [CrossRef]
105. Morel, D.; Jeffery, D.; Aspeslagh, S.; Almouzni, G.; Postel-Vinay, S. Combining epigenetic drugs with other therapies for solid tumours—Past lessons and future promise. *Nat. Rev. Clin. Oncol.* **2020**, *17*, 91–107. [CrossRef]
106. Lazaris, C.; Aifantis, I.; Tsirigos, A. On epigenetic plasticity and genome topology. *Trends Cancer* **2020**, *6*, 177–180. [CrossRef]
107. Segal, N.H.; Parsons, D.W.; Peggs, K.S.; Velculescu, V.; Kinzler, K.W.; Vogelstein, B.; Allison, J.P. Epitope landscape in breast and colorectal cancer. *Cancer Res.* **2008**, *68*, 889–892. [CrossRef]
108. Alexandrov, L.B.; Nik-Zainal, S.; Wedge, D.C.; Aparicio, S.A.; Behjati, S.; Biankin, A.V.; Bignell, G.R.; Bolli, N.; Borg, A.; Borresen-Dale, A.L.; et al. Signatures of mutational processes in human cancer. *Nature* **2013**, *500*, 415–421. [CrossRef] [PubMed]
109. Sanmamed, M.F.; LChe. A paradigm shift in cancer immunotherapy: From enhancement to normalization. *Cell* **2018**, *175*, 313–326. [CrossRef] [PubMed]
110. Zewde, M.; Kiyotani, K.; Park, J.H.; Fang, H.; Yap, K.L.; Yew, P.Y.; Alachkar, H.; Kato, T.; Mai, T.H.; Ikeda, Y.; et al. The era of immunogenomics/immunopharmacogenomics. *J. Hum. Genet.* **2018**, *63*, 865–875. [CrossRef]
111. Dennard, R.H.; Gaensslen, F.H.; Yu, H.N.; Rideout, V.L.; Bassous, E.; Leblanc, A.R. Design of ion-implanted MOSFET's with very small physical dimensions. *IEEE J. Solid State Circuits* **1974**, *9*, 256–268. [CrossRef]
112. Gorder, P.F. Multicore processors for science and engineering. *Comput. Sci. Eng.* **2007**, *9*, 3–7. [CrossRef]
113. Denning, P.J.; Lewis, T.G. Exponential laws of computing growth. *Commun. Acm* **2017**, *60*, 54–65. [CrossRef]
114. Thackray, A.; Brock, D.C. *Moore's Law: The Life of Gordon Moore, Silicon Valley's Quiet Revolutionary*; Basic Books: New York, NY, USA, 2015.
115. Koomey, J.G.; Berard, S.; Sanchez, M.; Wong, H. Implications of historical trends in the electrical efficiency of computing. *IEEE Comput. Soc.* **2011**, *33*, 46–54. [CrossRef]
116. Hill, M.D.; Marty, M.R. Amdahl's law in the multicore era. *Computer* **2008**, *41*, 33. [CrossRef]
117. Denning, P.J.; Tichy, W.F. Highly parallel computation. *Science* **1990**, *250*, 1217–1222. [CrossRef]

118. Hinkson, I.V.; Davidsen, T.M.; Klemm, J.D.; Kerlavage, A.R.; Kibbe, W.A.; Chandramouliswaran, I. A comprehensive infrastructure for big data in cancer research: Accelerating cancer research and precision medicine. *Front. Cell. Dev. Biol.* **2017**, *5*, 83. [CrossRef]
119. Wing, J.M. Computational thinking. *Commun. Acm* **2006**, *49*, 33–35. [CrossRef]
120. Regev, A.; Shapiro, E. Cellular abstractions: Cells as computation. *Nature* **2002**, *419*, 343-343. [CrossRef] [PubMed]
121. Searls, D.B. The roots of bioinformatics. *PLoS Comput. Biol.* **2010**, *6*. [CrossRef]
122. Moorthie, S.; Hall, A.; Wright, C.F. Informatics and clinical genome sequencing: Opening the black box. *Genet. Med.* **2013**, *15*, 165–171. [CrossRef] [PubMed]
123. Funari, V.; Canosa, S. The importance of bioinformatics in NGS: Breaking the bottleneck in data interpretation. *Science* **2014**, *344*, 653-653. [CrossRef]
124. Oliver, G.R.; Hart, S.N.; Klee, E.W. Bioinformatics for clinical next generation sequencing. *Clin. Chem.* **2015**, *61*, 124–135. [CrossRef] [PubMed]
125. Gullapalli, R.R.; Lyons-Weiler, M.; Petrosko, P.; Dhir, R.; Becich, M.J.; LaFramboise, W.A. Clinical integration of next-generation sequencing technology. *Clin. Lab. Med.* **2012**, *32*, 585–599. [CrossRef]
126. Hundal, J.; Miller, C.A.; Griffith, M.; Griffith, O.L.; Walker, J.; Kiwala, S.; Graubert, A.; McMichael, J.; Coffman, A.; Mardis, E.R. Cancer immunogenomics: computational neoantigen identification and vaccine design. *Cold Spring Harb. Symp. Quant. Biol.* **2016**, *81*, 105–111. [CrossRef]
127. Tenenbaum, J.D. Translational bioinformatics: Past, present, and future. *Genom. Proteomics Bioinform.* **2016**, *14*, 31–41. [CrossRef]
128. Weissenbach, J. The rise of genomics. *C R Biol.* **2016**, *339*, 231–239. [CrossRef]
129. Morganti, S.; Tarantino, P.; Ferraro, E.; D'Amico, P.; Viale, G.; Trapani, D.; Duso, B.A.; Curigliano, G. Complexity of genome sequencing and reporting: Next generation sequencing (NGS) technologies and implementation of precision medicine in real life. *Crit. Rev. Oncol. Hematol.* **2019**, *133*, 171–182. [CrossRef] [PubMed]
130. Koboldt, D.C.; Steinberg, K.M.; Larson, D.E.; Wilson, R.K.; Mardis, E.R. The next-generation sequencing revolution and its impact on genomics. *Cell* **2013**, *155*, 27–38. [CrossRef] [PubMed]
131. Nowell, P.C.; Rowley, J.D.; Knudson, A.G., Jr. Cancer genetics, cytogenetics—Defining the enemy within. *Nat. Med.* **1998**, *4*, 1107–1111. [CrossRef]
132. Druker, B.J.; Lydon, N.B. Lessons learned from the development of an abl tyrosine kinase inhibitor for chronic myelogenous leukemia. *J. Clin. Invest.* **2000**, *105*, 3–7. [CrossRef] [PubMed]
133. Rossari, F.; Minutolo, F.; Orciuolo, E. Past, present, and future of Bcr-Abl inhibitors: From chemical development to clinical efficacy. *J. Hematol. Oncol.* **2018**, *11*, 84. [CrossRef]
134. Druker, B.J.; Talpaz, M.; Resta, D.J.; Peng, B.; Buchdunger, E.; Ford, J.M.; Lydon, N.B.; Kantarjian, H.; Capdeville, R.; Ohno-Jones, S.; et al. Efficacy and safety of a specific inhibitor of the BCR-ABL tyrosine kinase in chronic myeloid leukemia. *N. Engl. J. Med.* **2001**, *344*, 1031–1037. [CrossRef]
135. Savage, D.G.; Antman, K.H. Imatinib mesylate—A new oral targeted therapy. *N. Engl. J. Med.* **2002**, *346*, 683–693. [CrossRef]
136. Lee, Y.T.; Tan, Y.J.; Oon, C.E. Molecular targeted therapy: Treating cancer with specificity. *Eur. J. Pharmacol.* **2018**, *834*, 188–196. [CrossRef]
137. Scholl, C.; Frohling, S. Exploiting rare driver mutations for precision cancer medicine. *Curr. Opin. Genet. Dev.* **2019**, *54*, 1–6. [CrossRef]
138. Jackson, S.E.; Chester, J.D. Personalised cancer medicine. *Int. J. Cancer* **2015**, *137*, 262–266. [CrossRef]
139. Neal, J.W.; Sledge, G.W. Decade in review-targeted therapy: Successes, toxicities and challenges in solid tumours. *Nat. Rev. Clin. Oncol.* **2014**, *11*, 627–628. [CrossRef] [PubMed]
140. Prasad, V.; Fojo, T.; MBrad. Precision oncology: Origins, optimism, and potential. *Lancet Oncol.* **2016**, *17*, e81–e86. [CrossRef]
141. El-Deiry, W.S.; Goldberg, R.M.; Lenz, H.J.; Shields, A.F.; Gibney, G.T.; Tan, A.R.; Brown, J.; Eisenberg, B.; Heath, E.I.; Phuphanich, S.; et al. The current state of molecular testing in the treatment of patients with solid tumors, 2019. *Cancer J. Clin.* **2019**, *69*, 305–343. [CrossRef] [PubMed]
142. National Cancer Institute. Targeted Cancer Therapies. Available online: https://www.cancer.gov/about-cancer/treatment/types/targeted-therapies/targeted-therapies-fact-sheet (accessed on 2 July 2020).

143. Khotskaya, Y.B.; Mills, G.B.; Mills Shaw, K.R. Next-Generation Sequencing and Result Interpretation in Clinical Oncology: Challenges of Personalized Cancer Therapy. *Annu. Rev. Med.* **2017**, *68*, 113–125. [CrossRef]
144. Buchanan, M. The law of accelerating returns. *Nat. Phys.* **2008**, *4*, 507-507. [CrossRef]
145. Kurzweil, R. The Law of Accelerating Returns. 2001. Available online: https://www.kurzweilai.net/the-law-of-accelerating-returns (accessed on 12 April 2020).
146. Blazer, K.R.; Nehoray, B.; Solomon, I.; Niell-Swiller, M.; Culver, J.O.; Uman, G.C.; Weitzel, J.N. Next-generation testing for cancer risk: Perceptions, experiences, and needs among early adopters in community healthcare settings. *Genet. Test. Mol. Biomarkers* **2015**, *19*, 657–665. [CrossRef]
147. Mauer, C.B.; Pirzadeh-Miller, S.M.; Robinson, L.D.; Euhus, D.M. The integration of next-generation sequencing panels in the clinical cancer genetics practice: An. institutional experience. *Genet. Med.* **2014**, *16*, 407–412. [CrossRef]
148. Sabour, L.; Sabour, M.; Ghorbian, S. Clinical applications of next-generation sequencing in cancer diagnosis. *Pathol. Oncol. Res.* **2017**, *23*, 225–234. [CrossRef]
149. Sylvester, D.E.; Chen, Y.; Jamieson, R.V.; Dalla-Pozza, L.; Byrne, J.A. Investigation of clinically relevant germline variants detected by next-generation sequencing in patients with childhood cancer: A review of the literature. *J. Med. Genet.* **2018**, *55*, 785–793. [CrossRef]
150. Obrochta, E.; Godley, L.A. Identifying patients with genetic predisposition to acute myeloid leukemia. *Best Pract. Res. Clin. Haematol.* **2018**, *31*, 373–378. [CrossRef]
151. Gomy, I.; Mdel, P.D. Hereditary cancer risk assessment: Insights and perspectives for the next-generation sequencing era. *Genet. Mol. Biol.* **2016**, *39*, 184–188. [CrossRef] [PubMed]
152. Pensabene, M.; Spagnoletti, I.; Capuano, I.; Condello, C.; Pepe, S.; Contegiacomo, A.; Lombardi, G.; Bevilacqua, G.; Caligo, M.A. Two mutations of BRCA2 gene at exon and splicing site in a woman who underwent oncogenetic counseling. *Ann. Oncol.* **2009**, *20*, 874–878. [CrossRef] [PubMed]
153. Kamps, R.; Brandao, R.D.; Bosch, B.J.; Paulussen, A.D.; Xanthoulea, S.; Blok, M.J.; Romano, A. Next-generation sequencing in oncology: Genetic diagnosis, risk prediction and cancer classification. *Int. J. Mol. Sci.* **2017**, *18*, 308. [CrossRef] [PubMed]
154. Domchek, S.M.; Bradbury, A.; Garber, J.E.; Offit, K.; Robson, M.E. Multiplex genetic testing for cancer susceptibility: Out on the high wire without a net? *J. Clin. Oncol.* **2013**, *31*, 1267–1270. [CrossRef]
155. Weitzel, J.N.; Blazer, K.R.; MacDonald, D.J.; Culver, J.O.; Offit, K. Genetics, genomics, and cancer risk assessment: State of the Art and future directions in the era of personalized medicine. *Cancer J. Clin.* **2011**, *61*, 327–359. [CrossRef] [PubMed]
156. Lynce, F.; Isaacs, C. How far do we go with genetic evaluation. *Am. Soc. Clin. Oncol. Educ. Book.* **2016**, *35*, e72–e78. [CrossRef]
157. Lui, S.T.; Shuch, B. Genetic testing in kidney cancer patients: Who, when, and how? *Eur. Urol. Focus* **2019**, *5*, 973–976. [CrossRef]
158. Piccinin, C.; Panchal, S.; Watkins, N.; Kim, R.H. An update on genetic risk assessment and prevention: The role of genetic testing panels in breast cancer. *Expert Rev. Anticancer Ther.* **2019**, *19*, 787–801. [CrossRef]
159. Plichta, J.K.; Sebastian, M.L.; Smith, L.A.; Menendez, C.S.; Johnson, A.T.; Bays, S.M.; Euhus, D.M.; Clifford, E.J.; Jalali, M.; Kurtzman, S.H.; et al. Germline genetic testing: What the breast surgeon needs to know. *Ann. Surg. Oncol.* **2019**, *26*, 2184–2190. [CrossRef]
160. Valle, L.; Vilar, E.; Tavtigian, S.V.; Stoffel, E.M. Genetic predisposition to colorectal cancer: Syndromes, genes, classification of genetic variants and implications for precision medicine. *J. Pathol.* **2019**, *247*, 574–588. [CrossRef]
161. Suszynska, M.; Klonowska, K.; Jasinska, A.J.; Kozlowski, P. Large-scale meta-analysis of mutations identified in panels of breast/ovarian cancer-related genes—Providing evidence of cancer predisposition genes. *Gynecol. Oncol.* **2019**, *153*, 452–462. [CrossRef] [PubMed]
162. Muskens, I.S.; de Smith, A.J.; Zhang, C.; Hansen, H.M.; Morimoto, L.; Metayer, C.; Ma, X.; Walsh, K.M.; Wiemels, J.L. Germline cancer predisposition variants and pediatric glioma: A population-based study in California. *Neuro. Oncol.* **2020**, *22*, 864–874. [CrossRef] [PubMed]
163. Abdel-Rahman, M.H.; Sample, K.M.; Pilarski, R.; Walsh, T.; Grosel, T.; Kinnamon, D.; Boru, G.; Massengill, J.B.; Schoenfield, L.; Kelly, B.; et al. Whole exome sequencing identifies candidate genes associated with hereditary predisposition to uveal melanoma. *Ophthalmology* **2020**, *127*, 668–678. [CrossRef] [PubMed]

164. Johansson, P.A.; Nathan, V.; Bourke, L.M.; Palmer, J.M.; Zhang, T.; Symmons, J.; Howlie, M.; Patch, A.M.; Read, J.; Holland, E.A.; et al. Evaluation of the contribution of germline variants in BRCA1 and BRCA2 to uveal and cutaneous melanoma. *Melanoma Res.* **2019**, *29*, 483–490. [CrossRef] [PubMed]
165. Shivakumar, M.; Miller, J.E.; Dasari, V.R.; Gogoi, R.; Kim, D. Exome-wide rare variant analysis from the discovEHR study identifies novel candidate predisposition genes for endometrial cancer. *Front. Oncol.* **2019**, *9*, 574. [CrossRef]
166. Bertelsen, B.; Tuxen, I.V.; Yde, C.W.; Gabrielaite, M.; Torp, M.H.; Kinalis, S.; Oestrup, O.; Rohrberg, K.; Spangaard, I.; Santoni-Rugiu, E.; et al. High. frequency of pathogenic germline variants within homologous recombination repair in patients with advanced cancer. *NPJ Genom. Med.* **2019**, *4*, 13. [CrossRef]
167. Akhavanfard, S.; Padmanabhan, R.; Yehia, L.; Cheng, F.; Eng, C. Comprehensive germline genomic profiles of children, adolescents and young adults with solid tumors. *Nat. Commun.* **2020**, *11*, 2206. [CrossRef]
168. Jin, Z.B.; Li, Z.; Liu, Z.; Jiang, Y.; Cai, X.B.; Wu, J. Identification of de novo germline mutations and causal genes for sporadic diseases using trio-based whole-exome/genome sequencing. *Biol. Rev. Camb. Philos. Soc.* **2018**, *93*, 1014–1031. [CrossRef]
169. Johnson, L.M.; Hamilton, K.V.; Valdez, J.M.; Knapp, E.; Baker, J.N.; Nichols, K.E. Ethical considerations surrounding germline next-generation sequencing of children with cancer. *Expert Rev. Mol. Diagn.* **2017**, *17*, 523–534. [CrossRef]
170. Stadler, Z.K.; Schrader, K.A.; Vijai, J.; Robson, M.E.; Offit, K. Cancer genomics and inherited risk. *J. Clin. Oncol.* **2014**, *32*, 687–698. [CrossRef]
171. Backman, S.; Bajic, D.; Crona, J.; Hellman, P.; Skogseid, B.; Stalberg, P. Whole genome sequencing of apparently mutation-negative MEN1 patients. *Eur. J. Endocrinol.* **2020**, *182*, 35–45. [CrossRef] [PubMed]
172. Nissim, S.; Leshchiner, I.; Mancias, J.D.; Greenblatt, M.B.; Maertens, O.; Cassa, C.A.; Rosenfeld, J.A.; Cox, A.G.; Hedgepeth, J.; Wucherpfennig, J.I.; et al. Mutations in RABL3 alter KRAS prenylation and are associated with hereditary pancreatic cancer. *Nat. Genet.* **2019**, *51*, 1308–1314. [CrossRef] [PubMed]
173. Okur, V.; Chung, W.K. The impact of hereditary cancer gene panels on clinical care and lessons learned. *Cold Spring Harb. Mol. Case Stud.* **2017**, *3*. [CrossRef] [PubMed]
174. Lumish, H.S.; Steinfeld, H.; Koval, C.; Russo, D.; Levinson, E.; Wynn, J.; Duong, J.; Chung, W.K. Impact of panel gene testing for hereditary breast and ovarian cancer on patients. *J. Genet. Couns.* **2017**, *26*, 1116–1129. [CrossRef] [PubMed]
175. Rosenthal, E.T.; Bernhisel, R.; Brown, K.; Kidd, J.; Manley, S. Clinical testing with a panel of 25 genes associated with increased cancer risk results in a significant increase in clinically significant findings across a broad range of cancer histories. *Cancer Genet.* **2017**, *218–219*, 58–68. [CrossRef]
176. Foley, S.B.; Rios, J.J.; Mgbemena, V.E.; Robinson, L.S.; Hampel, H.L.; Toland, A.E.; Durham, L.; Ross, T.S. Use of whole genome sequencing for diagnosis and discovery in the cancer genetics clinic. *Ebiomedicine* **2015**, *2*, 74–81. [CrossRef]
177. Fewings, E.; Larionov, A.; Redman, J.; Goldgraben, M.A.; Scarth, J.; Richardson, S.; Brewer, C.; Davidson, R.; Ellis, I.; Evans, D.G.; et al. Germline pathogenic variants in PALB2 and other cancer-predisposing genes in families with hereditary diffuse gastric cancer without CDH1 mutation: A whole-exome sequencing study. *Lancet Gastroenterol. Hepatol.* **2018**, *3*, 489–498. [CrossRef]
178. Richards, S.; Aziz, N.; Bale, S.; Bick, D.; Das, S.; Gastier-Foster, J.; Grody, W.W.; Hegde, M.; Lyon, E.; Spector, E.; et al. Standards and guidelines for the interpretation of sequence variants: A joint consensus recommendation of the American College of Medical Genetics and Genomics and the Association for Molecular Pathology. *Genet. Med.* **2015**, *17*, 405–424. [CrossRef]
179. Eccles, D.M.; Mitchell, G.; Monteiro, A.N.; Schmutzler, R.; Couch, F.J.; Spurdle, A.B.; Gomez-Garcia, E.B.; ENIGMA Clinical Working Group. BRCA1 and BRCA2 genetic testing-pitfalls and recommendations for managing variants of uncertain clinical significance. *Ann. Oncol.* **2015**, *26*, 2057–2065. [CrossRef]
180. Li, M.M.; Datto, M.; Duncavage, E.J.; Kulkarni, S.; Lindeman, N.I.; Roy, S.; Tsimberidou, A.M.; Vnencak-Jones, C.L.; Wolff, D.J.; Younes, A.; et al. Standards and guidelines for the interpretation and reporting of sequence variants in cancer: A joint consensus recommendation of the Association for Molecular Pathology, American Society of Clinical Oncology, and College of American Pathologists. *J. Mol. Diagn.* **2017**, *19*, 4–23. [CrossRef]
181. Hoffman-Andrews, L. The known unknown: The challenges of genetic variants of uncertain significance in clinical practice. *J. Law Biosci.* **2017**, *4*, 648–657. [CrossRef] [PubMed]

182. Cheon, J.Y.; Mozersky, J.; Cook-Deegan, R. Variants of uncertain significance in BRCA: A harbinger of ethical and policy issues to come? *Genome. Med.* **2014**, *6*, 121. [CrossRef] [PubMed]
183. Welsh, J.L.; Hoskin, T.L.; Day, C.N.; Thomas, A.S.; Cogswell, J.A.; Couch, F.J.; Boughey, J.C. Clinical decision-making in patients with variant of uncertain significance in BRCA1 or BRCA2 Genes. *Ann. Surg. Oncol.* **2017**, *24*, 3067–3072. [CrossRef] [PubMed]
184. Voelker, R. Quick uptakes: Taking the uncertainty out of interpreting BRCA variants. *J. Am. Med. Assoc.* **2019**, *321*, 1340–1341. [CrossRef]
185. Domchek, S.; Weber, B.L. Genetic variants of uncertain significance: Flies in the ointment. *J. Clin. Oncol.* **2008**, *26*, 16–17. [PubMed]
186. Medendorp, N.M.; Hillen, M.A.; Murugesu, L.; Aalfs, C.M.; Stiggelbout, A.M.; Smets, E.M.A. Uncertainty related to multigene panel testing for cancer: A qualitative study on counsellors' and counselees' views. *J. Community Genet.* **2019**, *10*, 303–312. [CrossRef]
187. Medendorp, N.M.; Hillen, M.A.; van Maarschalkerweerd, P.E.A.; Aalfs, C.M.; Ausems, M.; Verhoef, S.; van der Kolk, L.E.; Berger, L.P.V.; Wevers, M.R.; Wagner, A.; et al. "We don't know for sure": Discussion of uncertainty concerning multigene panel testing during initial cancer genetic consultations. *Fam. Cancer* **2020**, *19*, 65–76. [CrossRef]
188. Hamilton, J.G.; Robson, M.E. Psychosocial effects of multigene panel testing in the context of cancer genomics. *Hastings Cent. Rep.* **2019**, *49*, S44–S52. [CrossRef]
189. Afghahi, A.; AWKuria. The changing landscape of genetic testing for inherited breast cancer predisposition. *Curr. Treat Option Oncol.* **2017**, *18*, 27. [CrossRef]
190. Richter, S.; Haroun, I.; Graham, T.C.; Eisen, A.; Kiss, A.; Warner, E. Variants of unknown significance in BRCA testing: Impact on risk perception, worry, prevention and counseling. *Ann. Oncol.* **2013**, *24*, viii69–viii74. [CrossRef]
191. Idos, G.E.; Kurian, A.W.; Ricker, C.; Sturgeon, D.; Culver, J.O.; Kingham, K.E.; Koff, R.; Chun, N.M.; Rowe-Teeter, C.; Lebensohn, A.P.; et al. Multicenter prospective cohort study of the diagnostic yield and patient experience of multiplex gene panel testing for hereditary cancer risk. *JCO Precis. Oncol.* **2019**. [CrossRef]
192. Federici, G.; Soddu, S. Variants of uncertain significance in the era of high-throughput genome sequencing: A lesson from breast and ovary cancers. *J. Exp. Clin. Cancer Res.* **2020**, *39*, 46. [CrossRef] [PubMed]
193. Valencia, C.A.; Husami, A.; Holle, J.; Johnson, J.A.; Qian, Y.; Mathur, A.; Wei, C.; Indugula, S.R.; Zou, F.; Meng, H.; et al. Clinical impact and cost-effectiveness of whole exome sequencing as a diagnostic tool: A pediatric center's experience. *Front. Pediatr.* **2015**, *3*, 67. [CrossRef] [PubMed]
194. Gieldon, L.; Mackenroth, L.; Kahlert, A.K.; Lemke, J.R.; Porrmann, J.; Schallner, J.; von der Hagen, M.; Markus, S.; Weidensee, S.; Novotna, B.; et al. Diagnostic value of partial exome sequencing in developmental disorders. *PLoS ONE* **2018**, *13*, e0201041. [CrossRef] [PubMed]
195. Maxwell, K.N.; Hart, S.N.; Vijai, J.; Schrader, K.A.; Slavin, T.P.; Thomas, T.; Wubbenhorst, B.; Ravichandran, V.; Moore, R.M.; Hu, C.; et al. Evaluation of ACMG-guideline-based variant classification of cancer susceptibility and non-cancer-associated genes in families affected by breast cancer. *Am. J. Hum. Genet.* **2016**, *98*, 801–817. [CrossRef]
196. Eggington, J.M.; Bowles, K.R.; Moyes, K.; Manley, S.; Esterling, L.; Sizemore, S.; Rosenthal, E.; Theisen, A.; Saam, J.; Arnell, C.; et al. A comprehensive laboratory-based program for classification of variants of uncertain significance in hereditary cancer genes. *Clin. Genet.* **2014**, *86*, 229–237. [CrossRef]
197. Sud, A.; Kinnersley, B.; Houlston, R.S. Genome-wide association studies of cancer: Current insights and future perspectives. *Nat. Rev. Cancer* **2017**, *17*, 692–704. [CrossRef]
198. Turnbull, C.; Sud, A.; Houlston, R.S. Cancer genetics, precision prevention and a call to action. *Nat. Genet.* **2018**, *50*, 1212–1218. [CrossRef]
199. Kurian, A.W.; Hare, E.E.; Mills, M.A.; Kingham, K.E.; McPherson, L.; Whittemore, A.S.; McGuire, V.; Ladabaum, U.; Kobayashi, Y.; Lincoln, S.E.; et al. Clinical evaluation of a multiple-gene sequencing panel for hereditary cancer risk assessment. *J. Clin. Oncol.* **2014**, *32*, 2001–2009. [CrossRef]
200. Grissom, A.A.; Friend, P.J. Multigene panel testing for hereditary cancer risk. *J. Adv. Pract. Oncol.* **2016**, *7*, 394–407.
201. Kurian, A.W.; Ford, J.M. Multigene panel testing in oncology practice: How should we respond? *JAMA Oncol.* **2015**, *1*, 277–278. [CrossRef] [PubMed]

202. Secretary's Advisory Committee on Genetics, Health and Society. *Genetics Education and Training*; The Honorable Kathleen Sebelius Secretary of Health and Human Services: Washington, DC, USA, 2011.
203. Campion, M.; Goldgar, C.; Hopkin, R.J.; Prows, C.A.; Dasgupta, S. Genomic education for the next generation of health-care providers. *Genet. Med.* **2019**, *21*, 2422–2430. [CrossRef] [PubMed]
204. Guttmacher, A.E.; Porteous, M.E.; McInerney, J.D. Educating health-care professionals about genetics and genomics. *Nat. Rev. Genet.* **2007**, *8*, 151–157. [CrossRef] [PubMed]
205. Douma, K.F.; Smets, E.M.; Allain, D.C. Non-genetic health professionals' attitude towards, knowledge of and skills in discussing and ordering genetic testing for hereditary cancer. *Fam. Cancer* **2016**, *15*, 341–350. [CrossRef] [PubMed]
206. Maiese, D.R.; Keehn, A.; Lyon, M.; Flannery, D.; Watson, M.; Working Groups of the National Coordinating Center for Seven Regional Genetics Service Collaboratives. Current conditions in medical genetics practice. *Genet. Med.* **2019**, *21*, 1874–1877. [CrossRef] [PubMed]
207. Salari, K. The dawning era of personalized medicine exposes a gap in medical education. *PLoS Med.* **2009**, *6*, e1000138. [CrossRef]
208. Stoll, K.; Kubendran, S.; Cohen, S.A. The past, present and future of service delivery in genetic counseling: Keeping up in the era of precision medicine. *Am. J. Med. Genet. C Semin. Med. Genet.* **2018**, *178*, 24–37. [CrossRef]
209. Daly, M.B.; Stearman, B.; Masny, A.; Sein, E.; Mazzoni, S. How to establish a high-risk cancer genetics clinic: Limitations and successes. *Curr. Oncol. Rep.* **2005**, *7*, 469–474. [CrossRef]
210. Cohen, S.A.; Bradbury, A.; Henderson, V.; Hoskins, K.; Bednar, E.; Arun, B.K. Genetic counseling and testing in a community setting: Quality, access, and efficiency. *Am. Soc. Clin. Oncol. Educ. Book.* **2019**, *39*, e34–e44. [CrossRef]
211. Stopfer, J.E. Genetic counseling and clinical cancer genetics services. *Semin. Surg. Oncol.* **2000**, *18*, 347–357. [CrossRef]
212. Anderson, B.; McLosky, J.; Wasilevich, E.; Lyon-Callo, S.; Duquette, D.; Copeland, G. Barriers and facilitators for utilization of genetic counseling and risk assessment services in young female breast cancer survivors. *J. Cancer Epidemiol.* **2012**, *2012*, 298745. [CrossRef] [PubMed]
213. Cohen, S.A.; Marvin, M.L.; Riley, B.D.; Vig, H.S.; Rousseau, J.A.; Gustafson, S.L. Identification of genetic counseling service delivery models in practice: A report from the NSGC service delivery model task force. *J. Genet. Couns.* **2013**, *22*, 411–421. [CrossRef] [PubMed]
214. Ricker, C.; Lagos, V.; Feldman, N.; Hiyama, S.; Fuentes, S.; Kumar, V.; Farwell Hagman, K.; Palomares, M.; Blazer, K.; Lowstuter, K.; et al. If we build it ... will they come?—Establishing a cancer genetics services clinic for an underserved predominantly Latina cohort. *J. Genet. Couns.* **2007**, *15*, 505–514. [CrossRef]
215. Epstein, C.J.; Erickson, R.P.; Hall, B.D.; Golbus, M.S. The center-satellite system for the wide-scale distribution of genetic counseling services. *Am. J. Hum. Genet.* **1975**, *27*, 322–332. [PubMed]
216. Reid, K.J.; Sakati, N.; Prichard, L.L.; Schneiderman, L.J.; Jones, O.W.; Dixson, B.K. Genetic counseling: An evaluation of public health genetic clinics. *West. J. Med.* **1976**, *124*, 6–12. [PubMed]
217. Riccardi, V.M. Health care and disease prevention through genetic counseling: A regional approach. *Am. J. Public Health* **1976**, *66*, 268–272. [CrossRef]
218. Weissman, S.M.; Zellmer, K.; Gill, N.; Wham, D. Implementing a virtual health telemedicine program. in a community setting. *J. Genet. Couns.* **2018**, *27*, 323–325. [CrossRef]
219. Brown, J.; Athens, A.; Tait, D.L.; Crane, E.K.; Higgins, R.V.; Naumann, R.W.; Gusic, L.H.; Amacker-North, L. A comprehensive program: Enabling effective delivery of regional genetic counseling. *Int. J. Gynecol. Cancer* **2018**, *28*, 996–1002. [CrossRef]
220. Fournier, D.M.; Bazzell, A.F.; Dains, J.E. Comparing outcomes of genetic counseling options in breast and ovarian cancer: An integrative review. *Oncol. Nurs. Forum* **2018**, *45*, 96–105. [CrossRef]
221. Buchanan, A.H.; Rahm, A.K.; Williams, J.L. Alternate service delivery models in cancer genetic counseling: A mini-review. *Front. Oncol.* **2016**, *6*, 120. [CrossRef]
222. McDonald, E.; Lamb, A.; Grillo, B.; Lucas, L.; Miesfeldt, S. Acceptability of telemedicine and other cancer genetic counseling models of service delivery in geographically remote settings. *J. Genet. Couns.* **2014**, *23*, 221–228. [CrossRef] [PubMed]

223. MacDonald, D.J.; KRBlazer; JNWeitze. Extending comprehensive cancer center expertise in clinical cancer genetics and genomics to diverse communities: The power of partnership. *J. Natl. Compr. Canc. Netw.* **2010**, *8*, 615–624. [CrossRef] [PubMed]
224. Solomon, I.B.; McGraw, S.; Shen, J.; Albayrak, A.; Alterovitz, G.; Davies, M.; Fitz, C.D.V.; Freedman, R.A.; Lopez, L.N.; Sholl, L.M. Engaging patients in precision oncology: development and usability of a web-based patient-facing genomic sequencing report. *JCO Precis. Oncol.* **2020**, *4*, 307–318. [CrossRef]
225. Blazer, K.R.; Macdonald, D.J.; Culver, J.O.; Huizenga, C.R.; Morgan, R.J.; Uman, G.C.; Weitzel, J.N. Personalized cancer genetics training for personalized medicine: Improving community-based healthcare through a genetically literate workforce. *Genet. Med.* **2011**, *13*, 832–840. [CrossRef] [PubMed]
226. Whitworth, P.; Beitsch, P.; Arnell, C.; Cox, H.C.; Brown, K.; Kidd, J.; Lancaster, J.M. Impact of payer constraints on access to genetic testing. *J. Oncol. Pract.* **2017**, *13*, e47–e56. [CrossRef] [PubMed]
227. Karlovich, C.A.; Williams, P.M. Clinical applications of next-generation sequencing in precision oncology. *Cancer J.* **2019**, *25*, 264–271. [CrossRef]
228. Wadapurkar, R.; Vyas, R. Computational analysis of next generation sequencing data and its applications in clinical oncology. *Inform. Med. Unlocked* **2018**, *11*, 75–82. [CrossRef]
229. Hyman, D.M.; Taylor, B.S.; Baselga, J. Implementing genome-driven oncology. *Cell* **2017**, *168*, 584–599. [CrossRef]
230. Nangalia, J.; Campbell, P.J. Genome sequencing during a patient's journey through cancer. *N. Engl. J. Med.* **2019**, *381*, 2145–2156. [CrossRef]
231. Pleasance, E.D.; Cheetham, R.K.; Stephens, P.J.; McBride, D.J.; Humphray, S.J.; Greenman, C.D.; Varela, I.; Lin, M.L.; Ordonez, G.R.; Bignell, G.R.; et al. A comprehensive catalogue of somatic mutations from a human cancer genome. *Nature* **2010**, *463*, 191–196. [CrossRef]
232. Campbell, P.J.; Getz, G.; Korbel, J.O.; Stuart, J.M.; Jennings, J.L.; Stein, L.D.; Perry, M.D.; Nahal-Bose, H.K.; Ouellette, B.F.F.; Li, C.H.; et al. Pan-cancer analysis of whole genomes. *Nature* **2020**, *578*, 82–93.
233. Demircioglu, D.; Cukuroglu, E.; Kindermans, M.; Nandi, T.; Calabrese, C.; Fonseca, N.A.; Kahles, A.; Lehmann, K.V.; Stegle, O.; Brazma, A.; et al. A pan-cancer transcriptome analysis reveals pervasive regulation through alternative promoters. *Cell* **2019**, *178*, 1465–1477. [CrossRef] [PubMed]
234. Nagahashi, M.; Shimada, Y.; Ichikawa, H.; Kameyama, H.; Takabe, K.; Okuda, S.; Wakai, T. Next generation sequencing-based gene panel tests for the management of solid tumors. *Cancer Sci.* **2019**, *110*, 6–15. [CrossRef] [PubMed]
235. El Achi, H.; Khoury, J.D.; Loghavi, S. Liquid biopsy by next-generation sequencing: A multimodality test for management of cancer. *Curr. Hematol. Malig. Rep.* **2019**, *14*, 358–367. [CrossRef] [PubMed]
236. Kancherla, J.; Rao, S.; Bhuvaneshwar, K.; Riggins, R.B.; Beckman, R.A.; Madhavan, S.; Bravo, H.C.; Boca, S.M. Evidence-based network approach to recommending targeted cancer therapies. *JCO Clin. Cancer Inform.* **2020**, *4*, 71–88. [CrossRef]
237. Zhang, W.; Chien, J.; Yong, J.; Kuang, R. Network-based machine learning and graph theory algorithms for precision oncology. *NPJ Precis. Oncol.* **2017**, *1*, 25. [CrossRef]
238. Jiang, X.L.; Martinez-Ledesma, E.; Morcos, F. Revealing protein networks and gene-drug connectivity in cancer from direct information. *Sci. Rep.* **2017**, *7*, 3739. [CrossRef]
239. Zhang, Y.; Tao, C. Network analysis of cancer-focused association network reveals distinct network association patterns. *Cancer Inform.* **2014**, *13*, 45–51.
240. Cheng, F.; Liu, C.; Jiang, J.; Lu, W.; Li, W.; Liu, G.; Zhou, W.; Huang, J.; Tang, Y. Prediction of drug-target interactions and drug repositioning via network-based inference. *PLoS Comput. Biol.* **2012**, *8*, e1002503. [CrossRef]
241. Garber, K. In a major shift, cancer drugs go "tissue-agnostic". *Science* **2017**, *356*, 1111–1112. [CrossRef]
242. Luoh, S.W.; Flaherty, K.T. When tissue is no longer the issue: tissue-agnostic cancer therapy comes of age. *Ann. Intern. Med.* **2018**, *169*, 233–239. [CrossRef] [PubMed]
243. Mullard, A. FDA approves landmark tissue-agnostic cancer drug. *Nat. Rev. Drug Discov.* **2018**, *1*, 87. [CrossRef] [PubMed]
244. Torres-Ayuso, P.; Sahoo, S.; Ashton, G.; An, E.; Simms, N.; Galvin, M.; Leong, H.S.; Frese, K.K.; Simpson, K.; Cook, N.; et al. Signaling pathway screening platforms are an efficient approach to identify therapeutic targets in cancers that lack known driver mutations: A case report for a cancer of unknown primary origin. *NPJ Genom. Med.* **2018**, *3*, 15. [CrossRef] [PubMed]

245. Siu, L.L.; Conley, B.A.; Boerner, S.; LoRusso, P.M. Next-generation sequencing to guide clinical trials. *Clin. Cancer Res.* **2015**, *21*, 4536–4544. [CrossRef] [PubMed]
246. Beaubier, N.; Bontrager, M.; Huether, R.; Igartua, C.; Lau, D.; Tell, R.; Bobe, A.M.; Bush, S.; Chang, A.L.; Hoskinson, D.C.; et al. Integrated genomic profiling expands clinical options for patients with cancer. *Nat. Biotechnol.* **2019**, *37*, 1351–1360. [CrossRef]
247. Lih, C.J.; Harrington, R.D.; Sims, D.J.; Harper, K.N.; Bouk, C.H.; Datta, V.; Yau, J.; Singh, R.R.; Routbort, M.J.; Luthra, R.; et al. Analytical validation of the next-generation sequencing assay for a nationwide signal—Finding clinical trial: Molecular analysis for therapy choice clinical trial. *J. Mol. Diagn.* **2017**, *19*, 313–327. [CrossRef]
248. Bitzer, M.; Ostermann, L.; Horger, M.; Biskup, S.; Schulze, M.; Ruhm, K.; Hilke, F.; Öner, Ö.; Nikolaou, K.; Schroeder, C.; et al. Next-generation sequencing of advanced gi tumors reveals individual treatment options. *JCO Precis. Oncol.* **2020**, *4*, 258–271. [CrossRef]
249. Sicklick, J.K.; Kato, S.; Okamura, R.; Schwaederle, M.; Hahn, M.E.; Williams, C.B.; De, P.; Krie, A.; Piccioni, D.E.; Miller, V.A.; et al. Molecular profiling of cancer patients enables personalized combination therapy: The I-PREDICT study. *Nat. Med.* **2019**, *25*, 744–750. [CrossRef]
250. Rodon, J.; Soria, J.C.; Berger, R.; Miller, W.H.; Rubin, E.; Kugel, A.; Tsimberidou, A.; Saintigny, P.; Ackerstein, A.; Brana, I.; et al. Genomic and transcriptomic profiling expands precision cancer medicine: The WINTHER trial. *Nat. Med.* **2019**, *25*, 751–758. [CrossRef]
251. Rothwell, D.G.; Ayub, M.; Cook, N.; Thistlethwaite, F.; Carter, L.; Dean, E.; Smith, N.; Villa, S.; Dransfield, J.; Clipson, A.; et al. Utility of ctDNA to support patient selection for early phase clinical trials: The TARGET study. *Nat. Med.* **2019**, *25*, 738–743. [CrossRef]
252. Reitsma, M.; Fox, J.; Vanden Borre, P.; Cavanaugh, M.; Chudnovsky, Y.; Erlich, R.L.; Gribbin, T.E.; Anhorn, R. Effect of a collaboration between a health plan, oncology practice, and comprehensive genomic profiling company from the payer perspective. *J. Manag. Care Spec. Pharm.* **2019**, *25*, 601–611. [CrossRef] [PubMed]
253. Luh, F.; Yen, Y. Benefits and harms of the centers for medicare & medicaid services ruling on next-generation sequencing. *JAMA Oncol.* **2018**, *4*, 1171–1172. [PubMed]
254. Phillips, K.A.; Trosman, J.R.; Deverka, P.A.; Quinn, B.; Tunis, S.; Neumann, P.J.; Chambers, J.D.; Garrison, L.P., Jr.; Douglas, M.P.; Weldon, C.B. Insurance coverage for genomic tests. *Science* **2018**, *360*, 278–279.
255. Trosman, J.R.; Weldon, C.B.; Gradishar, W.J.; Benson, A.; Cristofanilli, M.; Kurian, A.W.; Ford, J.M.; Balch, A.; Watkins, J.; Phillips, K.A. From the past to the present: Insurer coverage frameworks for next-generation tumor sequencing. *Value Health* **2018**, *21*, 1062–1068. [CrossRef] [PubMed]
256. Freedman, A.N.; Klabunde, C.N.; Wiant, K.; Enewold, L.; Gray, S.W.; Filipski, K.K.; Keating, N.L.; Leonard, D.G.B.; Lively, T.; McNeel, T.S.; et al. Use of next-generation sequencing tests to guide cancer treatment: Results from a nationally representative survey of oncologists in the United States. *JCO Precision Oncol.* **2018**, *13*, 1–13. [CrossRef]
257. Miller, F.A.; Krueger, P.; Christensen, R.J.; Ahern, C.; Carter, R.F.; Kamel-Reid, S. Postal survey of physicians and laboratories: Practices and perceptions of molecular oncology testing. *BMC Health Serv. Res.* **2009**, *9*, 131. [CrossRef]
258. Gray, S.W.; Hicks-Courant, K.; Cronin, A.; Rollins, B.J.; Weeks, J.C. Physicians' attitudes about multiplex tumor genomic testing. *J. Clin. Oncol.* **2014**, *32*, 1317–1323. [CrossRef]
259. Gray, S.W.; Park, E.R.; Najita, J.; Martins, Y.; Traeger, L.; Bair, E.; Gagne, J.; Garber, J.; Janne, P.A.; Lindeman, N.; et al. Oncologists' and cancer patients' views on whole-exome sequencing and incidental findings: Results from the CanSeq study. *Genet. Med.* **2016**, *18*, 1011–1019. [CrossRef]
260. Malone, E.R.; Oliva, M.; Sabatini, P.J.B.; Stockley, T.L.; Siu, L.L. Molecular profiling for precision cancer therapies. *Genome Med.* **2020**, *12*, 8. [CrossRef]
261. Bieg-Bourne, C.C.; Millis, S.Z.; Piccioni, D.E.; Fanta, P.T.; Goldberg, M.E.; Chmielecki, J.; Parker, B.A.; Kurzrock, R. Next-generation sequencing in the clinical setting clarifies patient characteristics and potential actionability. *Cancer Res.* **2017**, *77*, 6313–6320. [CrossRef]
262. Clark, D.F.; Maxwell, K.N.; Powers, J.; Lieberman, D.B.; Ebrahimzadeh, J.; Long, J.M.; McKenna, D.; Shah, P.; Bradbury, A.; Morrissette, J.J.D.; et al. Identification and confirmation of potentially actionable germline mutations in tumor-only genomic sequencing. *JCO Precis. Oncol.* **2019**, *3*. [CrossRef]

263. Madhavan, S.; Subramaniam, S.; Brown, T.D.; Chen, J.L. Art and challenges of precision medicine: Interpreting and integrating genomic data into clinical practice. *Am. Soc. Clin. Oncol. Educ. Book. Educ. Book.* **2018**, *38*, 546–553. [CrossRef] [PubMed]
264. Gutierrez, M.E.; Choi, K.; Lanman, R.B.; Licitra, E.J.; Skrzypczak, S.M.; Pe Benito, R.; Wu, T.; Arunajadai, S.; Kaur, S.; Harper, H.; et al. Genomic profiling of advanced non-small cell lung cancer in community settings: Gaps and opportunities. *Clin. Lung. Cancer* **2017**, *18*, 651–659. [CrossRef]
265. Trosman, J.R.; Weldon, C.B.; Kelley, R.K.; Phillips, K.A. Challenges of coverage policy development for next-generation tumor sequencing panels: Experts and payers weigh in. *J. Natl. Compr. Canc. Netw.* **2015**, *13*, 311–318. [CrossRef] [PubMed]
266. Hughes, K.S.; Ambinder, E.P.; Hess, G.P.; Yu, P.P.; Bernstam, E.V.; Routbort, M.J.; Clemenceau, J.R.; Hamm, J.T.; Febbo, P.G.; Domchek, S.M.; et al. Identifying health information technology needs of oncologists to facilitate the adoption of genomic medicine: Recommendations from the 2016 American Society of Clinical Oncology Omics and Precision Oncology Workshop. *J. Clin. Oncol.* **2017**, *35*, 3153–3159. [CrossRef]
267. Griffith, M.; Spies, N.C.; Krysiak, K.; McMichael, J.F.; Coffman, A.C.; Danos, A.M.; Ainscough, B.J.; Ramirez, C.A.; Rieke, D.T.; Kujan, L.; et al. CIViC is a community knowledgebase for expert crowdsourcing the clinical interpretation of variants in cancer. *Nat. Genet.* **2017**, *49*, 170–174. [CrossRef] [PubMed]
268. Chakravarty, D.; Phillips, S.; Kundra, R.; Zhang, H.; Wang, J.; Rudolph, J.E.; Yaeger, R.; Soumerai, T.; Nissan, M.H.; Chang, M.T.; et al. OncoKB: A precision oncology knowledge base. *JCO Precis. Oncol.* **2017**. [CrossRef] [PubMed]
269. Kurnit, K.C.; Bailey, A.M.; Zeng, J.; Johnson, A.M.; Shufean, M.A.; Brusco, L.; Litzenburger, B.C.; Sanchez, N.S.; Khotskaya, Y.B.; Holla, V.; et al. "Personalized cancer therapy": A publicly available precision oncology resource. *Cancer Res.* **2017**, *77*, e123–e126. [CrossRef]
270. My Cancer Genome: Genetically Informed Cancer Medicine. Available online: https://www.mycancergenome.org/ (accessed on 25 April 2020).
271. Warner, J.L.; Prasad, I.; Bennett, M.; Arniella, M.; Beeghly-Fadiel, A.; Mandl, K.D.; Alterovitz, G. SMART cancer navigator: A framework for implementing ASCO workshop recommendations to enable precision cancer medicine. *JCO Precis. Oncol.* **2018**. [CrossRef]
272. City of Hope. Molecular Oncology. Available online: https://www.cityofhope.org/clinical-molecular-diagnostic-laboratory/list-of-cmdl-tests/molecular-oncology (accessed on 3 June 2020).
273. Ellis, P.G. Development and implementation of oncology care pathways in an integrated care network: The via oncology pathways experience. *J. Oncol. Pract.* **2013**, *9*, 171–173. [CrossRef]
274. Luchini, C.; Lawlor, R.T.; Milella, M.; Scarpa, A. Molecular tumor boards in clinical practice. *Trends Cancer* **2020**. [CrossRef]
275. Rolfo, C.; Manca, P.; Salgado, R.; Van Dam, P.; Dendooven, A.; Machado Coelho, A.; Ferri Gandia, J.; Rutten, A.; Lybaert, W.; Vermeij, J.; et al. Multidisciplinary molecular tumour board: A tool to improve clinical practice and selection accrual for clinical trials in patients with cancer. *ESMO Open.* **2018**, *3*, e000398. [CrossRef] [PubMed]
276. Remon, J.; Dienstmann, R. Precision oncology: Separating the wheat from the chaff. *ESMO Open* **2018**, *3*, e000446. [CrossRef] [PubMed]
277. Romero, D. Optimizing access to matched therapies. *Nat. Rev. Clin. Oncol.* **2019**, *16*, 401. [CrossRef] [PubMed]
278. Andre, F.; Mardis, E.; Salm, M.; Soria, J.C.; Siu, L.L.; Swanton, C. Prioritizing targets for precision cancer medicine. *Ann. Oncol.* **2014**, *25*, 2295–2303. [CrossRef] [PubMed]
279. Dalton, W.S.; Sullivan, D.; Ecsedy, J.; Caligiuri, M.A. Patient enrichment for precision-based cancer clinical trials: Using prospective cohort surveillance as an approach to improve clinical trials. *Clin. Pharmacol. Ther.* **2018**, *104*, 23–26. [CrossRef] [PubMed]
280. Chakradhar, S. Matching up. *Nat. Med.* **2018**, *24*, 882–884. [CrossRef]
281. Roychowdhury, S.; Iyer, M.K.; Robinson, D.R.; Lonigro, R.J.; Wu, Y.M.; Cao, X.; Kalyana-Sundaram, S.; Sam, L.; Balbin, O.A.; Quist, M.J.; et al. Personalized oncology through integrative high-throughput sequencing: A pilot study. *Sci. Transl. Med.* **2011**, *3*, 111ra121. [CrossRef]
282. Kurnit, K.C.; Dumbrava, E.E.I.; Litzenburger, B.; Khotskaya, Y.B.; Johnson, A.M.; Yap, T.A.; Rodon, J.; Zeng, J.; Shufean, M.A.; Bailey, A.M.; et al. Precision oncology decision support: Current approaches and strategies for the future. *Clin. Cancer Res.* **2018**, *24*, 2719–2731. [CrossRef]

283. Dalton, W.B.; Forde, P.M.; Kang, H.; Connolly, R.M.; Stearns, V.; Gocke, C.D.; Eshleman, J.R.; Axilbund, J.; Petry, D.; Geoghegan, C.; et al. Personalized medicine in the oncology clinic: Implementation and outcomes of the Johns Hopkins Molecular Tumor Board. *JCO Precis. Oncol.* **2017**. [CrossRef]
284. Meric-Bernstam, F.; Johnson, A.; Holla, V.; Bailey, A.M.; Brusco, L.; Chen, K.; Routbort, M.; Patel, K.P.; Zeng, J.; Kopetz, S.; et al. A decision support framework for genomically informed investigational cancer therapy. *J. Natl. Cancer Inst.* **2015**, *107*. [CrossRef]
285. Hyman, D.M.; Solit, D.B.; Arcila, M.E.; Cheng, D.T.; Sabbatini, P.; Baselga, J.; Berger, M.F.; Ladanyi, M. Precision medicine at Memorial Sloan Kettering Cancer Center: Clinical next-generation sequencing enabling next-generation targeted therapy trials. *Drug Discov. Today* **2015**, *20*, 1422–1428. [CrossRef] [PubMed]
286. Huang, L.D.; Fernandes, H.; Zia, H.; Tavassoli, P.; Rennert, H.; Pisapia, D.; Imielinski, M.; Sboner, A.; Rubin, M.A.; Kluk, M.; et al. The cancer precision medicine knowledge base for structured clinical-grade mutations and interpretations. *J. Am. Med. Inform. Assoc.* **2017**, *24*, 513–519. [CrossRef] [PubMed]
287. Beltran, H.; Eng, K.; Mosquera, J.M.; Sigaras, A.; Romanel, A.; Rennert, H.; Kossai, M.; Pauli, C.; Faltas, B.; Fontugne, J.; et al. Whole-exome sequencing of metastatic cancer and biomarkers of treatment response. *JAMA Oncol.* **2015**, *1*, 466–474. [CrossRef] [PubMed]
288. Schwaederle, M.; Parker, B.A.; Schwab, R.B.; Daniels, G.A.; Piccioni, D.E.; Kesari, S.; Helsten, T.L.; Bazhenova, L.A.; Romero, J.; Fanta, P.T.; et al. Precision oncology: The UC San Diego Moores Cancer Center PREDICT Experience. *Mol. Cancer Ther.* **2016**, *15*, 743–752. [CrossRef] [PubMed]
289. Said, R.; Tsimberidou, A.M. Basket trials and the MD Anderson Precision Medicine Clinical trials platform. *Cancer J.* **2019**, *25*, 282–286. [CrossRef] [PubMed]
290. Trivedi, H.; Acharya, D.; Chamarthy, U.; Meunier, J.; Ali-Ahmad, H.; Hamdan, M.; Herman, J.; Srkalovic, G. Implementation and outcomes of a molecular tumor board at Herbert-Herman Cancer Center, Sparrow Hospital. *Acta Med. Acad.* **2019**, *48*, 105–115.
291. Grandori, C.; Kemp, C.J. Personalized cancer models for target. discovery and precision medicine. *Trends Cancer* **2018**, *4*, 634–642. [CrossRef]
292. Pauli, C.; Hopkins, B.D.; Prandi, D.; Shaw, R.; Fedrizzi, T.; Sboner, A.; Sailer, V.; Augello, M.; Puca, L.; Rosati, R.; et al. Personalized in vitro and in vivo cancer models to guide precision medicine. *Cancer Discov.* **2017**, *7*, 462–477. [CrossRef]
293. Chen, H.Z.; Bonneville, R.; Roychowdhury, S. Implementing precision cancer medicine in the genomic era. *Semin. Cancer Biol.* **2019**, *55*, 16–27. [CrossRef]
294. Wong, C.H.; Siah, K.W.; Lo, A.W. Estimation of clinical trial success rates and related parameters. *Biostatistics* **2019**, *20*, 273–286. [CrossRef] [PubMed]
295. Sacks, L.V.; Shamsuddin, H.H.; Yasinskaya, Y.I.; Bouri, K.; Lanthier, M.L.; Sherman, R.E. Scientific and regulatory reasons for delay and denial of FDA approval of initial applications for new drugs, 2000–2012. *J. Am. Med. Assoc.* **2014**, *311*, 378–384. [CrossRef] [PubMed]
296. Hay, M.; Thomas, D.W.; Craighead, J.L.; Economides, C.; Rosenthal, J. Clinical development success rates for investigational drugs. *Nat. Biotechnol.* **2014**, *32*, 40–51. [CrossRef] [PubMed]
297. Fogel, D.B. Factors associated with clinical trials that fail and opportunities for improving the likelihood of success: A review. *Contemp. Clin. Trials Commun.* **2018**, *11*, 156–164. [CrossRef] [PubMed]
298. Khozin, S.; Liu, K.; Jarow, J.P.; Pazdur, R. Regulatory watch: Why do oncology drugs fail to gain US regulatory approval? *Nat. Rev. Drug. Discov.* **2015**, *14*, 450–451. [CrossRef]
299. Heneghan, C.; Goldacre, B.; Mahtani, K.R. Why clinical trial outcomes fail to translate into benefits for patients. *Trials* **2017**, *18*, 122. [CrossRef]
300. Seruga, B.; Ocana, A.; Amir, E.; Tannock, I.F. Failures in phase III: Causes and consequences. *Clin. Cancer Res.* **2015**, *21*, 4552–4560. [CrossRef]
301. Schmidt, C. The struggle to do no harm. *Nature* **2017**, *552*, S74–S75. [CrossRef]
302. Mullard, A. How much do phase III trials cost? *Nat. Rev. Drug Discov.* **2018**, *1*, 7777-7777. [CrossRef]
303. Vincent Rajkumar, S. The high cost of prescription drugs: Causes and solutions. *Blood Cancer J.* **2020**, *10*, 71. [CrossRef]
304. Sanders, A.B.; Fulginiti, J.V.; Witzke, D.B.; Bangs, K.A. Characteristics influencing career decisions of academic and nonacademic emergency physicians. *Ann. Emerg. Med.* **1994**, *23*, 81–87. [CrossRef]
305. Tsang, J.L.Y.; Ross, K. It's time to increase community hospital-based health research. *Acad. Med.* **2017**, *92*, 727. [CrossRef]

306. Dimond, E.P.; St Germain, D.; Nacpil, L.M.; Zaren, H.A.; Swanson, S.M.; Minnick, C.; Carrigan, A.; Denicoff, A.M.; Igo, K.E.; Acoba, J.D.; et al. Creating a "culture of research" in a community hospital: Strategies and tools from the National Cancer Institute Community Cancer Centers Program. *Clin. Trials* **2015**, *12*, 246–256. [CrossRef]
307. Boaz, A.; Hanney, S.; Jones, T.; Soper, B. Does the engagement of clinicians and organisations in research improve healthcare performance: A three-stage review. *BMJ Open* **2015**, *5*, e009415. [CrossRef]
308. Knepper, T.C.; Bell, G.C.; Hicks, J.K.; Padron, E.; Teer, J.K.; Vo, T.T.; Gillis, N.K.; Mason, N.T.; McLeod, H.L.; Walko, C.M. Key lessons learned from moffitt's molecular tumor board: The clinical genomics action committee experience. *Oncologist* **2017**, *22*, 144–151. [CrossRef] [PubMed]
309. Overman, M.J.; Morris, V.; Kee, B.; Fogelman, D.; Xiao, L.; Eng, C.; Dasari, A.; Shroff, R.; Mazard, T.; Shaw, K.; et al. Utility of a molecular prescreening program in advanced colorectal cancer for enrollment on biomarker-selected clinical trials. *Ann. Oncol.* **2016**, *27*, 1068–1074. [CrossRef] [PubMed]
310. Dienstmann, R.; Garralda, E.; Aguilar, S.; Sala, G.; Viaplana, C.; Ruiz-Pace, F.; González-Zorelle, J.; LoGiacco, D.G.; Ogbah, Z.; Masdeu, L.R.; et al. Evolving landscape of molecular prescreening strategies for oncology early clinical trials. *JCO Precis. Oncol.* **2020**, *4*, 505–513. [CrossRef]
311. Pishvaian, M.J.; Blais, E.M.; Bender, R.J.; Rao, S.; Boca, S.M.; Chung, V.; Hendifar, A.E.; Mikhail, S.; Sohal, D.P.S.; Pohlmann, P.R.; et al. A virtual molecular tumor board to improve efficiency and scalability of delivering precision oncology to physicians and their patients. *JAMIA Open* **2019**, *2*, 505–515. [CrossRef]
312. Schwaederle, M.; Zhao, M.; Lee, J.J.; Lazar, V.; Leyland-Jones, B.; Schilsky, R.L.; Mendelsohn, J.; Kurzrock, R. Association of biomarker-based treatment strategies with response rates and progression-free survival in refractory malignant neoplasms: A meta-analysis. *JAMA Oncol.* **2016**, *2*, 1452–1459. [CrossRef]
313. Schwaederle, M.; Zhao, M.; Lee, J.J.; Eggermont, A.M.; Schilsky, R.L.; Mendelsohn, J.; Lazar, V.; Kurzrock, R. Impact of precision medicine in diverse cancers: A meta-analysis of phase II clinical trials. *J. Clin. Oncol.* **2015**, *33*, 3817–3825. [CrossRef]
314. Stockley, T.L.; Oza, A.M.; Berman, H.K.; Leighl, N.B.; Knox, J.J.; Shepherd, F.A.; Chen, E.X.; Krzyzanowska, M.K.; Dhani, N.; Joshua, A.M.; et al. Molecular profiling of advanced solid tumors and patient outcomes with genotype-matched clinical trials: The Princess Margaret IMPACT/COMPACT trial. *Genome Med.* **2016**, *8*, 109. [CrossRef] [PubMed]
315. Haslem, D.S.; Van Norman, S.B.; Fulde, G.; Knighton, A.J.; Belnap, T.; Butler, A.M.; Rhagunath, S.; Newman, D.; Gilbert, H.; Tudor, B.P.; et al. A retrospective analysis of precision medicine outcomes in patients with advanced cancer reveals improved progression-free survival without increased health care costs. *J. Oncol. Pract.* **2017**, *13*, e108–e119. [CrossRef] [PubMed]
316. Radovich, M.; Kiel, P.J.; Nance, S.M.; Niland, E.E.; Parsley, M.E.; Ferguson, M.E.; Jiang, G.; Ammakkanavar, N.R.; Einhorn, L.H.; Cheng, L.; et al. Clinical benefit of a precision medicine based approach for guiding treatment of refractory cancers. *Oncotarget* **2016**, *7*, 56491–56500. [CrossRef]
317. Aust, S.; Schwameis, R.; Gagic, T.; Mullauer, L.; Langthaler, E.; Prager, G.; Grech, C.; Reinthaller, A.; Krainer, M.; Pils, D.; et al. Precision medicine tumor boards: Clinical applicability of personalized treatment concepts in ovarian cancer. *Cancers* **2020**, *12*, 548. [CrossRef] [PubMed]
318. Tafe, L.J.; Gorlov, I.P.; de Abreu, F.B.; Lefferts, J.A.; Liu, X.; Pettus, J.R.; Marotti, J.D.; Bloch, K.J.; Memoli, V.A.; Suriawinata, A.A.; et al. Implementation of a molecular tumor board: The impact on treatment decisions for 35 patients evaluated at Dartmouth-Hitchcock Medical Center. *Oncologist* **2015**, *20*, 1011–1018. [CrossRef]
319. Lamping, M.; Benary, M.; Leyvraz, S.; Messerschmidt, C.; Blanc, E.; Kessler, T.; Schutte, M.; Lenze, D.; Johrens, K.; Burock, S.; et al. Support of a molecular tumour board by an evidence-based decision management system for precision oncology. *Eur. J. Cancer* **2020**, *127*, 41–51. [CrossRef]
320. Boddu, S.; Walko, C.M.; Bienasz, S.; Bui, M.M.; Henderson-Jackson, E.; Naghavi, A.O.; Mullinax, J.E.; Joyce, D.M.; Binitie, O.; Letson, G.D.; et al. Clinical utility of genomic profiling in the treatment of advanced sarcomas: A single-center experience. *JCO Precis. Oncol.* **2018**, 1–8. [CrossRef]
321. Lane, B.R.; Bissonnette, J.; Waldherr, T.; Ritz-Holland, D.; Chesla, D.; Cottingham, S.L.; Alberta, S.; Liu, C.; Thompson, A.B.; Graveel, C.; et al. Development of a center for personalized cancer care at a regional cancer center: Feasibility trial of an institutional tumor sequencing advisory board. *J. Mol. Diagn.* **2015**, *17*, 695–704. [CrossRef]

322. Overton, L.C.; Corless, C.L.; Agrawal, M.; Assikis, V.J.; Beegle, N.L.; Blau, S.; Chernoff, M.; Divers, S.G.; Henry, D.H.; Nikolinakos, P.; et al. Impact of next-generation sequencing (NGS) on treatment decisions in the community oncology setting. *J. Clin. Oncol.* **2014**, *32*, 11028-11028. [CrossRef]
323. ASCO eLearning. Multidisciplinary Molecular Tumor Boards (MMTBs). Available online: https://elearning.asco.org/product-details/multidisciplinary-molecular-tumor-boards-mmtbs (accessed on 1 May 2020).
324. Healio Learn Genomics. Available online: https://www.healio.com/hematology-oncology/learn-genomics (accessed on 1 May 2020).
325. Pishvaian, M.J.; Bender, R.J.; Halverson, D.; Rahib, L.; Hendifar, A.E.; Mikhail, S.; Chung, V.; Picozzi, V.J.; Sohal, D.; Blais, E.M.; et al. Molecular profiling of patients with pancreatic cancer: Initial results from the know your tumor initiative. *Clin. Cancer Res.* **2018**, *24*, 5018–5027. [CrossRef]
326. Burkard, M.E.; Deming, D.A.; Parsons, B.M.; Kenny, P.A.; Schuh, M.R.; Leal, T.; Uboha, N.; Lang, J.M.; Thompson, M.A.; Warren, R.; et al. Implementation and clinical utility of an integrated academic-community regional molecular tumor board. *JCO Precis. Oncol.* **2017**, 1–10. [CrossRef]
327. Heifetz, L.J.; Christensen, S.D.; Devere-White, R.W.; Meyers, F.J. A model for rural oncology. *J. Oncol. Pract.* **2011**, *7*, 168–171. [CrossRef] [PubMed]
328. Shea, C.M.; Teal, R.; Haynes-Maslow, L.; McIntyre, M.; Weiner, B.J.; Wheeler, S.B.; Jacobs, S.R.; Mayer, D.K.; Young, M.; Shea, T.C. Assessing the feasibility of a virtual tumor board program: A case study. *J. Healthc. Manag.* **2014**, *59*, 177–193. [CrossRef] [PubMed]
329. Farhangfar, C. Utilization of consultative molecular tumor board in community setting. *J. Clin. Oncol.* **2017**, *35*, 6508. [CrossRef]
330. Marshall, C.L.; Petersen, N.J.; Naik, A.D.; Vander Velde, N.; Artinyan, A.; Albo, D.; Berger, D.H.; Anaya, D.A. Implementation of a regional virtual tumor board: A prospective study evaluating feasibility and provider acceptance. *Telemed. J. E Health* **2014**, *20*, 705–711. [CrossRef]
331. Nasser, S.; Kurdolgu, A.A.; Izatt, T.; Aldrich, J.; Russell, M.L.; Christoforides, A.; Tembe, W.; Keifer, J.A.; Corneveaux, J.J.; Byron, S.A.; et al. An Integrated framework for reporting clinically relevant biomarkers from paired tumor/normal genomic and transcriptomic sequencing data in support of clinical trials in personalized medicine. *Pac. Symp. Biocomput.* **2015**, *2015*, 56–67.
332. Von Hoff, D.; Han, H. *Precision Medicine in Cancer Therapy*; Springer International Publishing: New York, NY, USA, 2019.
333. Weiss, G.J.; Byron, S.A.; Aldrich, J.; Sangal, A.; Barilla, H.; Kiefer, J.A.; Carpten, J.D.; Craig, D.W.; Whitsett, T.G. A prospective pilot study of genome-wide exome and transcriptome profiling in patients with small cell lung cancer progressing after first-line therapy. *PLoS ONE* **2017**, *12*, e0179170. [CrossRef]
334. Byron, S.A.; Tran, N.L.; Halperin, R.F.; Phillips, J.J.; Kuhn, J.G.; de Groot, J.F.; Colman, H.; Ligon, K.L.; Wen, P.Y.; Cloughesy, T.F.; et al. Prospective feasibility trial for genomics-informed treatment in recurrent and progressive glioblastoma. *Clin. Cancer Res.* **2018**, *24*, 295–305. [CrossRef]
335. Mueller, S.; Jain, P.; Liang, W.S.; Kilburn, L.; Kline, C.; Gupta, N.; Panditharatna, E.; Magge, S.N.; Zhang, B.; Zhu, Y.; et al. A pilot precision medicine trial for children with diffuse intrinsic pontine glioma-PNOC003: A report from the Pacific Pediatric Neuro-Oncology Consortium. *Int. J. Cancer* **2019**, *145*, 1889–1901. [CrossRef]

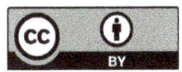

© 2020 by the authors. Licensee MDPI, Basel, Switzerland. This article is an open access article distributed under the terms and conditions of the Creative Commons Attribution (CC BY) license (http://creativecommons.org/licenses/by/4.0/).

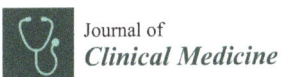

Review

Non-Small Cell Lung Cancer from Genomics to Therapeutics: A Framework for Community Practice Integration to Arrive at Personalized Therapy Strategies

Swapnil Rajurkar [†], Isa Mambetsariev [†], Rebecca Pharaon, Benjamin Leach, TingTing Tan, Prakash Kulkarni and Ravi Salgia *

Department of Medical Oncology and Therapeutics Research, City of Hope, Duarte, CA 91010, USA; srajurkar@coh.org (S.R.); Imambetsariev@coh.org (I.M.); rpharaon@coh.org (R.P.); bleach@coh.org (B.L.); titan@coh.org (T.T.); pkulkarni@coh.org (P.K.)
* Correspondence: rsalgia@coh.org
† These authors contributed equally to this work and should be considered co-first authors.

Received: 26 May 2020; Accepted: 12 June 2020; Published: 15 June 2020

Abstract: Non-small cell lung cancer (NSCLC) is a heterogeneous disease, and therapeutic management has advanced with the identification of various key oncogenic mutations that promote lung cancer tumorigenesis. Subsequent studies have developed targeted therapies against these oncogenes in the hope of personalizing therapy based on the molecular genomics of the tumor. This review presents approved treatments against actionable mutations in NSCLC as well as promising targets and therapies. We also discuss the current status of molecular testing practices in community oncology sites that would help to direct oncologists in lung cancer decision-making. We propose a collaborative framework between community practice and academic sites that can help improve the utilization of personalized strategies in the community, through incorporation of increased testing rates, virtual molecular tumor boards, vendor-based oncology clinical pathways, and an academic-type singular electronic health record system.

Keywords: non-small cell lung cancer; driver mutations; testing rates; receptor tyrosine kinases; team medicine

1. Introduction

Lung cancer remains the leading cause of cancer deaths in the United States and, in 2020, it will be responsible for an estimated 230,000 cases and 135,000 deaths in the US alone [1]. Non-small cell lung cancer (NSCLC) is the major histological subtype that accounts for approximately 85% of all lung cancer cases and encompasses several subtypes, including adenocarcinoma, squamous cell carcinoma, and large cell carcinoma [2]. Despite advances in screening and diagnosis, most patients still present with metastatic disease, at which point surgical intervention is no longer an option [3]. The advent of targeted therapy and immunotherapy has altered the course of treatment for the majority of patients—with molecular testing now a standard recommendation for late-stage lung adenocarcinoma patients. Tyrosine kinase inhibitors (TKIs) that target abnormalities in several genes, such as *ALK* and *EGFR*, have shown better progression-free survival (PFS) as compared with standard chemotherapy in a number of NSCLC trials [4–6]. More recently, other molecular markers, including ROS1, RET, NTRK, BRAF, and MET, have delivered similar clinical benefits to patients with late-stage NSCLC [7–12]. Furthermore, mature outcome data from second-generation TKIs is showing durable overall survival benefit for patients [13,14], a factor that was previously disputed with earlier TKIs [15].

Several molecular targets that were previously considered "unactionable", such as KRAS, now have several targeted therapies under consideration with promising early results [16,17]. Nevertheless, for patients without an actionable target or progression of disease, immune checkpoint inhibitors (ICIs) have resulted in durable outcomes and clinical benefit across several NSCLC trials in various lines of therapy [18–24]. Protein expression testing of programmed death-ligand 1 (PD-L1) has been identified as a potential, though not definitive, biomarker of predicting response to immunotherapy [21,25–27]. Beyond tumor response, recent results from KEYNOTE-001 showed that pembrolizumab monotherapy was associated with a 23.2% 5-year overall survival as compared to 15.5% for previously treated patients [28]. However, therapeutic advancements and outcome improvements have not been uniformly applied in practice, with the majority of trials and novel therapies being more prevalent in academic sites as compared to community practice. We previously showed in a retrospective study that in a cohort of 253 patients from nine community practice centers, the molecular testing rate for first-line treatment decisions was 81.75%, with testing for PD-L1 at only 56% [29]. This suggests that while community sites are on pace to improving their testing rates, the current results are inadequate and require more education and understanding of novel upcoming personalized therapies. The purpose of the current review is to shed light on the available and upcoming therapies in lung cancer, to report the gaps in community practice testing rates, and to identify the available tools that can assist in complex lung cancer management and decision-making.

2. Advances in Genomic Testing and Personalized Therapy

In the last 20 years, therapeutic management of lung cancer has progressed from cytotoxic chemotherapies to personalized targeted therapies that act upon specific genomic alterations. Prior to this, while cytotoxic therapies showed a benefit for early-stage disease [30,31], there was no reported outcome benefit in patients with late-stage lung cancer [32]. Following the completion of the multi-billion dollar endeavor of the Human Genome Project in 2003 [33], the development of next-generation sequencing with high-throughput has enabled large-scale parallel sequencing of the lung cancer genome revealing a plethora of genomic targets including EGFR (10–50%), KRAS (25%), ALK (2–7%), ROS1 (1–2%), RET (1%), BRAF (4%), and others [34,35]. Initially, EGFR tyrosine kinase inhibitors were evaluated in unselected populations with mixed responses due to inadequate selection of patients with EGFR alterations [36,37]. However, the results from randomized Phase III trials for EGFR and ALK tyrosine kinase inhibitors [5] led to the acceptance of genomic testing for ALK and EGFR alterations in routine clinical practice, and in turn, led to the development of faster and more efficient next-generation sequencing platforms that were Clinical Laboratory Improvement Amendments (CLIA)-certified and became widely accepted commercially and at academic sites [38]. While first-generation EGFR TKIs, including gefitinib and erlotinib, showed improved progression-free survival, retrospective studies and outcomes data failed to show improvements in overall survival outcomes [13,39–42]. In contrast to these results, the FLAURA trial for second-generation TKI, osimertinib, showed significant progression-free survival benefit (median PFS 18.9 vs. 10.2 months) and a considerable overall survival benefit of 35.8 months as compared to 27.0 months in the control [43]. The durable survival benefit of targeted therapies had previously been disputed, but recent results from the long-term survival of advanced ALK-rearranged patients treated with crizotinib showed an undisputable benefit of median OS of 6.8 years and a 5-year OS rate of 36% as compared to the historical 2% [44]. Moreover, advances in immunotherapy have yielded similar improvements and KEYNOTE-189 showed that patients who received immunotherapy resulted in a 20% improvement in the overall survival [45].

The promise of precision medicine and the arrival of personalized therapy has transformed lung cancer care with a number of genetic alterations that have come to fruition or are quickly rising with promising trial results, including EGFR, ALK, ROS1, MET, RET, NTRK, BRAF, KRAS, and immunotherapies (Table 1). However, the rapid and dynamic nature of emerging trial results has made lung cancer management difficult and while academic sites are familiar with trial results and the latest available therapies, a community oncologist, who may see a variety of solid tumors, may have difficulty grasping the complexity of these genomic alterations. In our experience at the academic site, actionable alterations were identified in 53.5% of patients with lung cancer, and the use of genomic-informed therapy was associated with improved survival benefit as compared to patients with no actionable alterations [46]. The use of genomic-informed therapy and selective immunotherapy must be standardized within community practice to ensure improved outcomes.

Table 1. Actionable targets in lung cancer and available therapeutics.

Biomarker Strategy	Approved and Investigational Therapies	Toxicities	Preferred Frontline Therapy	Incidence Rates in NSCLC
EGFR	Osimertinib, Erlotinib, Gefitinib, Afatinib, Dacomitinib	Cutaneous (acneiform rash), gastrointestinal (diarrhea)	Osimertinib	10–50%
ALK	Crizotinib, Ceritinib, Alectinib, Brigatinib, Lorlatinib	Gastrointestinal (nausea, diarrhea), transaminitis, visual changes, pneumonitis	Alectinib	1–7%
ROS1	Crizotinib, Ceritinib, Entrectinib, Lorlatinib	Gastrointestinal (nausea, diarrhea), transaminitis, visual changes, pneumonitis	Crizotinib or Entrectinib	1–2%
MET	Crizotinib, Capmatinib, Tepotinib, Telisotuzumab vedotin	Gastrointestinal, transaminitis	Crizotinib or Capmatinib	3–6%
RET	Cabozantinib, Vandetanib, Sunitinib, Selpercatinib, Pralsetnib(BLU-667) Selpercatinib (LOXO-292)	Fatigue, transaminitis, hypertension, diarrhea	Selpercatinib	1–2%
NTRK	Larotrectinib, Entrectinib, Loxo-195	Fatigue, edema, dizziness, constipation, diarrhea, liver abnormalities	Larotrectinib or Entrectinib	3–4%
BRAF	Dabrafenib, Trametinib, Vemurafenib	Rash, fever, headache, diarrhea	Dabrafenib+Trametinib	7%
PD-L1 expression	Pembrolizumab, Nivolumab, Ipilimumab, Atezolizumab, Durvalumab	Immune-mediated toxicities, including pulmonary and gastrointestinal	Various combination options of chemotherapy and immunotherapy or single-agent immunotherapy	~22–47% [47]

2.1. EGFR

The epidermal growth factor receptor is a transmembrane cell-surface receptor that is activated in 10–50% of patients with NSCLC, which varies based on populations and is more common in Asians and nonsmokers [34,48]. The receptors in the EGFR family exist as inactive monomers, but the binding of extracellular growth factors, such as epidermal growth factor (EGF), has been shown to cause receptor dimerization and induced autophosphorylation of the tyrosine kinase domain, with downstream and intercellular signaling cascades that in turn affect cell motility, invasion, proliferation, and angiogenesis [49]. Initial mutations in EGFR were first described in 2004 and activating mutations in EGFR occurring in exons 18–21 of the kinase domain were associated with sensitivity and response to gefitinib and erlotinib [50–52]. This led to the selection of patients with adenocarcinoma histology and EGFR alterations and, in 2009, a landmark Phase III Iressa Pan-Asia Study (IPASS) identified clinical responsiveness and increased progression-free survival in EGFR mutant patients who received gefitinib as compared to standard chemotherapy [50]. The landmark Phase III trial, EURTAC, evaluating erlotinib, an EGFR TKI, as a first-line therapy for patients with EGFR mutations, showed an increased median PFS of 9.7 months as compared to 5.2 months with standard chemotherapy [53]. Two other Phase III trials, the OPTIMAL and ENSURE trials, showed a similar improvement with erlotinib and the US Food and Drug Administration (FDA) approved erlotinib as a first-line cancer therapy for EGFR mutation-positive patients [4,53,54]. Similarly, afatinib, a second-generation TKI, received FDA approval in 2013 following two Phase III trials, Lux-Lung 3 and Lux-Lung 6, that both showed improved PFS of 11.1 months and 11 months respectively, as compared to standard chemotherapy in the first-line setting [55,56].

In 2015, efficacy results for patients with exon 19 deletions or exon 21 (L858R) mutations treated with gefitinib showed a 50% objective response rate (ORR) and led to the FDA approval of gefitinib as a first-line therapy for EGFR mutation-positive patients [57]. However, at that time erlotinib became the standard choice of therapy for many EGFR mutated patients, and mechanisms of primary and secondary resistance to TKI therapy began to emerge. The most commonly identified acquired resistance to early-generation TKIs was the T790M substitution, a secondary EGFR mutation in exon 20, that accounted for approximately 60% of cases [53,55,58,59]. The development of mutant selective pyrimidine-based third-generation TKIs that could block the T790M substitution led to the AURA3 trial evaluating osimertinib, a third-generation TKI, as second-line therapy following T790M EGFR TKI resistance [6]. In 2017, the results of the AURA3 trial showed a significantly improved PFS of 10.1 months and a response rate of 71% as compared to standard chemotherapy [6], and this led to the issuance of FDA approval for osimertinib in the second-line setting for EGFR T790M mutation-positive patients treated with first-line EGFR TKI. Compounding results also exhibited higher CNS response rates with osimertinib (40% vs. 17%) and a longer CNS PFS of 11.7 months vs. 5.6 months [60]. Brain metastases occur in approximately 20–40% of EGFR patients at presentation [61,62] and CNS activity of osimertinib hinted at its potential as a first-line therapy. Unsurprisingly, in 2018, the results of the FLAURA trial showed osimertinib as superior in the first-line setting as compared to first-generation TKIs, with a median PFS of 18.9 months (vs. 10.2 months), ORR of 77% (vs. 69%), and a median duration of response (DOR) at 17.6 months (vs. 9.6 months) [13]. This led to the issuance of FDA approval for osimertinib as the first-line therapy option for EGFR mutant lung cancer. Furthermore, mature data from the FLAURA trial also showed a medial overall survival benefit of 38.6 months over 31.8 months in the control and there was a significant improvement in quality of life, a clinical factor that was never previously achieved in first-generation TKIs [43].

However, despite advances in therapy, acquired resistance inevitably occurs, including EGFR-dependent resistance (6–10%), MET and HER2 amplifications (8–17%), small cell lung cancer (SCLC), and squamous cell carcinoma (SCC) transformation (15%), and others [63]. EGFR-dependent resistance includes S768I, L861Q, G719X, and other alterations that are resistant to most first-generation TKIs except for afatinib that was approved for first-line therapy for patients with rare EGFR alterations [64]. Additional TKIs such as poziotinib are currently under consideration for such alterations and Phase II preliminary data showed a response rate of 43% and a median PFS of 5.5 months in previously treated EGFR-mutant patients [65]. Additionally, other TKIs including TAK-788 (NCT03807778), TAS6417 (NCT04036682), and tarloxotinib (TH-4000) (NCT03805841) are currently under investigation in this setting. There are other trials available for less-frequent mutations of EGFR, such as exon 18 or exon 20 EGFR insertions. The availability of numerous EGFR TKIs in the first and refractory setting is strictly contingent upon appropriate assignment to therapy following reflex molecular testing. The improvements in survival are dependent on early identification of molecular markers and appropriate sequence of TKI therapy. In one retrospective study of rates of molecular testing in a community-based academic center, EGFR testing following the approval of reflex testing was only 62% [66]. In another larger cohort of 814 community practice patients, testing rates were similarly low, with only 69% of patients who were tested for EGFR mutations, and approximately 70% of patients who tested positive received appropriate targeted therapy [67]. In a retrospective evaluation of 1,203 advanced NSCLC patients from five community oncology practices, the testing rates of EGFR were at 54% [68]. A comprehensive retrospective cohort of 191 community oncology practices with 5688 patients performed by Flatiron Health, selected patients who were tested for EGFR alterations with either broad genomic sequencing or routine-testing and identified 154 EGFR-mutated patients in the broad-based sequencing group, but reported that only 25% of these patients received appropriate EGFR-targeted therapy [69]. The findings of the study concluded that there was no survival difference between broad-based and routine genomic sequencing, but this misrepresented the utility of broad-based genomic sequencing in the community, as better outcomes cannot be achieved without appropriate assignment to targeted therapy. Meanwhile, in our own community practice experience of 253 patients, we reported testing rates of 94% for EGFR and 96.2% of patients with an EGFR sensitizing mutation received a TKI therapy [29]. The translation of outcomes reported in clinical trials to real-world outcomes requires cooperation and acceptance of molecular testing within community practice and the integration of targeted therapies in community decision-making.

2.2. ALK

ALK, a receptor tyrosine kinase, was originally identified in lung cancer in 2007 with the detection of an echinoderm microtubule-associated protein-like 4 (EML4) gene and anaplastic lymphoma kinase (ALK) gene fusion from a surgically resected lung adenocarcinoma patient [70]. This gene rearrangement is largely independent of EGFR alterations and has been described as an actionable oncogene with incidence in 1–7% of lung cancer patients [71]. ALK-rearranged patients tend to be younger and—similar to EGFR—have a limited history of smoking. Crizotinib, while originally developed as a MET therapeutic, showed a preclinical efficacy for ALK [72]. The Phase I trial lead to the FDA approval of crizotinib in ALK-positive NSCLC [5]. In 2013, the results of the Phase III trial evaluating crizotinib compared to standard chemotherapy showed PFS of 7.7 months (vs. 3.0 months) and ORR of 65% (vs. 20%) [5], resulting in FDA approval of crizotinib for first-line therapy as a standard of care. As with other TKIs, while patients initially respond to ALK inhibitors, resistance invariably develops and one of the most common resistance mechanisms is an acquired ALK mutation (1151Tins, L1152R, C1156Y, F1174V/L, G1269A, and others) [73]. Other resistance mechanisms include EGFR activation, KIT activation, KRAS mutation, and IGF1R activation [74–79]. It was estimated that 25% of ALK-mutated patients do not respond to crizotinib in the first-line setting and, in response to these resistance mechanisms [77], other ALK TKIs have been developed. In 2014, the results from the Phase I trial evaluating ceritinib as a potential therapy in ALK-rearranged NSCLC patients with disease progression on crizotinib showed a median progression-free survival of 7.0 months and a response rate of 56% [80]. Based on only the Phase I trial results, the FDA approved ceritinib in patients who have progressed on crizotinib, and in 2017, it expanded its approval for first-line use. Alectinib received similar approval in 2015 in the refractory setting that was later expanded to first-line in 2017 [81–83]. In the first-line, alectinib showed a median PFS of 34.8 months with an OS rate of 62.5% as compared to crizotinib with 11 months and 52% [81–83]. Brigatinib, a second-generation ALK TKI, was initially identified to have preclinical efficacy and grater potency against all 17 ALK mutants as compared with crizotinib [84,85]. Initial results for brigatinib from a Phase II trial in the refractory setting showed promising responses and yielded FDA approval in 2017 [86]. While alectinib has been shown to be effective against L1196M, C1156Y, and F1174L ALK gatekeeper mutations [87], brigatinib has shown efficacy against ROS1, FLT3, and IGF-1 secondary mutations [88]. The results of the Phase III trial for brigatinib vs. crizotinib in the first-line showed an estimated PFS of 12 months as compared to 11 months with crizotinib, and two-year follow-up data showed brigatinib reduced the risk of progression or death by 76% [14,89]. Several other new generation ALK TKIs including lorlatinib and ensartinib demonstrated 73% and 72% ORR, respectively, following crizotinib and we are awaiting first-line results [90,91].

The availability of a number of ALK inhibitors has complicated management of ALK patients, but in a long-term assessment of 110 patients with an ALK inhibitor, a remarkable OS for advanced ALK NSCLC patients of 6.8 years was reported with 78.4% of patients receiving another ALK inhibitor after first-line progression [44]. Therefore, many studies are reporting that the success of ALK inhibition therapy may lie in the sequence of administrating ALK inhibitors based on metastatic progression and resistance profiles [92,93]. In a retrospective analysis of 31,483 patients with advanced NSCLC at community practices, ALK overall testing rates were 53.1% and rose to 62.1% in 2016, with 21.5% of patients who were initiated into non-targeted therapy before receiving test results [94]. Gierman et al. in 2019 evaluated 1,203 advanced NSCLC patients from five community practices and results showed that only 51% of patients were tested for ALK rearrangement, with approximately 45% of actionable patients receiving targeted therapy [68]. A concurrent study of 814 community practice patients showed that only 65% were tested for ALK alterations [67]. A retrospective study of advanced NSCLC across over 70 community sites in the US showed that only ~50% of patients were tested for ALK alterations during their cancer care [95], suggesting that advancements in liquid biopsies and testing are not translating to real-world practice. The use of liquid biopsies in a large cfDNA study showed that genomic results were concordant with tissue and utilizing cfDNA liquid biopsies increased detection and rates of testing by 48% [96]. The integration of liquid biopsy testing and further controls on tissue biopsy testing may improve the rates of ALK testing and translate the 6.8-year median survival benefit from academic site-wide studies into real-world efficacy.

2.3. ROS1

ROS1 has been identified as an oncogene in lung cancer and rearrangements have been reported in 1 to 2% of patients with NSCLC [34]. The fusion mutations lead to the dysregulation of the tyrosine-kinase dependent multi-use intracellular signaling pathway, which in turn accelerates growth, proliferation, and progression [97]. Similar to EGFR and ALK alterations, *ROS1* fusions and rearrangements are mutually exclusive and independent of other oncogenes such as KRAS or MET [98]. Following the discovery of *ROS1* fusions in 2007 and in part due to the high degree of homology between *ALK* and *ROS1*, the tyrosine kinase inhibitor crizotinib was explored as a therapeutic option [99,100]. Crizotinib was approved by the FDA in 2016 contingent upon clinical benefit from a PROFILE 1001 Phase I study, where patients had a median PFS of 19.2 months and an ORR of 72% [101]. A Phase II study of ceritinib with 32 patients showed an ORR response rate of 62% and a PFS of 19.3 months for crizotinib-naïve patients, but FDA approval is pending and ceritinib was ineffective against resistance mutations but had activity against CNS disease, as intracranial ORR was 25% and intracranial DCR was 63% [102]. Unlike ceritinib, entrectinib has been shown to be effective against some resistance mutations and had similar CNS activity with a median PFS of 13.6 months and ORR of 55% for patients with CNS disease [103]. This led to the FDA's approval of entrectinib in the management of ROS1-positive NSCLC. However, lorlatinib is currently the only inhibitor under consideration for *ROS1* that is effective against most resistance mutations and in a Phase II trial it induced an ORR of 26.5% with a PFS of 8.5, with considerable CNS activity inducing an ORR of 52.6% [104]. Other agents such as DS6051b (NCT02279433) and repotrectinib (NCT03093116) are also currently under investigation with results awaiting. A 2018 study by Friends of Cancer Research and Deerfield Institute announced the response of a survey of 157 oncologists and showed that ROS1 testing in the community centers was 32% [105]. However, a comprehensive study of 14,461 patients treated in the community showed testing rates for ROS1 were incrementally lower at 5.7% with 35.5% and 32.9% for *EGFR* and *ALK* respectively [106]. Of the three major approved alterations, ROS1 has the lowest testing rates in several studies [67,105,106]. While tissue biopsies remain the gold standard in detecting *ROS1* fusions and rearrangements, advances in liquid biopsy have shown that it is a viable option for *ROS1* and implementation of this practice may increase the testing rates within the community practice [29,107].

2.4. MET

MET oncogenic mutations and amplification has been noted in various solid tumor malignancies, including NSCLC, breast cancer, and head and neck cancer [108–112]. MET alterations or its ligand activation (hepatocyte growth factor) causes the activation of the tyrosine kinase which subsequently activates downstream signaling pathways related to cell growth, apoptosis, motility, and invasiveness [113]. Initially discovered in familial and sporadic papillary renal carcinomas [114], subsequent studies revealed the incidence of *MET* alterations in SCLC and NSCLC, especially MET exon 14 skipping as identified initially by our laboratory [115,116]. *MET* alterations have an incidence rate of 6% in lung adenocarcinoma and 3% of lung squamous cell carcinoma [117,118]. The most frequent alteration is the *MET* exon 14 skipping mutation, which has been identified in 4% of lung cancers. A 2015 study was the first to demonstrate clinical efficacy of crizotinib or cabozantinib in NSCLC patients with *MET* exon 14 skipping mutations [119]. A recent study enrolled 69 NSCLC patients harboring *MET* exon 14 alterations that were treated with crizotinib and reported an ORR of 32% and a median PFS of 7.3 months, suggesting antitumor activity with crizotinib treatment [120]. Several clinical trials, such as the GEOMETRY mono-1 trial and the VISION trial, are evaluating other TKIs like capmatinib and tepotinib in MET exon 14-mutated NSCLC and have shown promising results [12,121]. Interim results of the Phase II GEOMETRY mono-1 trial with 97 enrolled patients reported good ORR and a median PFS of 9.13 months in the treatment-naïve cohort [12]. Recently, capmantinib was granted accelerated FDA approval in metastatic NSCLC patients with *MET* exon 14 skipping mutation, the first TKI approved for MET NSCLC patients. MET amplification, which accounts for 1–4% of NSCLC patients who have not been treated with EGFR TKIs, is associated with a poor prognosis [122,123]. A Phase I trial investigated telisotuzumab vedotin, an antibody-drug conjugate, in NSCLC patients with MET overexpression and demonstrated safety and tolerability of the drug with promising antitumor efficacy [124]. In a study of NGS testing rates of genomic biomarkers in NSCLC patients treated at community sites, only 15% of the 814 patients underwent NGS testing for MET, a sharp decline compared to EGFR (69%) or ALK (65%) testing rates [67]. This testing rate was recapitulated in another community analysis [69], however, MET testing rates were reported as low as 6% in an analysis of NGS screening rates between private clinics, academic centers, and community sites [105].

2.5. RET

Activation of RET results in downstream pathway signaling including MAPK, JAK/STAT, and PI3K/AKT, leading to cell proliferation and migration. Alterations in *RET* are most frequently found in medullary thyroid carcinoma and NSCLC. In NSCLC, RET rearrangements are found in approximately 1–2% of cases [117]. These patients tend to be non- or former light smokers with adenocarcinoma histology and present with advanced disease [125]. Since its discovery, several targeted therapies have been investigated including multikinase inhibitors and selective RET inhibitors. A Phase II trial of RET fusion-positive NSCLC patients were treated with cabozantinib, a TKI targeting RET, VEGFR, and MET. The results demonstrated good clinical efficacy with an ORR of 28% and a median PFS of 5.5 months [126]. The most promising selective RET inhibitors currently under investigation are BLU-677 and selpercatinib (LOXO-292). Interim results from a Phase I clinical trial of 79 RET fusion-positive NSCLC patients treated with BLU-677 demonstrated an ORR of 56% among the 57 evaluable patients and encouraging central nervous system (CNS) activity against brain metastases [127]. The Phase I/II LIBRETTO-001 trial evaluating selpercatinib in a cohort of previously treated NSCLC patients with RET rearrangements (N = 105) also demonstrated marked antitumor efficacy with an ORR of 68%, a remarkable CNS response of 91%, and a median PFS of 18.4 months [8]. In the treatment-naïve cohort (N = 34) of the trial, the ORR was 85%, resulting in the FDA approval of selpercatinib for patients with RET-positive NSCLC. Like MET testing rates, RET demonstrated a 14–15% testing rate in community NSCLC patients [67,69]. Also similar to MET, RET testing rates were reported as low as 8% [105]. This is a staggeringly low rate considering the recent FDA approval and great antitumor activity of selective RET inhibitors.

2.6. NTRK

NTRK genes (*NTRK1, NTRK2,* and *NTRK3*) encode three TRK proteins (TRKA, TRKB, and TRKC), which play an important role in the cell growth, differentiation, and apoptosis of peripheral and CNS neurons [128]. *NTRK1* and *NTRK2* rearrangements account for 3–4% of NSCLC cases [129]. Several clinical trials have shown the efficacy of TRK inhibitor treatment in *TRK*-positive tumors. Larotrectinib (LOXO-101), a highly selective pan-TRK inhibitor, was first evaluated in a study of 55 pediatric and adult patients with various *TRK* fusion-positive malignancies, four of whom had lung cancer, and reported an ORR of 75% [10]. Remarkably, responses were shown to be durable with a response rate of 71% while 51% of patients stayed progression-free at one year. A multicenter analysis of three major Phase I/II clinical trials—STARTRK-1, STARTRK-2, and ALKA-372-001—investigating entrectinib in 54 patients diagnosed with advanced or metastatic *NTRK*-positive tumors demonstrated an ORR of 57%, a median PFS of 11.2 months, and a median OS of 20.9 months [130]. Larotrectinib and entrectinib are currently FDA-approved for the treatment of advanced *NTRK* fusion-positive NSCLC. Although these clinical trials have shown strong and durable responses to first-generation TRK TKIs, acquired resistance mutations have been identified in colorectal and mammary analogue secretory carcinomas, requiring the development of second-generation TKIs [131,132]. LOXO-195, a second-generation TRK-selective inhibitor, has shown preclinical efficacy and clinical activity in a Phase I trial of *NTRK* fusion-positive cancers previously treated with larotrectinib, demonstrating an ORR of 45% [133,134]. Despite the great clinical response elicited by NTRK-targeted therapies, NTRK testing rates were shown to range from 0–15% in several community site analyses [69,105].

2.7. BRAF

BRAF mutations represent 7% of NSCLC cases and are more commonly found in current or former smokers and female patients [117]. The most frequent *BRAF* activating mutation, V600E, carries a poorer prognosis and a shorter disease-free survival [135]. A Phase II trial investigated combination treatments of dabrafenib and trametinib in chemotherapy-pretreated patients diagnosed with *BRAF* V600E-mutated NSCLC and reported an ORR of 63% and a median PFS of 9.7 months in 52 evaluable patients [11]. In a Phase II trial of treatment-naïve patients with *BRAF* V600E-mutated NSCLC, treatment with dabrafenib and trametinib resulted in an ORR of 64% and a median PFS of 10.9 months, although 69% of patients experienced at least one grade 3/4 adverse event [136]. Currently, the combination of dabrafenib and trametinib is FDA approved for the treatment of advanced NSCLC harboring the *BRAF* V600E mutation regardless of the previous therapy. In an analysis by Gutierrez et al., BRAF NGS testing rates in 814 community site patients were reported to be 18%, similar to MET and RET NGS testing rates [67]. Other analyses demonstrated consistent rates of 12–29% [68,69,105]. Interestingly, rates of BRAF testing were shown to be as low as 0.1% in a larger analysis of 14,461 NSCLC patients treated in the community [106].

2.8. KRAS

Alterations in *KRAS*, one of the most frequent oncogenes in solid tumor malignancies, represent up to 32% of lung adenocarcinoma cases [117]. They are generally found in smokers [137] and are associated with a poor prognosis [138], although recent data have reported that it has a minimal effect on overall survival in early-stage NSCLC [139]. Therapeutic targeting of *KRAS* has been notoriously difficult, thus dubbing the molecular marker as an "undruggable" target. However, research into KRAS small molecule inhibitors targeting mutational variants of *KRAS* has shown preclinical and clinical efficacy. AMG-510, an inhibitor targeting KRAS G12C, which accounts for 13% of *KRAS* mutant NSCLC [140], is currently under investigation in a Phase I/II clinical trial of advanced *KRAS* mutant solid tumors. Interim results were recently presented and showed that out of the 29 patients, 10 were diagnosed with NSCLC, of which 90% ($N = 9$) of patients exhibited either a partial response or stable disease [16]. Although there are currently no FDA-approved drugs targeting *KRAS*, small molecule inhibitors like AMG-510 and JNJ-74699157 continue to demonstrate good clinical activity. Another drug, MRTX849, has also shown potent efficacy in vitro and in vivo for G12C positive lung cancer, with pronounced tumor regression in 17 of 26 (65%) KRAS G12C positive cell lines [141]. Preliminary data from the Phase I trial also showed a ~30% decrease in target lesions in heavily pre-treated lung cancer patients [141]. NGS testing of KRAS, although still important now, will become necessary once targeted therapies become approved. In several studies of molecular testing rates in community sites, KRAS testing has widely varied, ranging from 0–43% [66,67,69,105]. As more and more targets such as KRAS become clinically actionable, the landscape of lung cancer therapeutic management will continue to change. However, a number of actionable alterations are currently FDA approved and have distinct therapeutic strategies currently available (Figure 1).

The testing rates reported in the community have been rising over the years, and the main driver of this transformation has been education and dissemination of novel therapeutics available for the different oncogenes. However, more effort is required as the primary challenge remains that many newly approved targets face an astronomical hurdle in being implemented in daily community practice (Table 2). The most distinct example of this is the testing rates of BRAF reported in community practice at 0.1% in 14,445 patients—the lack of testing also poses a threat towards clinical trial enrollment and delivery of novel therapeutics to patients [106].

Table 2. Reported testing rates of clinically actionable and clinically relevant oncogenes in community practice.

Reported Study	EGFR	ALK	ROS1	MET	RET	NTRK	BRAF	KRAS	PD-L1 Expression
Inal et al. [66]	62%	23%	N/A	N/A	N/A	N/A	N/A	43%	N/A
Gutierrez et al. [67]	69%	65%	25%	15%	14%	N/A	18%	34%	N/A
Gierman et al. [68]	54%	51%	43%	N/A	N/A	N/A	29%	N/A	N/A
Presley et al. [69]	100%	95%	~15%	~15%	~15%	~15%	~15%	~15%	~15%
Illei et al. [94]	N/A	53.1%	N/A	N/A	N/A	N/A	N/A	N/A	N/A
Hussein et al. [95]	~60%	~50%	N/A	N/A	N/A	N/A	N/A	N/A	N/A
Mason et al. [29]	94%	92%	85%	N/A	N/A	N/A	N/A	N/A	56%
Audibert et al. [105]	68%	67%	32%	6%	8%	0%	12%	0%	N/A
Khozin et al. [142]	64%	61%	N/A	N/A	N/A	N/A	N/A	N/A	8.3%
Nadler et al. 2018 [143]	37%	35%	N/A	N/A	N/A	N/A	N/A	N/A	1.2%
Nadler et al. 2019 [106]	35.5%	32.9%	5.7%	N/A	N/A	N/A	0.1%	N/A	5.7%

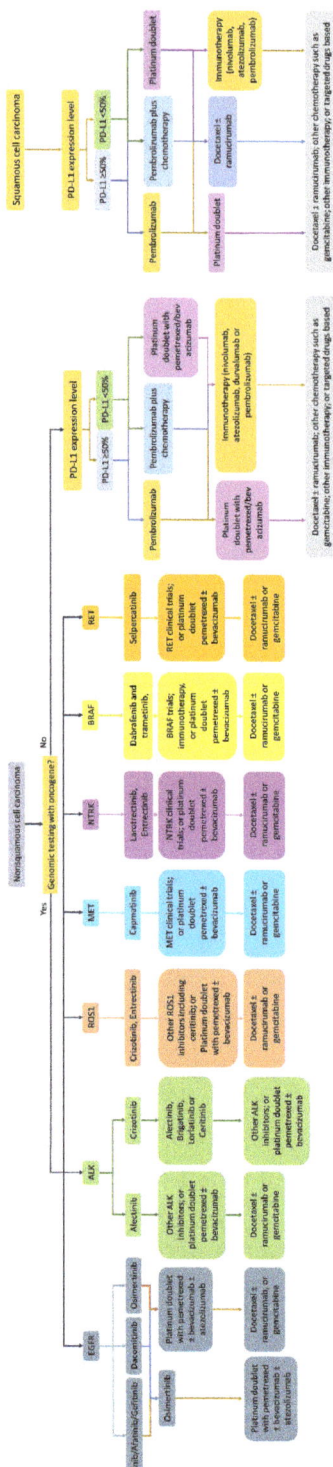

Figure 1. Genomic-informed and immunotherapy-focused management of NSCLC based on approved therapies. The role of immunotherapy is not clear in all of the actionable targets but is currently under investigation.

2.9. Immunotherapy

The availability and discovery of more and more targeted therapies makes it a priority that all advanced NSCLC patients are tested at presentation. However, when an actionable alteration is not available, treatment decisions may depend on PD-L1 expression, histology, or the onset of progressive disease. In these situations, immune checkpoint inhibitors have induced response through interaction with cytotoxic T cells, helper T cells, NK cells, macrophages, and other immune mechanisms. In 2015, the first results of monoclonal antibodies against programmed death ligand-1 (PD-1) in the refractory setting showed efficacy of nivolumab, PD-1 inhibitor, with OS (12.2 months) as compared to second-line chemotherapy (9.5 months) [18–20]. This led to the FDA approval of nivolumab in advanced NSCLC. Similar approval of pembrolizumab, a PD-1 inhibitor, was contingent upon results from KEYNOTE-001 that showed ORR of 19.4 in refractory NSCLC patients [21]. Soon after, two PD-L1 inhibitors, atezolizumab for stage IV metastatic disease and durvalumab for stage III disease, were also approved based on positive ORRs and OS [22,144]. However, the preliminary analysis reported that PD-L1 expression may be a potential biomarker of response and resistance with only 6.6% of patients whose tumors were negative to PD-L1 responding to durvalumab [22]. In the front-line setting, pembrolizumab was the first immune checkpoint inhibitor (ICI) to demonstrate median PFS of 10.3 months (vs. 6 months) and a response rate of 44.8% (vs. 27.8%) based on the results of KEYNOTE-024 as compared to chemotherapy [145], and it can be utilized as a monotherapy or in combination with chemotherapy depending on PD-L1 expression and the performance status of the patient at presentation [146]. The addition of chemotherapy to pembrolizumab resulted in an increased OS at 12 months of 69.2% (vs. 49.4%) and a median PFS of 8.8 months (vs. 4.9 months), with a comparable adverse event rate of 67.2% vs. 65.8% [147]. These results were surprisingly not recreated when nivolumab was evaluated as a monotherapy, showing a median PFS of 4.2 months with nivolumab vs. 5.9 months, and a similar OS benefit of 14.4 months vs. 13.2 months in the chemotherapy control group [23]. However, it did have success in combination with ipilimumab, showing an improvement in overall survival of 17.1 months vs. 13.9 months with chemotherapy, and a nominal duration of response of 23.3 months (vs. 6.2 months) for the front line setting [148].

Nivolumab plus ipilimumab remains a controversial choice due to grade 3 and 4 adverse events in 32.8% of patients [148]. Atezolizumab monotherapy achieved similar approval with incremental improvements in OS [24], but durvalumab in combination and alone failed to improve survival [149]. While the availability of therapies is beneficial to patients, pembrolizumab is slowly becoming the first-choice option for front-line immunotherapy, partially due to its favorable toxicity profile and versatility as a monotherapy and in combination therapy [150]. However, the availability of therapies has not translated into practice and a retrospective observational study of 55,969 NSCLC patients from the community showed that only 1,344 patients received nivolumab or pembrolizumab in the metastatic setting [142]. More surprisingly, only 8% of these patients were tested for PD-L1 expression [142]. More so, an outcomes study of 423 patients with high PD-L1 who received first-line pembrolizumab monotherapy in the community showed that community clinical outcomes were comparable to clinical trial results with a median PFS of 6.8 months vs. 6.1 months and a median OS of 19.1 months vs. 20 months [151]. A larger study of 10,689 patients in the community showed that utilization of immunotherapy in the first-line is not yet implemented, with <1% of patients treated with immunotherapy in the first-line, but rates were improved in the second and third-line setting [143]. PD-L1 expression was equally underperformed and was tested in <1% of patients [143]. Furthermore, in a quality improvement study of 100 patients who received immunotherapy in the community, only 61% fully completed immunotherapy as planned and 81% had immune-related adverse events [152]. While it is concerning that the reported use of immunotherapy in the community practice is limited, based on experience from melanoma and immunotherapy, the rates are anticipated to slowly increase over time with more education and acceptance of various immunotherapy options [153].

While PD-L1 remains an imperfect biomarker, several subgroup analyses in the trials mentioned above show an increased benefit in patients with PD-L1 ≥1% or ≥50%. Therefore, PD-L1 testing should be considered in everyday decision-making, and currently four PD-L1 testing types are available: 22C3, 28-8, SP263, and SP142 [154]. The 22C3 IHC assays were developed alongside pembrolizumab in the Phase I trial as a biomarker for patients who may benefit from treatment [155]. Meanwhile, IHC 28-8 test was developed to be used in conjunction with nivolumab, and SP142 was developed for trial use with atezolizumab [18,19,156,157]. SP263 is the most recent assay that was developed for use with durvalumab, especially in the Stage III setting in NSCLC [156]. All four assays are FDA approved in their individual setting and while testing is not required to initiate treatment, it may support clinical decision-making [156]. Meta-analysis reports show that there is high concordance between 22C3, 28-8, and SP263 assays, but SP142 detected significantly lower PD-L1 expression [154,156]. At the same time, evidence shows that non-commercial laboratory-developed tests (LDTs) used by academic centers detect similar overall percentages of PD-L1 (≥1%) at 63% (vs. 22C3 61%), but PD-L1 ≥50% were much lower at 23% (vs. 22C3 33%) suggesting LDTs are less sensitive than commercial tests [158]. LDTs are becoming more and more utilized in practice and offer a potential solution to the complexity of commercial PD-L1 tests. However, the lack of PD-L1 testing and the difficulty of immune-related toxicities is a challenge that is more difficult to address, and we believe that the integration of community practice with the academic site model is one solution to this grave issue.

3. Integration of Personalized Therapy and Molecular Testing in the Community through an Academic Site to Community Practice Network

Advances in targeted therapy and immunotherapy have lowered the costs of molecular testing, making it a viable practice in the academic sites and the community [159]. While academic sites have benefited from a close knowledge of clinical trials and novel therapies, the drive of personalized medicine has not been uniform, with the majority of patients in the community lacking appropriate testing and assignment to therapy [66–69,94,95,106,142,143,152]. This is especially concerning as the majority of patients or approximately 85% with cancer are treated in the community setting and 50% of collaborative group trial accruals occur in the community [160]. Several models have been proposed to integrate community oncologists into the academic paradigm of personalized medicine, with the most promising being the establishment of interpersonal relationships between community oncologists and academic site physicians through molecular tumor board (MTB) teams [161–165]. The establishment of an MTB team would allow for the proper evaluation of imaging, histopathology, and genomic information that is required to make the appropriate therapeutic decision [166]. One reported study involving 1725 patients who were evaluated through a cloud-based virtual molecular tumor board (VMTB) showed that oncologists chose the VMTB-derived therapies over others, resulting in an increase of matched therapies [165]. Such a model also allows for the dissemination of information regarding available CLIA-certified vendors and platforms for both tissue and liquid biopsy testing that are imperative to improving testing rates and outcomes [167]. The MTB model can be scaled into the community through virtual or physical collaboration, and would further improve collaboration between community sites and academic sites through the interactions between pathologists, oncologists, primary care physicians, radiologists, and pulmonologists in the decision-making process (Figure 2). This team-based approach can be utilized in all cancers, especially during crises such as the recent pandemic of novel coronavirus [168]. The improvement in the relationships with various experts and free-flow of information from the academic site to the community will invariably yield improvements in patient outcomes.

Another available tool in building the community and academic network is the incorporation of guidelines and pathways into everyday practice. As the majority of oncologists in the community see a number of patients with varying histologies, it is often difficult to keep track of various therapies available, especially for lung cancer. While guidelines such as the National Comprehensive Cancer Network (NCCN) and the American Society of Clinical Oncology provide guidelines regarding the use of immunotherapy and targeted therapy, as well as genomic testing for FDA approved alterations [169], the results in our review show that the gaps in testing rates still remain prevalent and these guidelines are often difficult to interpret during a busy community practice. One proposed solution to this challenge is the implementation of vendor-based oncology clinical pathways (OCPs) that guide physicians in their decision-making based on query questions regarding the patient case [170]. A number of studies have shown that the use of OCPs not only maintains or improves outcomes, but they lower overhead costs for community practice [171–174]. While guidelines offer multiple recommendations that are difficult to interpret, clinical pathways create a local structure and framework from guidelines or evidence, with the goal of providing the single best therapeutic decision that provides value to the patient (Figure 3) [175]. The advantage of OCPs is not only the availability of decision-making support but the collection of analytics data that can be analyzed for research purposes and continuous quality improvement [176]. An OCP implemented in the community not only evaluates the performance of the community practice, but gives the tools to the community to drive improvements in testing rates and personalized therapy. The wide majority of community practice patients do not consider enrollment in clinical trials, as they are unaware of the option [177]. The pathways incorporate the clinical trials open within the entire enterprise, where trial decisions are placed ahead of other recommendations and always count as on-pathway, which encourages trial enrollment and integrates clinical trials into community practice. Our community practice utilizes the ClinicaPath (formerly ViaOncology) pathway systems in the decision-making process, but there are several vendors available [170].

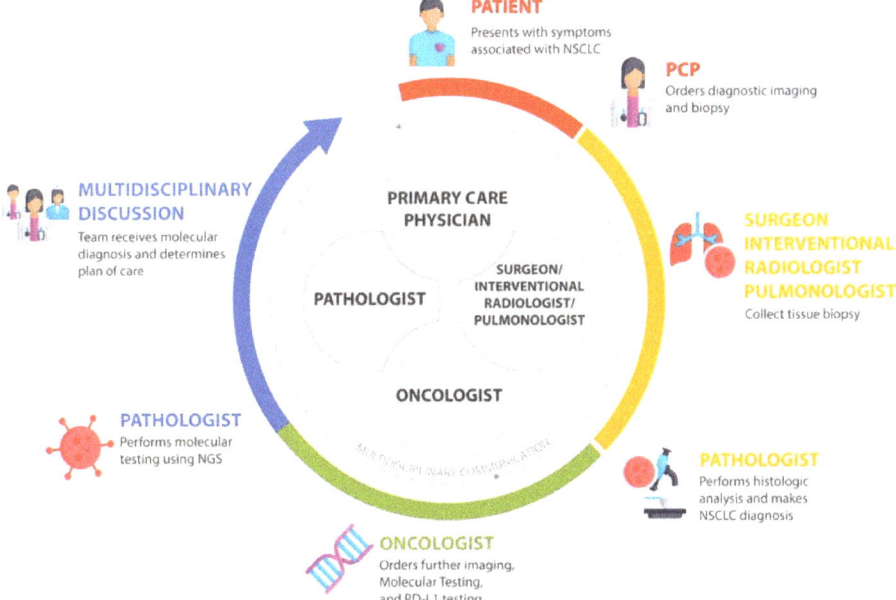

Figure 2. The multidisciplinary care model for community and academic practice integration for lung cancer decision-making.

One recent development in our enterprise is the implementation of a standardized electronic health record (EHR) system in the community that mirrors the academic site medical records in a single system and allows for optimization of testing results and physician referrals for clinical trials. The standardization of molecular testing results and reporting in a fast and reliable manner through the medical record is an important barrier for community oncology practice towards improving testing rates [178]. The cohesiveness of a singular EHR not only results in clinical decision support, but allows the community oncologists to participate in the clinical and translational research process through the evaluation of retrospective patient cohorts in a collaborative model that encompasses a multi-disciplinary team of pathologists, radiologists, and other specialties. The seamless amalgamation of high level genomic and treatment data from the community can be quickly extrapolated from the EHR and utilized in translational studies including evaluation of testing rates and therapy outcomes. This also helps in identifying patients that would be eligible for enrollment in clinical trials available at partnering academic sites, as evidenced by the top accrual rates of the adjuvant EVEREST study in renal cell carcinoma at City of Hope [179]. This is an especially significant strategy to implement in order to enroll and treat older cancer patients who are primarily seen at community sites [180]. Furthermore, the establishment of integrated clinical research has been shown to translate to wider awareness and acceptance of research results, and in 2013, the NCI formed the NCI Community Oncology Research Program (NCORP) [181]. First-cycle results showed that NCORP improved cancer care delivery and access in the community, but challenges remain in growing the program to more organizations across the nation [182]. The evolution of cancer care has to be met with advancements in cancer care and genomic testing access and delivery in community practice. However, the ultimate development of a successful community-based research program requires funding to empower local physicians, infrastructure to support implementation, collaboration between academic and community investigators, and flexibility in operations and organizations.

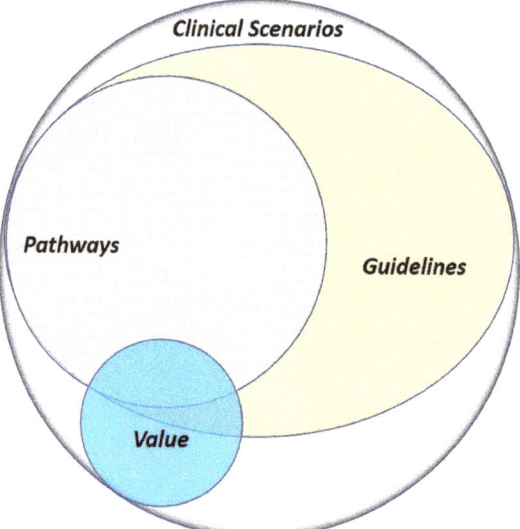

Figure 3. Advantage of guidelines and pathways in clinical scenarios. Patient outcomes are reliant on adherence to evidence-based medicine, which can be facilitated by guidelines and enhanced by pathways.

4. Conclusions

The advancements in lung cancer therapy and genomic testing have transformed the lung cancer decision-making process in the last decade. Next-generation sequencing has expanded from a few genes tested with routine testing to broad-based sequencing that has identified a plethora of oncogenes that are involved in driving the progression of NSCLC [183–185]. While targeted therapy was initially implemented in the first-line setting, the availability of a number of second- and third-generation TKIs has transitioned from a model of systemic therapy in the refractory setting to a framework of a number of TKIs administered in sequence based on resistance mechanisms and clinical progression of the individual patient [186]. The promise of personalized medicine continues to be realized through the development of ground-breaking immune checkpoint inhibitors and upcoming trials show promise for chimeric antigen receptor (CAR) T-cell therapy [187]. To further realize this mission of precision medicine and to deliver improved outcomes, rigorous clinical data science, and translational research of the care delivery model and access have to be expanded beyond academic sites and into community practice. As we have brought to attention in this review, the community practice, while currently lagging behind academic sites in delivery oncology care, can be systematically and procedurally integrated with academic centers in a unified model for lung cancer decision-making and clinical collaboration. Our identified tools and collaborative concepts, including pathways and MTBs, can be realized in any community setting to enhance communication and trial enrollment.

Author Contributions: Conceptualization, R.S., S.R., P.K, I.M.; Writing—original draft preparation, S.R., I.M., R.P., R.S., P.K.; Writing—review and editing, S.R., I.M., R.P., R.S., P.K., B.L. and T.T. All authors have read and agreed to the published version of the manuscript.

Funding: The work was supported by the National Cancer Institute of Health under award numbers P30CA033572, U54CA209978, R01CA247471 and R01CA218545

Acknowledgments: We would like to express our deepest gratitude for philanthropic funding by the Tenenblatt Family.

Conflicts of Interest: S.R: Speaker for Boehringer Ingelheim Pharmaceuticals Inc., Puma Biotechnology Inc.; I.M., R.P., B.L., T.T., P.K. and R.S. declare no conflict of interest.

References

1. Siegel, R.L.; Miller, K.D.; Jemal, A. Cancer statistics, 2020. *CA A Cancer J. Clin.* **2020**, *70*, 7–30. [CrossRef]
2. Molina, J.R.; Yang, P.; Cassivi, S.D.; Schild, S.E.; Adjei, A.A. Non-small cell lung cancer: Epidemiology, risk factors, treatment, and survivorship. *Mayo Clin. Proc.* **2008**, *83*, 584–594. [CrossRef]
3. Cancer Stat Facts: Lung and Bronchus Cancer, Statistics at a Glance. Available online: https://seer.cancer.gov/statfacts/html/lungb.html (accessed on 20 May 2020).
4. Zhou, C.; Wu, Y.L.; Chen, G.; Feng, J.; Liu, X.Q.; Wang, C.; Zhang, S.; Wang, J.; Zhou, S.; Ren, S.; et al. Erlotinib versus chemotherapy as first-line treatment for patients with advanced EGFR mutation-positive non-small-cell lung cancer (OPTIMAL, CTONG-0802): A multicentre, open-label, randomised, phase 3 study. *Lancet Oncol.* **2011**, *12*, 735–742. [CrossRef]
5. Shaw, A.T.; Kim, D.W.; Nakagawa, K.; Seto, T.; Crino, L.; Ahn, M.J.; De Pas, T.; Besse, B.; Solomon, B.J.; Blackhall, F.; et al. Crizotinib versus chemotherapy in advanced ALK-positive lung cancer. *N. Engl. J. Med.* **2013**, *368*, 2385–2394. [CrossRef] [PubMed]
6. Mok, T.S.; Wu, Y.-L.; Ahn, M.-J.; Garassino, M.C.; Kim, H.R.; Ramalingam, S.S.; Shepherd, F.A.; He, Y.; Akamatsu, H.; Theelen, W.S.M.E.; et al. Osimertinib or Platinum–Pemetrexed in EGFR T790M–Positive Lung Cancer. *N. Engl. J. Med.* **2016**, *376*, 629–640. [CrossRef]
7. Shaw, A.T.; Riely, G.J.; Bang, Y.J.; Kim, D.W.; Camidge, D.R.; Solomon, B.J.; Varella-Garcia, M.; Iafrate, A.J.; Shapiro, G.I.; Usari, T.; et al. Crizotinib in ROS1-rearranged advanced non-small-cell lung cancer (NSCLC): Updated results, including overall survival, from PROFILE 1001. *Ann. Oncol.* **2019**, *30*, 1121–1126. [CrossRef]
8. Drilon, A.; Oxnard, G.; Wirth, L.; Besse, B.; Gautschi, O.; Tan, S.W.D.; Loong, H.; Bauer, T.; Kim, Y.J.; Horiike, A.; et al. PL02.08 Registrational Results of LIBRETTO-001: A Phase 1/2 Trial of LOXO-292 in Patients with RET Fusion-Positive Lung Cancers. *J. Thoracic Oncol.* **2019**, *14*, S6–S7. [CrossRef]
9. Drilon, A.; Siena, S.; Dziadziuszko, R.; Barlesi, F.; Krebs, M.G.; Shaw, A.T.; de Braud, F.; Rolfo, C.; Ahn, M.-J.; Wolf, J.; et al. Entrectinib in ROS1 fusion-positive non-small-cell lung cancer: Integrated analysis of three phase 1–2 trials. *Lancet Oncol.* **2020**, *21*, 261–270. [CrossRef]
10. Drilon, A.; Laetsch, T.W.; Kummar, S.; DuBois, S.G.; Lassen, U.N.; Demetri, G.D.; Nathenson, M.; Doebele, R.C.; Farago, A.F.; Pappo, A.S.; et al. Efficacy of Larotrectinib in TRK Fusion–Positive Cancers in Adults and Children. *N. Engl. J. Med.* **2018**, *378*, 731–739. [CrossRef]
11. Planchard, D.; Besse, B.; Groen, H.J.M.; Souquet, P.J.; Quoix, E.; Baik, C.S.; Barlesi, F.; Kim, T.M.; Mazieres, J.; Novello, S.; et al. Dabrafenib plus trametinib in patients with previously treated BRAF(V600E)-mutant metastatic non-small cell lung cancer: An open-label, multicentre phase 2 trial. *Lancet Oncol.* **2016**, *17*, 984–993. [CrossRef]

12. Wolf, J.; Seto, T.; Han, J.-Y.; Reguart, N.; Garon, E.B.; Groen, H.J.M.; Tan, D.S.-W.; Hida, T.; Jonge, M.J.D.; Orlov, S.V.; et al. Capmatinib (INC280) in METΔex14-mutated advanced non-small cell lung cancer (NSCLC): Efficacy data from the phase II GEOMETRY mono-1 study. *J. Clin. Oncol.* **2019**, *37*, 9004. [CrossRef]
13. Soria, J.-C.; Ohe, Y.; Vansteenkiste, J.; Reungwetwattana, T.; Chewaskulyong, B.; Lee, K.H.; Dechaphunkul, A.; Imamura, F.; Nogami, N.; Kurata, T.; et al. Osimertinib in Untreated EGFR-Mutated Advanced Non–Small-Cell Lung Cancer. *N. Engl. J. Med.* **2017**, *378*, 113–125. [CrossRef] [PubMed]
14. Camidge, D.R.; Kim, H.R.; Ahn, M.-J.; Yang, J.C.-H.; Han, J.-Y.; Lee, J.-S.; Hochmair, M.J.; Li, J.Y.-C.; Chang, G.-C.; Lee, K.H.; et al. Brigatinib versus Crizotinib in ALK-Positive Non–Small-Cell Lung Cancer. *N. Engl. J. Med.* **2018**, *379*, 2027–2039. [CrossRef]
15. Kuan, F.-C.; Kuo, L.-T.; Chen, M.-C.; Yang, C.-T.; Shi, C.-S.; Teng, D.; Lee, K.-D. Overall survival benefits of first-line EGFR tyrosine kinase inhibitors in EGFR-mutated non-small-cell lung cancers: A systematic review and meta-analysis. *Br. J. Cancer* **2015**, *113*, 1519–1528. [CrossRef] [PubMed]
16. Govindan, R.; Fakih, M.; Price, T.; Falchook, G.; Desai, J.; Kuo, J.; Strickler, J.; Krauss, J.; Li, B.; Denlinger, C.; et al. Phase 1 Study of AMG 510, a Novel Molecule Targeting KRAS G12C Mutant Solid Tumors. *ESMO 2019 Congress* **2019**, *30* (Suppl. 5), 159–193. [CrossRef]
17. Jänne, P. A phase 1 clinical trial evaluating the pharmacokinetics (PK), safety, and clinical activity of MRTX849, a mutant-selective small molecule KRAS G12C inhibitor, in advanced solid tumors. In Proceedings of the AACR-NCI-EORTC International Conference on Molecular Targets and Cancer Therapeutics, Boston, MA, USA, 26–30 October 2019.
18. Brahmer, J.; Reckamp, K.L.; Baas, P.; Crinò, L.; Eberhardt, W.E.E.; Poddubskaya, E.; Antonia, S.; Pluzanski, A.; Vokes, E.E.; Holgado, E.; et al. Nivolumab versus Docetaxel in Advanced Squamous-Cell Non–Small-Cell Lung Cancer. *N. Engl. J. Med.* **2015**, *373*, 123–135. [CrossRef]
19. Borghaei, H.; Paz-Ares, L.; Horn, L.; Spigel, D.R.; Steins, M.; Ready, N.E.; Chow, L.Q.; Vokes, E.E.; Felip, E.; Holgado, E.; et al. Nivolumab versus Docetaxel in Advanced Nonsquamous Non-Small-Cell Lung Cancer. *N. Engl. J. Med.* **2015**, *373*, 1627–1639. [CrossRef] [PubMed]
20. Horn, L.; Spigel, D.R.; Vokes, E.E.; Holgado, E.; Ready, N.; Steins, M.; Poddubskaya, E.; Borghaei, H.; Felip, E.; Paz-Ares, L.; et al. Nivolumab Versus Docetaxel in Previously Treated Patients With Advanced Non-Small-Cell Lung Cancer: Two-Year Outcomes From Two Randomized, Open-Label, Phase III Trials (CheckMate 017 and CheckMate 057). *J. Clin. Oncol.* **2017**, *35*, 3924–3933. [CrossRef] [PubMed]
21. Herbst, R.S.; Baas, P.; Kim, D.W.; Felip, E.; Pérez-Gracia, J.L.; Han, J.Y.; Molina, J.; Kim, J.H.; Arvis, C.D.; Ahn, M.J.; et al. Pembrolizumab versus docetaxel for previously treated, PD-L1-positive, advanced non-small-cell lung cancer (KEYNOTE-010): A randomised controlled trial. *Lancet* **2016**, *387*, 1540–1550. [CrossRef]
22. Garassino, M.C.; Cho, B.C.; Kim, J.H.; Mazières, J.; Vansteenkiste, J.; Lena, H.; Corral Jaime, J.; Gray, J.E.; Powderly, J.; Chouaid, C.; et al. Durvalumab as third-line or later treatment for advanced non-small-cell lung cancer (ATLANTIC): An open-label, single-arm, phase 2 study. *Lancet Oncol.* **2018**, *19*, 521–536. [CrossRef]
23. Carbone, D.P.; Reck, M.; Paz-Ares, L.; Creelan, B.; Horn, L.; Steins, M.; Felip, E.; van den Heuvel, M.M.; Ciuleanu, T.-E.; Badin, F.; et al. First-Line Nivolumab in Stage IV or Recurrent Non–Small-Cell Lung Cancer. *N. Engl. J. Med.* **2017**, *376*, 2415–2426. [CrossRef] [PubMed]
24. Spigel, D.; de Marinis, F.; Giaccone, G.; Reinmuth, N.; Vergnenegre, A.; Barrios, C.H.; Morise, M.; Felip, E.; Andric, Z.G.; Geater, S.; et al. LBA78-IMpower110: Interim overall survival (OS) analysis of a phase III study of atezolizumab (atezo) vs platinum-based chemotherapy (chemo) as first-line (1L) treatment (tx) in PD-L1–selected NSCLC. *Ann. Oncol.* **2019**, *30*, v915. [CrossRef]
25. Cottrell, T.R.; Taube, J.M. PD-L1 and Emerging Biomarkers in Immune Checkpoint Blockade Therapy. *Cancer J.* **2018**, *24*, 41–46. [CrossRef] [PubMed]
26. Davis, A.A.; Patel, V.G. The role of PD-L1 expression as a predictive biomarker: An analysis of all US Food and Drug Administration (FDA) approvals of immune checkpoint inhibitors. *J. Immunother. Cancer* **2019**, *7*, 278. [CrossRef] [PubMed]
27. Lantuejoul, S.; Sound-Tsao, M.; Cooper, W.A.; Girard, N.; Hirsch, F.R.; Roden, A.C.; Lopez-Rios, F.; Jain, D.; Chou, T.-Y.; Motoi, N.; et al. PD-L1 Testing for Lung Cancer in 2019: Perspective From the IASLC Pathology Committee. *J. Thorac. Oncol.* **2020**, *15*, 499–519. [CrossRef]

28. Garon, E.B.; Hellmann, M.D.; Rizvi, N.A.; Carcereny, E.; Leighl, N.B.; Ahn, M.J.; Eder, J.P.; Balmanoukian, A.S.; Aggarwal, C.; Horn, L.; et al. Five-Year Overall Survival for Patients With Advanced Non-Small-Cell Lung Cancer Treated With Pembrolizumab: Results From the Phase I KEYNOTE-001 Study. *J. Clin. Oncol.* **2019**, *37*, 2518–2527. [CrossRef] [PubMed]
29. Mason, C.; Ellis, P.G.; Lokay, K.; Barry, A.; Dickson, N.; Page, R.; Polite, B.; Salgia, R.; Savin, M.; Shamah, C.; et al. Patterns of Biomarker Testing Rates and Appropriate Use of Targeted Therapy in the First-Line, Metastatic Non-Small Cell Lung Cancer Treatment Setting. *J. Clin. Pathw.* **2018**, *4*, 49–54. [CrossRef]
30. Dillman, R.O.; Seagren, S.L.; Propert, K.J.; Guerra, J.; Eaton, W.L.; Perry, M.C.; Carey, R.W.; Frei, E.F., 3rd; Green, M.R. A randomized trial of induction chemotherapy plus high-dose radiation versus radiation alone in stage III non-small-cell lung cancer. *N. Engl. J. Med.* **1990**, *323*, 940–945. [CrossRef] [PubMed]
31. Curran, W.J., Jr.; Paulus, R.; Langer, C.J.; Komaki, R.; Lee, J.S.; Hauser, S.; Movsas, B.; Wasserman, T.; Rosenthal, S.A.; Gore, E.; et al. Sequential vs. concurrent chemoradiation for stage III non-small cell lung cancer: Randomized phase III trial RTOG 9410. *J. Natl. Cancer Inst.* **2011**, *103*, 1452–1460. [CrossRef] [PubMed]
32. Schiller, J.H.; Harrington, D.; Belani, C.P.; Langer, C.; Sandler, A.; Krook, J.; Zhu, J.; Johnson, D.H. Comparison of four chemotherapy regimens for advanced non-small-cell lung cancer. *N. Engl. J. Med.* **2002**, *346*, 92–98. [CrossRef]
33. Evans, J.P. The Human Genome Project at 10 years: A teachable moment. *Genet. Med.* **2010**, *12*, 477. [CrossRef] [PubMed]
34. Salgia, R. Mutation testing for directing upfront targeted therapy and post-progression combination therapy strategies in lung adenocarcinoma. *Expert Rev. Mol. Diagn.* **2016**, *16*, 737–749. [CrossRef] [PubMed]
35. Ashley, E.A. Towards precision medicine. *Nat. Rev. Genet.* **2016**, *17*, 507–522. [CrossRef] [PubMed]
36. Kris, M.G.; Natale, R.B.; Herbst, R.S.; Lynch, T.J., Jr.; Prager, D.; Belani, C.P.; Schiller, J.H.; Kelly, K.; Spiridonidis, H.; Sandler, A.; et al. Efficacy of gefitinib, an inhibitor of the epidermal growth factor receptor tyrosine kinase, in symptomatic patients with non-small cell lung cancer: A randomized trial. *Jama* **2003**, *290*, 2149–2158. [CrossRef]
37. Fukuoka, M.; Yano, S.; Giaccone, G.; Tamura, T.; Nakagawa, K.; Douillard, J.Y.; Nishiwaki, Y.; Vansteenkiste, J.; Kudoh, S.; Rischin, D.; et al. Multi-institutional randomized phase II trial of gefitinib for previously treated patients with advanced non-small-cell lung cancer (The IDEAL 1 Trial) [corrected]. *J. Clin. Oncol.* **2003**, *21*, 2237–2246. [CrossRef] [PubMed]
38. Lindeman, N.I.; Cagle, P.T.; Beasley, M.B.; Chitale, D.A.; Dacic, S.; Giaccone, G.; Jenkins, R.B.; Kwiatkowski, D.J.; Saldivar, J.S.; Squire, J.; et al. Molecular testing guideline for selection of lung cancer patients for EGFR and ALK tyrosine kinase inhibitors: Guideline from the College of American Pathologists, International Association for the Study of Lung Cancer, and Association for Molecular Pathology. *J. Thorac. Oncol.* **2013**, *8*, 823–859. [CrossRef]
39. Blumenthal, G.M.; Karuri, S.W.; Zhang, H.; Zhang, L.; Khozin, S.; Kazandjian, D.; Tang, S.; Sridhara, R.; Keegan, P.; Pazdur, R. Overall response rate, progression-free survival, and overall survival with targeted and standard therapies in advanced non-small-cell lung cancer: US Food and Drug Administration trial-level and patient-level analyses. *J. Clin. Oncol.* **2015**, *33*, 1008–1014. [CrossRef]
40. Simeone, J.C.; Nordstrom, B.L.; Patel, K.; Klein, A.B. Treatment patterns and overall survival in metastatic non-small-cell lung cancer in a real-world, US setting. *Future Oncol.* **2019**, *15*, 3491–3502. [CrossRef]
41. Arbour, K.C.; Riely, G.J. Systemic Therapy for Locally Advanced and Metastatic Non-Small Cell Lung Cancer: A Review. *Jama* **2019**, *322*, 764–774. [CrossRef]
42. Buyse, M.E.; Squifflet, P.; Laporte, S.; Fossella, F.V.; Georgoulias, V.; Pujol, J.; Kubota, K.; Monnier, A.; Kudoh, S.; Douillard, J. Prediction of survival benefits from progression-free survival in patients with advanced non small cell lung cancer: Evidence from a pooled analysis of 2,838 patients randomized in 7 trials. *J. Clin. Oncol.* **2008**, *26*, 8019. [CrossRef]
43. Ramalingam, S.S.; Vansteenkiste, J.; Planchard, D.; Cho, B.C.; Gray, J.E.; Ohe, Y.; Zhou, C.; Reungwetwattana, T.; Cheng, Y.; Chewaskulyong, B.; et al. Overall Survival with Osimertinib in Untreated, EGFR-Mutated Advanced NSCLC. *N. Engl. J. Med.* **2020**, *382*, 41–50. [CrossRef] [PubMed]
44. Pacheco, J.M.; Gao, D.; Smith, D.; Purcell, T.; Hancock, M.; Bunn, P.; Robin, T.; Liu, A.; Karam, S.; Gaspar, L.; et al. Natural History and Factors Associated with Overall Survival in Stage IV ALK-Rearranged Non-Small Cell Lung Cancer. *J. Thorac Oncol.* **2019**, *14*, 691–700. [CrossRef] [PubMed]

45. Gadgeel, S.; Rodríguez-Abreu, D.; Speranza, G.; Esteban, E.; Felip, E.; Dómine, M.; Hui, R.; Hochmair, M.J.; Clingan, P.; Powell, S.F.; et al. Updated Analysis From KEYNOTE-189: Pembrolizumab or Placebo Plus Pemetrexed and Platinum for Previously Untreated Metastatic Nonsquamous Non-Small-Cell Lung Cancer. *J. Clin. Oncol.* **2020**, *38*, 1505–1517. [CrossRef] [PubMed]
46. Mambetsariev, I.; Wang, Y.; Chen, C.; Nadaf, S.; Pharaon, R.; Fricke, J.; Amanam, I.; Amini, A.; Bild, A.; Chu, P.; et al. Precision medicine and actionable alterations in lung cancer: A single institution experience. *PLoS ONE* **2020**, *15*, e0228188. [CrossRef] [PubMed]
47. Dietel, M.; Savelov, N.; Salanova, R.; Micke, P.; Bigras, G.; Hida, T.; Piperdi, B.; Burke, T.; Khambata-Ford, S.; Deitz, A. 130O Real-world prevalence of PD-L1 expression in locally advanced or metastatic non-small cell lung cancer (NSCLC): The global, multicentre EXPRESS study. *J. Thorac. Oncol.* **2018**, *13*, S74–S75. [CrossRef]
48. Gómez, X.E.; Soto, A.; Gómez, M.A. Survival and prognostic factors in non-small cell lung cancer patients with mutation of the EGFR gene treated with tyrosine kinase inhibitors in a peruvian hospital. *Am. J. Cancer Res.* **2019**, *9*, 1009–1016.
49. Ciardiello, F.; Tortora, G. EGFR Antagonists in Cancer Treatment. *N. Engl. J. Med.* **2008**, *358*, 1160–1174. [CrossRef]
50. Lynch, T.J.; Bell, D.W.; Sordella, R.; Gurubhagavatula, S.; Okimoto, R.A.; Brannigan, B.W.; Harris, P.L.; Haserlat, S.M.; Supko, J.G.; Haluska, F.G.; et al. Activating mutations in the epidermal growth factor receptor underlying responsiveness of non-small-cell lung cancer to gefitinib. *N. Engl. J. Med.* **2004**, *350*, 2129–2139. [CrossRef]
51. Paez, J.G.; Jänne, P.A.; Lee, J.C.; Tracy, S.; Greulich, H.; Gabriel, S.; Herman, P.; Kaye, F.J.; Lindeman, N.; Boggon, T.J.; et al. EGFR mutations in lung cancer: Correlation with clinical response to gefitinib therapy. *Science* **2004**, *304*, 1497–1500. [CrossRef]
52. Pao, W.; Miller, V.; Zakowski, M.; Doherty, J.; Politi, K.; Sarkaria, I.; Singh, B.; Heelan, R.; Rusch, V.; Fulton, L.; et al. EGF receptor gene mutations are common in lung cancers from "never smokers" and are associated with sensitivity of tumors to gefitinib and erlotinib. *Proc. Natl. Acad. Sci. USA* **2004**, *101*, 13306–13311. [CrossRef]
53. Rosell, R.; Carcereny, E.; Gervais, R.; Vergnenegre, A.; Massuti, B.; Felip, E.; Palmero, R.; Garcia-Gomez, R.; Pallares, C.; Sanchez, J.M.; et al. Erlotinib versus standard chemotherapy as first-line treatment for European patients with advanced EGFR mutation-positive non-small-cell lung cancer (EURTAC): A multicentre, open-label, randomised phase 3 trial. *Lancet Oncol.* **2012**, *13*, 239–246. [CrossRef]
54. Wu, Y.L.; Zhou, C.; Liam, C.K.; Wu, G.; Liu, X.; Zhong, Z.; Lu, S.; Cheng, Y.; Han, B.; Chen, L.; et al. First-line erlotinib versus gemcitabine/cisplatin in patients with advanced EGFR mutation-positive non-small-cell lung cancer: Analyses from the phase III, randomized, open-label, ENSURE study. *Ann. Oncol.* **2015**, *26*, 1883–1889. [CrossRef] [PubMed]
55. Wu, Y.L.; Zhou, C.; Hu, C.P.; Feng, J.; Lu, S.; Huang, Y.; Li, W.; Hou, M.; Shi, J.H.; Lee, K.Y.; et al. Afatinib versus cisplatin plus gemcitabine for first-line treatment of Asian patients with advanced non-small-cell lung cancer harbouring EGFR mutations (LUX-Lung 6): An open-label, randomised phase 3 trial. *Lancet Oncol.* **2014**, *15*, 213–222. [CrossRef]
56. Yang, J.C.; Wu, Y.L.; Schuler, M.; Sebastian, M.; Popat, S.; Yamamoto, N.; Zhou, C.; Hu, C.P.; O'Byrne, K.; Feng, J.; et al. Afatinib versus cisplatin-based chemotherapy for EGFR mutation-positive lung adenocarcinoma (LUX-Lung 3 and LUX-Lung 6): Analysis of overall survival data from two randomised, phase 3 trials. *Lancet Oncol.* **2015**, *16*, 141–151. [CrossRef]
57. Kazandjian, D.; Blumenthal, G.M.; Yuan, W.; He, K.; Keegan, P.; Pazdur, R. FDA Approval of Gefitinib for the Treatment of Patients with Metastatic EGFR Mutation-Positive Non-Small Cell Lung Cancer. *Clin. Cancer Res.* **2016**, *22*, 1307–1312. [CrossRef]
58. Han, J.Y.; Park, K.; Kim, S.W.; Lee, D.H.; Kim, H.Y.; Kim, H.T.; Ahn, M.J.; Yun, T.; Ahn, J.S.; Suh, C.; et al. First-SIGNAL: First-line single-agent iressa versus gemcitabine and cisplatin trial in never-smokers with adenocarcinoma of the lung. *J. Clin. Oncol.* **2012**, *30*, 1122–1128. [CrossRef]
59. Sequist, L.V.; Yang, J.C.; Yamamoto, N.; O'Byrne, K.; Hirsh, V.; Mok, T.; Geater, S.L.; Orlov, S.; Tsai, C.M.; Boyer, M.; et al. Phase III study of afatinib or cisplatin plus pemetrexed in patients with metastatic lung adenocarcinoma with EGFR mutations. *J. Clin. Oncol.* **2013**, *31*, 3327–3334. [CrossRef]

60. Mok, T.; Ahn, M.-J.; Han, J.-Y.; Kang, J.H.; Katakami, N.; Kim, H.; Hodge, R.; Ghiorghiu, D.C.; Cantarini, M.; Wu, Y.-L.; et al. CNS response to osimertinib in patients (pts) with T790M-positive advanced NSCLC: Data from a randomized phase III trial (AURA3). *J. Clin. Oncol.* **2017**, *35*, 9005. [CrossRef]
61. Sun, M.; Behrens, C.; Feng, L.; Ozburn, N.; Tang, X.; Yin, G.; Komaki, R.; Varella-Garcia, M.; Hong, W.K.; Aldape, K.D.; et al. HER family receptor abnormalities in lung cancer brain metastases and corresponding primary tumors. *Clin. Cancer Res.* **2009**, *15*, 4829–4837. [CrossRef]
62. Daniele, L.; Cassoni, P.; Bacillo, E.; Cappia, S.; Righi, L.; Volante, M.; Tondat, F.; Inghirami, G.; Sapino, A.; Scagliotti, G.V.; et al. Epidermal growth factor receptor gene in primary tumor and metastatic sites from non-small cell lung cancer. *J. Thorac Oncol.* **2009**, *4*, 684–688. [CrossRef]
63. Leonetti, A.; Sharma, S.; Minari, R.; Perego, P.; Giovannetti, E.; Tiseo, M. Resistance mechanisms to osimertinib in EGFR-mutated non-small cell lung cancer. *Br. J. Cancer* **2019**, *121*, 725–737. [CrossRef] [PubMed]
64. Yang, J.C.; Schuler, M.; Popat, S.; Miura, S.; Heeke, S.; Park, K.; Märten, A.; Kim, E.S. Afatinib for the Treatment of NSCLC Harboring Uncommon EGFR Mutations: A Database of 693 Cases. *J. Thorac Oncol.* **2020**, *15*, 803–815. [CrossRef] [PubMed]
65. Heymach, J.; Negrao, M.; Robichaux, J.; Carter, B.; Patel, A.; Altan, M.; Gibbons, D.; Fossella, F.; Simon, G.; Lam, V.; et al. OA02.06 A Phase II Trial of Poziotinib in EGFR and HER2 exon 20 Mutant Non-Small Cell Lung Cancer (NSCLC). *J. Thoracic Oncol.* **2018**, *13*, S323–S324. [CrossRef]
66. Inal, C.; Yilmaz, E.; Cheng, H.; Zhu, C.; Pullman, J.; Gucalp, R.A.; Keller, S.M.; Perez-Soler, R.; Piperdi, B. Effect of reflex testing by pathologists on molecular testing rates in lung cancer patients: Experience from a community-based academic center. *J. Clin. Oncol.* **2014**, *32*, 8098. [CrossRef]
67. Gutierrez, M.E.; Choi, K.; Lanman, R.B.; Licitra, E.J.; Skrzypczak, S.M.; Pe Benito, R.; Wu, T.; Arunajadai, S.; Kaur, S.; Harper, H.; et al. Genomic Profiling of Advanced Non-Small Cell Lung Cancer in Community Settings: Gaps and Opportunities. *Clin. Lung Cancer* **2017**, *18*, 651–659. [CrossRef]
68. Gierman, H.J.; Goldfarb, S.; Labrador, M.; Weipert, C.M.; Getty, B.; Skrzypczak, S.M.; Catasus, C.; Carbral, S.; Singaraju, M.; Singleton, N.; et al. Genomic testing and treatment landscape in patients with advanced non-small cell lung cancer (aNSCLC) using real-world data from community oncology practices. *J. Clin. Oncol.* **2019**, *37*, 1585. [CrossRef]
69. Presley, C.J.; Tang, D.; Soulos, P.R.; Chiang, A.C.; Longtine, J.A.; Adelson, K.B.; Herbst, R.S.; Zhu, W.; Nussbaum, N.C.; Sorg, R.A.; et al. Association of Broad-Based Genomic Sequencing With Survival Among Patients With Advanced Non-Small Cell Lung Cancer in the Community Oncology Setting. *Jama* **2018**, *320*, 469–477. [CrossRef]
70. Soda, M.; Choi, Y.L.; Enomoto, M.; Takada, S.; Yamashita, Y.; Ishikawa, S.; Fujiwara, S.; Watanabe, H.; Kurashina, K.; Hatanaka, H.; et al. Identification of the transforming EML4-ALK fusion gene in non-small-cell lung cancer. *Nature* **2007**, *448*, 561–566. [CrossRef]
71. Shaw, A.T.; Yeap, B.Y.; Mino-Kenudson, M.; Digumarthy, S.R.; Costa, D.B.; Heist, R.S.; Solomon, B.; Stubbs, H.; Admane, S.; McDermott, U.; et al. Clinical features and outcome of patients with non-small-cell lung cancer who harbor EML4-ALK. *J. Clin. Oncol.* **2009**, *27*, 4247–4253. [CrossRef]
72. Koivunen, J.P.; Mermel, C.; Zejnullahu, K.; Murphy, C.; Lifshits, E.; Holmes, A.J.; Choi, H.G.; Kim, J.; Chiang, D.; Thomas, R.; et al. EML4-ALK fusion gene and efficacy of an ALK kinase inhibitor in lung cancer. *Clin. Cancer Res.* **2008**, *14*, 4275–4283. [CrossRef]
73. Liao, B.C.; Lin, C.C.; Shih, J.Y.; Yang, J.C. Treating patients with ALK-positive non-small cell lung cancer: Latest evidence and management strategy. *Ther. Adv. Med. Oncol.* **2015**, *7*, 274–290. [CrossRef] [PubMed]
74. Choi, Y.L.; Soda, M.; Yamashita, Y.; Ueno, T.; Takashima, J.; Nakajima, T.; Yatabe, Y.; Takeuchi, K.; Hamada, T.; Haruta, H.; et al. EML4-ALK mutations in lung cancer that confer resistance to ALK inhibitors. *N. Engl. J. Med.* **2010**, *363*, 1734–1739. [CrossRef] [PubMed]
75. Sasaki, T.; Koivunen, J.; Ogino, A.; Yanagita, M.; Nikiforow, S.; Zheng, W.; Lathan, C.; Marcoux, J.P.; Du, J.; Okuda, K.; et al. A novel ALK secondary mutation and EGFR signaling cause resistance to ALK kinase inhibitors. *Cancer Res.* **2011**, *71*, 6051–6060. [CrossRef]
76. Lovly, C.M.; Pao, W. Escaping ALK inhibition: Mechanisms of and strategies to overcome resistance. *Sci. Transl. Med.* **2012**, *4*, 120ps122. [CrossRef] [PubMed]
77. Katayama, R.; Shaw, A.T.; Khan, T.M.; Mino-Kenudson, M.; Solomon, B.J.; Halmos, B.; Jessop, N.A.; Wain, J.C.; Yeo, A.T.; Benes, C.; et al. Mechanisms of acquired crizotinib resistance in ALK-rearranged lung Cancers. *Sci. Transl. Med.* **2012**, *4*, 120ra117. [CrossRef]

78. Katayama, R.; Khan, T.M.; Benes, C.; Lifshits, E.; Ebi, H.; Rivera, V.M.; Shakespeare, W.C.; Iafrate, A.J.; Engelman, J.A.; Shaw, A.T. Therapeutic strategies to overcome crizotinib resistance in non-small cell lung cancers harboring the fusion oncogene EML4-ALK. *Proc. Natl. Acad. Sci. USA* **2011**, *108*, 7535–7540. [CrossRef]
79. Doebele, R.C.; Pilling, A.B.; Aisner, D.L.; Kutateladze, T.G.; Le, A.T.; Weickhardt, A.J.; Kondo, K.L.; Linderman, D.J.; Heasley, L.E.; Franklin, W.A.; et al. Mechanisms of resistance to crizotinib in patients with ALK gene rearranged non-small cell lung cancer. *Clin. Cancer Res.* **2012**, *18*, 1472–1482. [CrossRef]
80. Shaw, A.T.; Kim, D.-W.; Mehra, R.; Tan, D.S.W.; Felip, E.; Chow, L.Q.M.; Camidge, D.R.; Vansteenkiste, J.; Sharma, S.; De Pas, T.; et al. Ceritinib in ALK-Rearranged Non–Small-Cell Lung Cancer. *N. Engl. J. Med.* **2014**, *370*, 1189–1197. [CrossRef]
81. Camidge, D.R.; Dziadziuszko, R.; Peters, S.; Mok, T.; Noe, J.; Nowicka, M.; Gadgeel, S.M.; Cheema, P.; Pavlakis, N.; de Marinis, F.; et al. Updated Efficacy and Safety Data and Impact of the EML4-ALK Fusion Variant on the Efficacy of Alectinib in Untreated ALK-Positive Advanced Non-Small Cell Lung Cancer in the Global Phase III ALEX Study. *J. Thorac Oncol.* **2019**, *14*, 1233–1243. [CrossRef]
82. Hida, T.; Nokihara, H.; Kondo, M.; Kim, Y.H.; Azuma, K.; Seto, T.; Takiguchi, Y.; Nishio, M.; Yoshioka, H.; Imamura, F.; et al. Alectinib versus crizotinib in patients with ALK-positive non-small-cell lung cancer (J-ALEX): An open-label, randomised phase 3 trial. *Lancet* **2017**, *390*, 29–39. [CrossRef]
83. Peters, S.; Camidge, D.R.; Shaw, A.T.; Gadgeel, S.; Ahn, J.S.; Kim, D.-W.; Ou, S.-H.I.; Pérol, M.; Dziadziuszko, R.; Rosell, R.; et al. Alectinib versus Crizotinib in Untreated ALK-Positive Non–Small-Cell Lung Cancer. *N. Engl. J. Med.* **2017**, *377*, 829–838. [CrossRef] [PubMed]
84. Zhang, S.; Anjum, R.; Squillace, R.; Nadworny, S.; Zhou, T.; Keats, J.; Ning, Y.; Wardwell, S.D.; Miller, D.; Song, Y.; et al. The Potent ALK Inhibitor Brigatinib (AP26113) Overcomes Mechanisms of Resistance to First- and Second-Generation ALK Inhibitors in Preclinical Models. *Clin. Cancer Res.* **2016**, *22*, 5527–5538. [CrossRef] [PubMed]
85. Amanam, I.; Gupta, R.; Mambetsariev, I.; Salgia, R. The brigatinib experience: A new generation of therapy for ALK-positive non-small-cell lung cancer. *Future Oncol.* **2018**, *14*, 1897–1908. [CrossRef]
86. Kim, D.W.; Tiseo, M.; Ahn, M.J.; Reckamp, K.L.; Hansen, K.H.; Kim, S.W.; Huber, R.M.; West, H.L.; Groen, H.J.M.; Hochmair, M.J.; et al. Brigatinib in Patients With Crizotinib-Refractory Anaplastic Lymphoma Kinase-Positive Non-Small-Cell Lung Cancer: A Randomized, Multicenter Phase II Trial. *J. Clin. Oncol.* **2017**, *35*, 2490–2498. [CrossRef] [PubMed]
87. Sakamoto, H.; Tsukaguchi, T.; Hiroshima, S.; Kodama, T.; Kobayashi, T.; Fukami, T.A.; Oikawa, N.; Tsukuda, T.; Ishii, N.; Aoki, Y. CH5424802, a selective ALK inhibitor capable of blocking the resistant gatekeeper mutant. *Cancer Cell.* **2011**, *19*, 679–690. [CrossRef]
88. Rivera, V.M.; Wang, F.; Anjum, R.; Zhang, S.; Squillace, R.; Keats, J.; Miller, D.; Ning, Y.; Wardwell, S.D.; Moran, L.; et al. Abstract 1794: AP26113 is a dual ALK/EGFR inhibitor: Characterization against EGFR T790M in cell and mouse models of NSCLC. *Cancer Res.* **2012**, *72*, 1794. [CrossRef]
89. Camidge, R.; Kim, H.R.; Ahn, M.J.; Yang, J.C.H.; Han, J.Y.; Hochmair, M.J.; Lee, K.H.; Delmonte, A.; Garcia Campelo, M.R.; Kim, D.W.; et al. Brigatinib vs crizotinib in patients with ALK inhibitor-naive advanced ALK+ NSCLC: Updated results from the phase III ALTA-1L trial. *Ann. Oncol.* **2019**, *30*, ix195–ix196. [CrossRef]
90. Horn, L.; Infante, J.R.; Reckamp, K.L.; Blumenschein, G.R.; Leal, T.A.; Waqar, S.N.; Gitlitz, B.J.; Sanborn, R.E.; Whisenant, J.G.; Du, L.; et al. Ensartinib (X-396) in ALK-Positive Non–Small Cell Lung Cancer: Results from a First-in-Human Phase I/II, Multicenter Study. *Clin. Cancer Res.* **2018**, *24*, 2771–2779. [CrossRef]
91. Shaw, A.T.; Solomon, B.J.; Besse, B.; Bauer, T.M.; Lin, C.C.; Soo, R.A.; Riely, G.J.; Ou, S.I.; Clancy, J.S.; Li, S.; et al. ALK Resistance Mutations and Efficacy of Lorlatinib in Advanced Anaplastic Lymphoma Kinase-Positive Non-Small-Cell Lung Cancer. *J. Clin. Oncol.* **2019**, *37*, 1370–1379. [CrossRef]
92. Barrows, S.M.; Wright, K.; Copley-Merriman, C.; Kaye, J.A.; Chioda, M.; Wiltshire, R.; Torgersen, K.M.; Masters, E.T. Systematic review of sequencing of ALK inhibitors in ALK-positive non-small-cell lung cancer. *Lung Cancer (Auckl)* **2019**, *10*, 11–20. [CrossRef]
93. Xu, H.; Ma, D.; Yang, G.; Li, J.; Hao, X.; Xing, P.; Yang, L.; Xu, F.; Wang, Y. Sequential therapy according to distinct disease progression patterns in advanced ALK-positive non-small-cell lung cancer after crizotinib treatment. *Chin. J. Cancer Res.* **2019**, *31*, 349–356. [CrossRef]
94. Illei, P.B.; Wong, W.; Wu, N.; Chu, L.; Gupta, R.; Schulze, K.; Gubens, M.A. ALK Testing Trends and Patterns Among Community Practices in the United States. *JCO Precis. Oncol.* **2018**, *2*, 1–11. [CrossRef]

95. Hussein, M.; Richards, D.A.; Ulrich, B.; Korytowsky, B.; Pandya, D.; Cogswell, J.; Batenchuk, C.; Burns, V. ORAL01.02: Biopsies in Initial Diagnosis of Non–Small Cell Lung Cancer in US Community Oncology Practices: Implications for First-Line Immunotherapy: Topic: Medical Oncology. *J. Thorac. Oncol.* **2016**, *11*, S249–S250. [CrossRef]
96. Leighl, N.B.; Page, R.D.; Raymond, V.M.; Daniel, D.B.; Divers, S.G.; Reckamp, K.L.; Villalona-Calero, M.A.; Dix, D.; Odegaard, J.I.; Lanman, R.B.; et al. Clinical Utility of Comprehensive Cell-Free DNA Analysis to Identify Genomic Biomarkers in Patients with Newly Diagnosed Metastatic Non-Small Cell Lung Cancer. *Clin. Cancer Res.* **2019**. [CrossRef] [PubMed]
97. Rikova, K.; Guo, A.; Zeng, Q.; Possemato, A.; Yu, J.; Haack, H.; Nardone, J.; Lee, K.; Reeves, C.; Li, Y.; et al. Global survey of phosphotyrosine signaling identifies oncogenic kinases in lung cancer. *Cell* **2007**, *131*, 1190–1203. [CrossRef] [PubMed]
98. Korpanty, G.J.; Graham, D.M.; Vincent, M.D.; Leighl, N.B. Biomarkers That Currently Affect Clinical Practice in Lung Cancer: EGFR, ALK, MET, ROS-1, and KRAS. *Front. Oncol.* **2014**, *4*, 204. [CrossRef] [PubMed]
99. Gainor, J.F.; Tseng, D.; Yoda, S.; Dagogo-Jack, I.; Friboulet, L.; Lin, J.J.; Hubbeling, H.G.; Dardaei, L.; Farago, A.F.; Schultz, K.R.; et al. Patterns of Metastatic Spread and Mechanisms of Resistance to Crizotinib in ROS1-Positive Non-Small-Cell Lung Cancer. *JCO Precis Oncol.* **2017**, *2017*. [CrossRef] [PubMed]
100. Dagogo-Jack, I.; Shaw, A.T. Expanding the Roster of ROS1 Inhibitors. *J. Clin. Oncol.* **2017**, *35*, 2595–2597. [CrossRef]
101. Shaw, A.T.; Ou, S.H.; Bang, Y.J.; Camidge, D.R.; Solomon, B.J.; Salgia, R.; Riely, G.J.; Varella-Garcia, M.; Shapiro, G.I.; Costa, D.B.; et al. Crizotinib in ROS1-rearranged non-small-cell lung cancer. *N. Engl. J. Med.* **2014**, *371*, 1963–1971. [CrossRef]
102. Lim, S.M.; Kim, H.R.; Lee, J.S.; Lee, K.H.; Lee, Y.G.; Min, Y.J.; Cho, E.K.; Lee, S.S.; Kim, B.S.; Choi, M.Y.; et al. Open-Label, Multicenter, Phase II Study of Ceritinib in Patients With Non-Small-Cell Lung Cancer Harboring ROS1 Rearrangement. *J. Clin. Oncol.* **2017**, *35*, 2613–2618. [CrossRef]
103. Doebele, R.; Ahn, M.; Siena, S.; Drilon, A.; Krebs, M.; Lin, C.; De Braud, F.; John, T.; Tan, D.; Seto, T.; et al. OA02.01 Efficacy and Safety of Entrectinib in Locally Advanced or Metastatic ROS1 Fusion-Positive Non-Small Cell Lung Cancer (NSCLC). *J. Thorac. Oncol.* **2018**, *13*, S321–S322. [CrossRef]
104. Ou, S.; Shaw, A.; Riely, G.; Chiari, R.; Bauman, J.; Clancy, J.; Thurm, H.; Peltz, G.; Abbattista, A.; Solomon, B. OA02.03 Clinical Activity of Lorlatinib in Patients with ROS1+ Advanced Non-Small Cell Lung Cancer: Phase 2 Study Cohort EXP-6. *J. Thorac. Oncol.* **2018**, *13*, S322–S323. [CrossRef]
105. Research, F.o.C. Trends in the Molecular Diagnosis of Lung Cancer, Results from an Online Market Research Survey. Available online: https://www.focr.org/sites/default/files/pdf/FINAL%202017%20Friends%20NSCLC%20White%20Paper.pdf (accessed on 20 May 2020).
106. Nadler, E.; Pavilack, M.; Clark, J.; Espirito, J.; Fernandes, A. Biomarker Testing Rates in Patients with Advanced Non-Small Cell Lung Cancer Treated in the Community. *J. Cancer Ther.* **2019**, *10*, 971–984. [CrossRef]
107. Rijavec, E.; Coco, S.; Genova, C.; Rossi, G.; Longo, L.; Grossi, F. Liquid Biopsy in Non-Small Cell Lung Cancer: Highlights and Challenges. *Cancers (Basel)* **2019**, *12*, 17. [CrossRef] [PubMed]
108. de Melo Gagliato, D.; Jardim, D.L.F.; Falchook, G.; Tang, C.; Zinner, R.; Wheler, J.J.; Janku, F.; Subbiah, V.; Piha-Paul, S.A.; Fu, S.; et al. Analysis of MET genetic aberrations in patients with breast cancer at MD Anderson Phase I unit. *Clin. Breast Cancer* **2014**, *14*, 468–474. [CrossRef] [PubMed]
109. Cappuzzo, F.; Marchetti, A.; Skokan, M.; Rossi, E.; Gajapathy, S.; Felicioni, L.; Del Grammastro, M.; Sciarrotta, M.G.; Buttitta, F.; Incarbone, M.; et al. Increased MET gene copy number negatively affects survival of surgically resected non-small-cell lung cancer patients. *J. Clin. Oncol. Off. J. Am. Soc. Clin. Oncol.* **2009**, *27*, 1667–1674. [CrossRef] [PubMed]
110. Carracedo, A.; Egervari, K.; Salido, M.; Rojo, F.; Corominas, J.M.; Arumi, M.; Corzo, C.; Tusquets, I.; Espinet, B.; Rovira, A.; et al. FISH and immunohistochemical status of the hepatocyte growth factor receptor (c-Met) in 184 invasive breast tumors. *Breast Cancer Res.* **2009**, *11*, 402. [CrossRef]
111. Drilon, A.; Cappuzzo, F.; Ou, S.-H.I.; Camidge, D.R. Targeting MET in Lung Cancer: Will Expectations Finally Be MET? *J. Thorac. Oncol.* **2017**, *12*, 15–26. [CrossRef]
112. Ghadjar, P.; Blank-Liss, W.; Simcock, M.; Hegyi, I.; Beer, K.T.; Moch, H.; Aebersold, D.M.; Zimmer, Y. MET Y1253D-activating point mutation and development of distant metastasis in advanced head and neck cancers. *Clin. Exp. Metastasis* **2009**, *26*, 809–815. [CrossRef]

113. Cipriani, N.A.; Abidoye, O.O.; Vokes, E.; Salgia, R. MET as a target for treatment of chest tumors. *Lung Cancer* **2009**, *63*, 169–179. [CrossRef]
114. Schmidt, L.; Duh, F.M.; Chen, F.; Kishida, T.; Glenn, G.; Choyke, P.; Scherer, S.W.; Zhuang, Z.; Lubensky, I.; Dean, M.; et al. Germline and somatic mutations in the tyrosine kinase domain of the MET proto-oncogene in papillary renal carcinomas. *Nat. Genet.* **1997**, *16*, 68–73. [CrossRef] [PubMed]
115. Ma, P.C.; Jagadeeswaran, R.; Jagadeesh, S.; Tretiakova, M.S.; Nallasura, V.; Fox, E.A.; Hansen, M.; Schaefer, E.; Naoki, K.; Lader, A.; et al. Functional expression and mutations of c-Met and its therapeutic inhibition with SU11274 and small interfering RNA in non-small cell lung cancer. *Cancer Res.* **2005**, *65*, 1479–1488. [CrossRef]
116. Ma, P.C.; Kijima, T.; Maulik, G.; Fox, E.A.; Sattler, M.; Griffin, J.D.; Johnson, B.E.; Salgia, R. c-MET mutational analysis in small cell lung cancer: Novel juxtamembrane domain mutations regulating cytoskeletal functions. *Cancer Res.* **2003**, *63*, 6272–6281. [PubMed]
117. Comprehensive molecular profiling of lung adenocarcinoma. *Nature* **2014**, *511*, 543–550. [CrossRef] [PubMed]
118. Comprehensive genomic characterization of squamous cell lung cancers. *Nature* **2012**, *489*, 519–525. [CrossRef]
119. Paik, P.K.; Drilon, A.; Fan, P.-D.; Yu, H.; Rekhtman, N.; Ginsberg, M.S.; Borsu, L.; Schultz, N.; Berger, M.F.; Rudin, C.M.; et al. Response to MET Inhibitors in Patients with Stage IV Lung Adenocarcinomas Harboring MET Mutations Causing Exon 14 Skipping. *Cancer Discov.* **2015**, *5*, 842–849. [CrossRef]
120. Drilon, A.; Clark, J.W.; Weiss, J.; Ou, S.I.; Camidge, D.R.; Solomon, B.J.; Otterson, G.A.; Villaruz, L.C.; Riely, G.J.; Heist, R.S.; et al. Antitumor activity of crizotinib in lung cancers harboring a MET exon 14 alteration. *Nat. Med.* **2020**, *26*, 47–51. [CrossRef]
121. Felip, E.; Horn, L.; Patel, J.D.; Sakai, H.; Scheele, J.; Bruns, R.; Paik, P.K. Tepotinib in patients with advanced non-small cell lung cancer (NSCLC) harboring MET exon 14-skipping mutations: Phase II trial. *J. Clin. Oncol.* **2018**, *36*, 9016. [CrossRef]
122. Nakamura, Y.; Niki, T.; Goto, A.; Morikawa, T.; Miyazawa, K.; Nakajima, J.; Fukayama, M. c-Met activation in lung adenocarcinoma tissues: An immunohistochemical analysis. *Cancer Sci* **2007**, *98*, 1006–1013. [CrossRef]
123. Cappuzzo, F.; Janne, P.A.; Skokan, M.; Finocchiaro, G.; Rossi, E.; Ligorio, C.; Zucali, P.A.; Terracciano, L.; Toschi, L.; Roncalli, M.; et al. MET increased gene copy number and primary resistance to gefitinib therapy in non-small-cell lung cancer patients. *Ann. Oncol.* **2009**, *20*, 298–304. [CrossRef]
124. Strickler, J.H.; Weekes, C.D.; Nemunaitis, J.; Ramanathan, R.K.; Heist, R.S.; Morgensztern, D.; Angevin, E.; Bauer, T.M.; Yue, H.; Motwani, M.; et al. First-in-Human Phase I, Dose-Escalation and -Expansion Study of Telisotuzumab Vedotin, an Antibody-Drug Conjugate Targeting c-Met, in Patients With Advanced Solid Tumors. *J. Clin. Oncol.* **2018**, *36*, 3298–3306. [CrossRef] [PubMed]
125. Wang, R.; Hu, H.; Pan, Y.; Li, Y.; Ye, T.; Li, C.; Luo, X.; Wang, L.; Li, H.; Zhang, Y.; et al. RET fusions define a unique molecular and clinicopathologic subtype of non-small-cell lung cancer. *J. Clin. Oncol.* **2012**, *30*, 4352–4359. [CrossRef] [PubMed]
126. Drilon, A.; Rekhtman, N.; Arcila, M.; Wang, L.; Ni, A.; Albano, M.; Van Voorthuysen, M.; Somwar, R.; Smith, R.S.; Montecalvo, J.; et al. Cabozantinib in patients with advanced RET-rearranged non-small-cell lung cancer: An open-label, single-centre, phase 2, single-arm trial. *Lancet Oncol.* **2016**, *17*, 1653–1660. [CrossRef]
127. Gainor, J.F.; Lee, D.H.; Curigliano, G.; Doebele, R.C.; Kim, D.-W.; Baik, C.S.; Tan, D.S.-W.; Lopes, G.; Gadgeel, S.M.; Cassier, P.A.; et al. Clinical activity and tolerability of BLU-667, a highly potent and selective RET inhibitor, in patients (pts) with advanced RET-fusion+ non-small cell lung cancer (NSCLC). *J. Clin. Oncol.* **2019**, *37*, 9008. [CrossRef]
128. Nakagawara, A. Trk receptor tyrosine kinases: A bridge between cancer and neural development. *Cancer Lett.* **2001**, *169*, 107–114. [CrossRef]
129. Vaishnavi, A.; Capelletti, M.; Le, A.T.; Kako, S.; Butaney, M.; Ercan, D.; Mahale, S.; Davies, K.D.; Aisner, D.L.; Pilling, A.B.; et al. Oncogenic and drug-sensitive NTRK1 rearrangements in lung cancer. *Nat. Med.* **2013**, *19*, 1469–1472. [CrossRef]
130. Doebele, R.C.; Drilon, A.; Paz-Ares, L.; Siena, S.; Shaw, A.T.; Farago, A.F.; Blakely, C.M.; Seto, T.; Cho, B.C.; Tosi, D.; et al. Entrectinib in patients with advanced or metastatic NTRK fusion-positive solid tumours: Integrated analysis of three phase 1-2 trials. *Lancet Oncol.* **2020**, *21*, 271–282. [CrossRef]

131. Drilon, A.; Li, G.; Dogan, S.; Gounder, M.; Shen, R.; Arcila, M.; Wang, L.; Hyman, D.M.; Hechtman, J.; Wei, G.; et al. What hides behind the MASC: Clinical response and acquired resistance to entrectinib after ETV6-NTRK3 identification in a mammary analogue secretory carcinoma (MASC). *Ann. Oncol.* **2016**, *27*, 920–926. [CrossRef]
132. Russo, M.; Misale, S.; Wei, G.; Siravegna, G.; Crisafulli, G.; Lazzari, L.; Corti, G.; Rospo, G.; Novara, L.; Mussolin, B.; et al. Acquired Resistance to the TRK Inhibitor Entrectinib in Colorectal Cancer. *Cancer Discov.* **2016**, *6*, 36–44. [CrossRef]
133. Drilon, A.; Nagasubramanian, R.; Blake, J.F.; Ku, N.; Tuch, B.B.; Ebata, K.; Smith, S.; Lauriault, V.; Kolakowski, G.R.; Brandhuber, B.J.; et al. A Next-Generation TRK Kinase Inhibitor Overcomes Acquired Resistance to Prior TRK Kinase Inhibition in Patients with TRK Fusion–Positive Solid Tumors. *Cancer Discov.* **2017**, *7*, 963–972. [CrossRef]
134. Hyman, D.; Kummar, S.; Farago, A.; Geoerger, B.; Mau-Sorensen, M.; Taylor, M.; Garralda, E.; Nagasubramanian, R.; Natheson, M.; Song, L.; et al. Abstract CT127: Phase I and expanded access experience of LOXO-195 (BAY 2731954), a selective next-generation TRK inhibitor (TRKi). *Cancer Res.* **2019**, *79*, CT127. [CrossRef]
135. Marchetti, A.; Felicioni, L.; Malatesta, S.; Sciarrotta, M.G.; Guetti, L.; Chella, A.; Viola, P.; Pullara, C.; Mucilli, F.; Buttitta, F. Clinical Features and Outcome of Patients With Non–Small-Cell Lung Cancer Harboring BRAF Mutations. *J. Clin. Oncol.* **2011**, *29*, 3574–3579. [CrossRef] [PubMed]
136. Planchard, D.; Smit, E.F.; Groen, H.J.M.; Mazieres, J.; Besse, B.; Helland, Å.; Giannone, V.; D'Amelio, A.M., Jr.; Zhang, P.; Mookerjee, B.; et al. Dabrafenib plus trametinib in patients with previously untreated BRAF(V600E)-mutant metastatic non-small-cell lung cancer: An open-label, phase 2 trial. *Lancet Oncol.* **2017**, *18*, 1307–1316. [CrossRef]
137. Mao, C.; Qiu, L.X.; Liao, R.Y.; Du, F.B.; Ding, H.; Yang, W.C.; Li, J.; Chen, Q. KRAS mutations and resistance to EGFR-TKIs treatment in patients with non-small cell lung cancer: A meta-analysis of 22 studies. *Lung Cancer* **2010**, *69*, 272–278. [CrossRef] [PubMed]
138. Johnson, M.L.; Sima, C.S.; Chaft, J.; Paik, P.K.; Pao, W.; Kris, M.G.; Ladanyi, M.; Riely, G.J. Association of KRAS and EGFR mutations with survival in patients with advanced lung adenocarcinomas. *Cancer* **2013**, *119*, 356–362. [CrossRef]
139. Shepherd, F.A.; Lacas, B.; Le Teuff, G.; Hainaut, P.; Janne, P.A.; Pignon, J.P.; Le Chevalier, T.; Seymour, L.; Douillard, J.Y.; Graziano, S.; et al. Pooled Analysis of the Prognostic and Predictive Effects of TP53 Comutation Status Combined With KRAS or EGFR Mutation in Early-Stage Resected Non-Small-Cell Lung Cancer in Four Trials of Adjuvant Chemotherapy. *J. Clin. Oncol.* **2017**, *35*, 2018–2027. [CrossRef]
140. AACR Project GENIE: Powering Precision Medicine through an International Consortium. *Cancer Discov.* **2017**, *7*, 818–831. [CrossRef]
141. Christensen, J.G.; Hallin, J.; Engstrom, L.D.; Hargis, L.; Calinisan, A.; Aranda, R.; Briere, D.M.; Sudhakar, N.; Bowcut, V.; Baer, B.R.; et al. The KRASG12C Inhibitor, MRTX849, Provides Insight Toward Therapeutic Susceptibility of KRAS Mutant Cancers in Mouse Models and Patients. *Cancer Discov.* **2019**, *10*, 54–71. [CrossRef]
142. Khozin, S.; Abernethy, A.P.; Nussbaum, N.C.; Zhi, J.; Curtis, M.D.; Tucker, M.; Lee, S.E.; Light, D.E.; Gossai, A.; Sorg, R.A.; et al. Characteristics of Real-World Metastatic Non-Small Cell Lung Cancer Patients Treated with Nivolumab and Pembrolizumab During the Year Following Approval. *Oncologist* **2018**, *23*, 328–336. [CrossRef]
143. Nadler, E.; Espirito, J.L.; Pavilack, M.; Boyd, M.; Vergara-Silva, A.; Fernandes, A. Treatment Patterns and Clinical Outcomes Among Metastatic Non-Small-Cell Lung Cancer Patients Treated in the Community Practice Setting. *Clin. Lung Cancer* **2018**, *19*, 360–370. [CrossRef] [PubMed]
144. Fehrenbacher, L.; Spira, A.; Ballinger, M.; Kowanetz, M.; Vansteenkiste, J.; Mazieres, J.; Park, K.; Smith, D.; Artal-Cortes, A.; Lewanski, C.; et al. Atezolizumab versus docetaxel for patients with previously treated non-small-cell lung cancer (POPLAR): A multicentre, open-label, phase 2 randomised controlled trial. *Lancet* **2016**, *387*, 1837–1846. [CrossRef]
145. Reck, M.; Rodríguez-Abreu, D.; Robinson, A.G.; Hui, R.; Csőszi, T.; Fülöp, A.; Gottfried, M.; Peled, N.; Tafreshi, A.; Cuffe, S.; et al. Updated Analysis of KEYNOTE-024: Pembrolizumab Versus Platinum-Based Chemotherapy for Advanced Non-Small-Cell Lung Cancer With PD-L1 Tumor Proportion Score of 50% or Greater. *J. Clin. Oncol.* **2019**, *37*, 537–546. [CrossRef] [PubMed]

146. Zhou, Y.; Lin, Z.; Zhang, X.; Chen, C.; Zhao, H.; Hong, S.; Zhang, L. First-line treatment for patients with advanced non-small cell lung carcinoma and high PD-L1 expression: Pembrolizumab or pembrolizumab plus chemotherapy. *J. Immunother. Cancer* **2019**, *7*, 120. [CrossRef] [PubMed]
147. Gandhi, L.; Rodríguez-Abreu, D.; Gadgeel, S.; Esteban, E.; Felip, E.; De Angelis, F.; Domine, M.; Clingan, P.; Hochmair, M.J.; Powell, S.F.; et al. Pembrolizumab plus Chemotherapy in Metastatic Non–Small-Cell Lung Cancer. *N. Engl. J. Med.* **2018**, *378*, 2078–2092. [CrossRef]
148. Hellmann, M.D.; Paz-Ares, L.; Bernabe Caro, R.; Zurawski, B.; Kim, S.-W.; Carcereny Costa, E.; Park, K.; Alexandru, A.; Lupinacci, L.; de la Mora Jimenez, E.; et al. Nivolumab plus Ipilimumab in Advanced Non–Small-Cell Lung Cancer. *N. Engl. J. Med.* **2019**, *381*, 2020–2031. [CrossRef]
149. Rizvi, N.A.; Cho, B.C.; Reinmuth, N.; Lee, K.H.; Luft, A.; Ahn, M.J.; van den Heuvel, M.M.; Cobo, M.; Vicente, D.; Smolin, A.; et al. Durvalumab With or Without Tremelimumab vs Standard Chemotherapy in First-line Treatment of Metastatic Non-Small Cell Lung Cancer: The MYSTIC Phase 3 Randomized Clinical Trial. *JAMA Oncol.* **2020**, *6*, 661–674. [CrossRef]
150. Theelen, W.S.M.E.; Baas, P. Pembrolizumab monotherapy for PD-L1 ≥50% non-small cell lung cancer, undisputed first choice? *Ann. Transl. Med.* **2019**, *7*, S140. [CrossRef]
151. Velcheti, V.; Chandwani, S.; Chen, X.; Pietanza, M.C.; Piperdi, B.; Burke, T. Outcomes of first-line pembrolizumab monotherapy for PD-L1-positive (TPS ≥50%) metastatic NSCLC at US oncology practices. *Immunotherapy* **2019**, *11*, 1541–1554. [CrossRef]
152. Shivakumar, L.; Weldon, C.B.; Lucas, L.; Perloff, T. Identifying obstacles to optimal integration of cancer immunotherapies in the community setting. *J. Clin. Oncol.* **2019**, *37*, 87. [CrossRef]
153. Krimphove, M.J.; Tully, K.H.; Friedlander, D.F.; Marchese, M.; Ravi, P.; Lipsitz, S.R.; Kilbridge, K.L.; Kibel, A.S.; Kluth, L.A.; Ott, P.A.; et al. Adoption of immunotherapy in the community for patients diagnosed with metastatic melanoma. *J. Immunother. Cancer* **2019**, *7*, 289. [CrossRef]
154. Ancevski Hunter, K.; Socinski, M.A.; Villaruz, L.C. PD-L1 Testing in Guiding Patient Selection for PD-1/PD-L1 Inhibitor Therapy in Lung Cancer. *Mol. Diagn. Ther.* **2018**, *22*, 1–10. [CrossRef] [PubMed]
155. Roach, C.; Zhang, N.; Corigliano, E.; Jansson, M.; Toland, G.; Ponto, G.; Dolled-Filhart, M.; Emancipator, K.; Stanforth, D.; Kulangara, K. Development of a Companion Diagnostic PD-L1 Immunohistochemistry Assay for Pembrolizumab Therapy in Non-Small-cell Lung Cancer. *Appl. Immunohistochem. Mol. Morphol. AIMM* **2016**, *24*, 392–397. [CrossRef] [PubMed]
156. Büttner, R.; Gosney, J.R.; Skov, B.G.; Adam, J.; Motoi, N.; Bloom, K.J.; Dietel, M.; Longshore, J.W.; López-Ríos, F.; Penault-Llorca, F.; et al. Programmed Death-Ligand 1 Immunohistochemistry Testing: A Review of Analytical Assays and Clinical Implementation in Non-Small-Cell Lung Cancer. *J. Clin. Oncol.* **2017**, *35*, 3867–3876. [CrossRef]
157. Rittmeyer, A.; Barlesi, F.; Waterkamp, D.; Park, K.; Ciardiello, F.; von Pawel, J.; Gadgeel, S.M.; Hida, T.; Kowalski, D.M.; Dols, M.C.; et al. Atezolizumab versus docetaxel in patients with previously treated non-small-cell lung cancer (OAK): A phase 3, open-label, multicentre randomised controlled trial. *Lancet* **2017**, *389*, 255–265. [CrossRef]
158. Velcheti, V.; Patwardhan, P.D.; Liu, F.X.; Chen, X.; Cao, X.; Burke, T. Real-world PD-L1 testing and distribution of PD-L1 tumor expression by immunohistochemistry assay type among patients with metastatic non-small cell lung cancer in the United States. *PLoS ONE* **2018**, *13*, e0206370. [CrossRef]
159. Gong, J.; Pan, K.; Fakih, M.; Pal, S.; Salgia, R. Value-based genomics. *Oncotarget Adv. Publ.* **2018**, *9*, 15792. [CrossRef] [PubMed]
160. Ellis, L.M.; Bernstein, D.S.; Voest, E.E.; Berlin, J.D.; Sargent, D.; Cortazar, P.; Garrett-Mayer, E.; Herbst, R.S.; Lilenbaum, R.C.; Sima, C.; et al. American Society of Clinical Oncology perspective: Raising the bar for clinical trials by defining clinically meaningful outcomes. *J. Clin. Oncol.* **2014**, *32*, 1277–1280. [CrossRef]
161. Chu, L.; Kelly, K.; Gandara, D.; Lara, P.; Borowsky, A.; Meyers, F.; McPherson, J.; Erlich, R.; Almog, N.; Schrock, A.; et al. P3.13-26 Outcomes of Patients with Metastatic Lung Cancer Presented in a Multidisciplinary Molecular Tumor Board. *J. Thoracic Oncol.* **2018**, *13*, S986. [CrossRef]
162. Koopman, B.; Wekken, A.J.v.d.; Elst, A.t.; Hiltermann, T.J.N.; Vilacha, J.F.; Groves, M.R.; Berg, A.v.d.; Hiddinga, B.I.; Hijmering-Kappelle, L.B.M.; Stigt, J.A.; et al. Relevance and Effectiveness of Molecular Tumor Board Recommendations for Patients With Non–Small-Cell Lung Cancer With Rare or Complex Mutational Profiles. *JCO Precis. Oncol.* **2020**, *4*, 393–410. [CrossRef]

163. Planchard, D.; Faivre, L.; Sullivan, I.; Kahn-charpy, V.; Lacroix, L.; Auger, N.; Adam, J.; De Montpreville, V.T.; Dorfmuller, P.; Pechoux, C.L.; et al. 3081 Molecular Tumor Board (MTB) in non-small cell lung cancers (NSCLC) to optimize targeted therapies: 4 years' experience at Gustave Roussy. *Eur. J. Cancer* **2015**, *51*, S624. [CrossRef]
164. Rolfo, C.; Manca, P.; Salgado, R.; Van Dam, P.; Dendooven, A.; Machado Coelho, A.; Ferri Gandia, J.; Rutten, A.; Lybaert, W.; Vermeij, J.; et al. Multidisciplinary molecular tumour board: A tool to improve clinical practice and selection accrual for clinical trials in patients with cancer. *ESMO Open* **2018**, *3*, e000398. [CrossRef]
165. Pishvaian, M.J.; Blais, E.M.; Bender, R.J.; Rao, S.; Boca, S.M.; Chung, V.; Hendifar, A.E.; Mikhail, S.; Sohal, D.P.S.; Pohlmann, P.R.; et al. A virtual molecular tumor board to improve efficiency and scalability of delivering precision oncology to physicians and their patients. *JAMIA Open* **2019**, *2*, 505–515. [CrossRef]
166. Lesslie, M.; Parikh, J.R. Implementing a Multidisciplinary Tumor Board in the Community Practice Setting. *Diagnostics (Basel)* **2017**, *7*, 55. [CrossRef] [PubMed]
167. El-Deiry, W.S.; Goldberg, R.M.; Lenz, H.-J.; Shields, A.F.; Gibney, G.T.; Tan, A.R.; Brown, J.; Eisenberg, B.; Heath, E.I.; Phuphanich, S.; et al. The current state of molecular testing in the treatment of patients with solid tumors, 2019. *CA A Cancer J. Clin.* **2019**, *69*, 305–343. [CrossRef] [PubMed]
168. Wang, T.; Liu, S.; Joseph, T.; Lyou, Y. Managing Bladder Cancer Care during the COVID-19 Pandemic Using a Team-Based Approach. *J. Clin. Med.* **2020**, *9*, 1574. [CrossRef] [PubMed]
169. Bironzo, P.; Di Maio, M. A review of guidelines for lung cancer. *J. Thorac Dis.* **2018**, *10*, S1556–S1563. [CrossRef]
170. Daly, B.; Zon, R.T.; Page, R.D.; Edge, S.B.; Lyman, G.H.; Green, S.R.; Wollins, D.S.; Bosserman, L.D. Oncology Clinical Pathways: Charting the Landscape of Pathway Providers. *J. Oncol. Pract.* **2018**, *14*, e194–e200. [CrossRef]
171. Neubauer, M.A.; Hoverman, J.R.; Kolodziej, M.; Reisman, L.; Gruschkus, S.K.; Hoang, S.; Alva, A.A.; McArthur, M.; Forsyth, M.; Rothermel, T.; et al. Cost effectiveness of evidence-based treatment guidelines for the treatment of non-small-cell lung cancer in the community setting. *J. Oncol. Pract.* **2010**, *6*, 12–18. [CrossRef]
172. Hoverman, J.R.; Cartwright, T.H.; Patt, D.A.; Espirito, J.L.; Clayton, M.P.; Garey, J.S.; Kopp, T.J.; Kolodziej, M.; Neubauer, M.A.; Fitch, K.; et al. Pathways, outcomes, and costs in colon cancer: Retrospective evaluations in two distinct databases. *J. Oncol. Pract.* **2011**, *7*, 52s–59s. [CrossRef]
173. Kreys, E.D.; Koeller, J.M. Documenting the benefits and cost savings of a large multistate cancer pathway program from a payer's perspective. *J. Oncol. Pract.* **2013**, *9*, e241–e247. [CrossRef] [PubMed]
174. Jackman, D.M.; Zhang, Y.; Dalby, C.; Nguyen, T.; Nagle, J.; Lydon, C.A.; Rabin, M.S.; McNiff, K.K.; Fraile, B.; Jacobson, J.O. Cost and Survival Analysis Before and After Implementation of Dana-Farber Clinical Pathways for Patients With Stage IV Non-Small-Cell Lung Cancer. *J. Oncol. Pract.* **2017**, *13*, e346–e352. [CrossRef]
175. Lawal, A.K.; Rotter, T.; Kinsman, L.; Machotta, A.; Ronellenfitsch, U.; Scott, S.D.; Goodridge, D.; Plishka, C.; Groot, G. What is a clinical pathway? Refinement of an operational definition to identify clinical pathway studies for a Cochrane systematic review. *BMC Med.* **2016**, *14*, 35. [CrossRef] [PubMed]
176. Zon, R.T.; Edge, S.B.; Page, R.D.; Frame, J.N.; Lyman, G.H.; Omel, J.L.; Wollins, D.S.; Green, S.R.; Bosserman, L.D. American Society of Clinical Oncology Criteria for High-Quality Clinical Pathways in Oncology. *J. Oncol. Pract.* **2017**, *13*, 207–210. [CrossRef] [PubMed]
177. Comis, R.L.; Miller, J.D.; Aldigé, C.R.; Krebs, L.; Stoval, E. Public attitudes toward participation in cancer clinical trials. *J. Clin. Oncol.* **2003**, *21*, 830–835. [CrossRef] [PubMed]
178. Ohno-Machado, L.; Kim, J.; Gabriel, R.A.; Kuo, G.M.; Hogarth, M.A. Genomics and electronic health record systems. *Hum. Mol. Genet.* **2018**, *27*, R48–R55. [CrossRef] [PubMed]
179. Salgia, N.; Philip, E.; Ziari, M.; Yap, K.; Pal, S. Advancing the Science and Management of Renal Cell Carcinoma: Bridging the Divide between Academic and Community Practices. *J. Clin. Med.* **2020**, *9*, 1508. [CrossRef]
180. Liu, J.; Gutierrez, E.; Tiwari, A.; Padam, S.; Li, D.; Dale, W.; Pal, S.; Stewart, D.; Subbiah, S.; Bosserman, L.; et al. Strategies to Improve Participation of Older Adults in Cancer Research. *J. Clin. Med.* **2020**, *9*, 1571. [CrossRef]
181. Zon, R.T.; Bruinooge, S.S.; Lyss, A.P. The Changing Face of Research in Community Practice. *J. Oncol. Pract.* **2014**, *10*, 155–160. [CrossRef] [PubMed]

182. Geiger, A.M.; O'Mara, A.M.; McCaskill-Stevens, W.J.; Adjei, B.; Tuovenin, P.; Castro, K.M. Evolution of Cancer Care Delivery Research in the NCI Community Oncology Research Program. *JNCI J. Natl. Cancer Inst.* **2019**. [CrossRef]
183. Herbst, R.S.; Morgensztern, D.; Boshoff, C. The biology and management of non-small cell lung cancer. *Nature* **2018**, *553*, 446–454. [CrossRef]
184. Aggarwal, C.; Thompson, J.C.; Black, T.A.; Katz, S.I.; Fan, R.; Yee, S.S.; Chien, A.L.; Evans, T.L.; Bauml, J.M.; Alley, E.W.; et al. Clinical Implications of Plasma-Based Genotyping With the Delivery of Personalized Therapy in Metastatic Non-Small Cell Lung Cancer. *JAMA Oncol.* **2019**, *5*, 173–180. [CrossRef] [PubMed]
185. Jonna, S.; Subramaniam, D.S. Molecular diagnostics and targeted therapies in non-small cell lung cancer (NSCLC): An update. *Discov. Med.* **2019**, *27*, 167–170. [PubMed]
186. Doroshow, D.B.; Herbst, R.S. Treatment of Advanced Non-Small Cell Lung Cancer in 2018. *JAMA Oncol.* **2018**, *4*, 569–570. [CrossRef] [PubMed]
187. Zeltsman, M.; Dozier, J.; McGee, E.; Ngai, D.; Adusumilli, P.S. CAR T-cell therapy for lung cancer and malignant pleural mesothelioma. *Transl. Res.* **2017**, *187*, 1–10. [CrossRef] [PubMed]

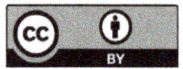

© 2020 by the authors. Licensee MDPI, Basel, Switzerland. This article is an open access article distributed under the terms and conditions of the Creative Commons Attribution (CC BY) license (http://creativecommons.org/licenses/by/4.0/).

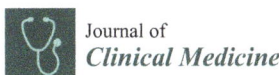

Review

Integrating Academic and Community Practices in the Management of Colorectal Cancer: The City of Hope Model

Misagh Karimi [1], Chongkai Wang [1], Bahareh Bahadini [2], George Hajjar [2] and Marwan Fakih [1,*]

1. Department of Medical Oncology and Therapeutic Research, City of Hope Comprehensive Cancer Center, Duarte, CA 91010, USA; mkarimi@coh.org (M.K.); chowang@coh.org (C.W.)
2. Department of Medical Oncology and Hematology, City of Hope National Medical Center, Mission Hills, CA 91345, USA; bbahadini@coh.org (B.B.); ghajjar@coh.org (G.H.)
* Correspondence: mfakih@coh.org

Received: 27 March 2020; Accepted: 26 May 2020; Published: 2 June 2020

Abstract: Colorectal cancer (CRC) management continues to evolve. In metastatic CRC, several clinical and molecular biomarkers are now recommended to guide treatment decisions. Primary tumor location (right versus left) has been shown to predict benefit from anti-epidermal growth factor receptors (EGFRs) in rat sarcoma viral oncogene homologue (*RAS*) and v-raf murine sarcoma viral oncogene homolog B1 (*BRAF*) wild-type patients. Anti-EGFR therapy has not resulted in any benefit in *RAS*-mutated tumors, irrespective of the primary tumor location. *BRAF-V600E* mutations have been associated with poor prognosis and treatment resistance but may benefit from a combination of anti-EGFR therapy and BRAF inhibitors. Human epidermal growth factor receptor 2 (*HER-2*) amplification was recently shown to predict relative resistance to anti-EGFR therapy but a response to dual HER-2 targeting within the *RAS* wild-type population. Finally, the mismatch repair (MMR)-deficient subgroup benefits significantly from immunotherapeutic strategies. In addition to the increasingly complex biomarker landscape in CRC, metastatic CRC remains one of the few malignancies that benefits from metastasectomies, ablative therapies, and regional hepatic treatments. This treatment complexity requires a multi-disciplinary approach to treatment and close collaborations between various stakeholders in large cancer center networks. Here, we describe the City of Hope experience and strategy to enhance colorectal cancer care across its network.

Keywords: colorectal cancer; precisian medicine; academic and community oncology

---

1. Introduction

Colorectal cancer is the second most common cause of cancer-related death in the United States, with an annual incidence of 145,000 cases in 2019 and 51,000 deaths according to the American Cancer Society [1]. The life-time risk of developing colorectal cancer in men and women is 4.6% and 4.2%, respectively, according to 2014–2016 data [2]. The five-year survival rate for metastatic disease and regional disease are 14.2% and 71.3%, respectively [3,4]. Therefore, significant progress is still needed, especially in metastatic colorectal cancer settings.

In this report, we will review the latest approaches in the treatment of metastatic disease. We will also explore the City of Hope approach to delivering optimized care with partnership between academic researchers and community clinicians in cancer care.

2. Our Path to Precision Medicine in the Treatment of Metastatic CRC

The management of metastatic colorectal cancer must take into consideration sidedness, as well as molecular biomarkers including *RAS*, *BRAF*, *HER-2*, and MMR status. We have previously extensively reviewed this topic [5,6]. In short, it is now well-established that the benefits of anti-EGFR therapy appear to be limited to *RAS* and *BRAF* wild-type tumors that originate from the left colon [7–9]. For this group of patients, the addition of anti-EGFR therapy to combination chemotherapy in the first-line setting is better than bevacizumab according to subgroup analyses from two large randomized trials [10,11]. On the other hand, right-sided tumors as well as *RAS* mutated tumors benefit from the addition of bevacizumab to combination first-line chemotherapy. Second-line treatments are typically shaped by first-line treatment decisions and are addressed in our prior reviews [6].

BRAF-V600E-mutated colorectal cancers constitute approximately 8% of metastatic colorectal cancers. These tumors are associated with a poor prognosis and relative chemotherapeutic resistance [12–14]. Given their aggressive histology, and based on subgroup analyses from the TRIBE clinical trial, we advocate a combination of 5-FU, irinotecan, and oxaliplatin (FOLFOXIRI) with bevacizumab in the first-line treatment for those deemed to be fit enough to tolerate this regimen [15]. Otherwise, the first-line treatment of *BRAF-V600E*-mutated colorectal cancer is typically managed in a similar fashion as that of *RAS*-mutated metastatic colorectal cancer. A ray of hope has finally emerged in the targeted therapy of these *BRAF*-mutated patients. The BEACON trial has recently demonstrated that in the second-line and third-line settings, a combination of a BRAF inhibitor (encorafenib) and EGFR inhibitor (cetuximab) is better than a combination of chemotherapy (irinotecan with or without 5-FU) and cetuximab [16,17]. Encorafenib plus cetuximab is now to be considered a standard second-line therapy in these patients.

HER-2 amplification occurs in 2% of colorectal cancers and is enriched in left-sided and *RAS* and *BRAF* wild-type tumors [18]. These tumors exhibit a relative resistance to anti-EGFR therapy and respond well to lapatinib and trastuzumab or trastuzumab and pertuzumab, based on the HERACLES and MYPATHWAY trials, respectively [19,20]. This has prompted the National Comprehensive Cancer Network (NCCN) to recommend these treatments in the later lines of treatment for this molecular subgroup. The value of anti-EGFR therapy in these patients is still under investigation. We hope that the ongoing SWOG trial (S1613) will finally shed some light on this issue [21].

Finally, MMR deficiency has emerged as a predictive biomarker of response to PD-1 inhibitors, with or without CTLA-4 inhibitors, in colorectal cancer [22,23]. Nivolumab and pembrolizumab have shown remarkably durable responses in the second- and third-line treatment of these patients [24,25]. The addition of ipilimumab to nivolumab appears to enhance the responses and disease control rates, with promising first-line and beyond outcomes being reported from the CHECKMATE 142 trial [26,27]. Therefore, the NCCN has recommended the integration of these agents (monotherapy or combination) in the second-line (and beyond) treatment of MMR-deficient patients. In addition, the NCCN has recommended the consideration of immunotherapy in MMR-deficient frail metastatic colorectal cancer in first-line settings.

In addition to systemic therapies, one must acknowledge an important role for metastasectomies and ablative therapies in colorectal cancer. These should be important considerations for patients with oligometastatic disease—where surgical intervention can result in a curative outcome and/or improved survival [28,29]. Ablative therapies include microwave or radiofrequency ablation as well as stereotactic body radiation therapy. These are typically used in conjunction with or in lieu of surgery in an individualized fashion. Additional regional therapies in patients with liver-only or liver-predominant metastatic disease include radioembolization and hepatic arterial infusion. The discussion around surgery, ablative therapy, and regional therapy is beyond the scope of this manuscript. However, the above highlights the multi-disciplinary needs in the management of metastatic colorectal cancer.

3. Integration of Academic and Community Oncology

Achieving the best outcome in patient care has been the long-standing desire at City of Hope. While academicians design and conduct clinical trials, community physicians provide care to most patients and are critical to clinical trial enrollment and the application of standard of care therapy. The optimal partnership requires significant planning and efforts on both sides. A multimodality approach is becoming exceedingly important in the care of colorectal cancer and should be integrated seamlessly across academic and community practices. Here, we describe our efforts to enhance partnerships between our City of Hope Cancer Center and our associated Community Practice Satellites.

3.1. Integrating Community Practices in Tumor Board Discussions

Increasingly, the management of colorectal cancer requires the involvement of a multidisciplinary team including medical oncologists, radiation oncologists, pathologists, gastroenterologists, cancer geneticists, colorectal cancer surgeons, thoracic surgeons, and surgical oncologists. At City of Hope, we have conducted Gastrointestinal Oncology Tumor Boards on a twice-weekly basis (Mondays and Thursdays) with representative members from each of the disciplines above. **Tumor boards are disease specific and are run on a weekly basis, with email invitations generated to all interested community physicians. In general, community practices participate when they have an interesting case that requires input in a multidisciplinary setting.**

During these meetings, complex colorectal cases are discussed to determine the best treatment options. The recommendations made span from chemotherapy/immunotherapy/targeted-therapy refinement to decisions regarding metastasectomy, adjuvant therapy, radiation therapy, stereotactic body radiation therapy (SBRT), radioembolization, and hepatic artery infusion therapy. Community practice physicians present their cases remotely to these conferences, providing them with the opportunity to benefit from a multidisciplinary review of their cases and the receipt of a multispecialty input regarding a comprehensive approach towards colorectal cancer. **Such participation has altered treatment management in select cases (such as recommendations regarding adjuvant or neoadjuvant therapy or complex surgery), in allowing to link them to certain cases with appropriate clinical trials in our Duarte campus.**

3.2. Integrating Clinical Trials in Community Practices

Clinical trial access has become increasingly important for our colorectal cancer patients. However, the proximity of patients to a main center that provides these treatments has been and remains a main problem that has hindered patient enrollment. City of Hope is supporting a strong initiative to activate clinical trials in our various community centers as part of our mission to enhance research and improve patient access to novel therapeutics. We have partnered with our Community Practices to activate studies of interest to the community, with a strong focus on Phase II and III studies, early-phase investigator-initiated studies, and cooperative group trials. **The end result has been an increase in the accrual rate in community practices, where 70–100 patients have been enrolled in therapeutic clinical trials on a yearly basis.** This has particularly applied to colorectal cancer, where we have activated therapeutic trials that span first-line, second-line, and third-line studies (examples are listed in Table 1).

Table 1. Selection of colorectal cancer trials activated in City of Hope Community Practices.

NCT Number	Line of Treatment	Title
NCT04094688	First Line	Vitamin D3 With Chemotherapy and Bevacizumab in Treating Patients With Advanced or Metastatic Colorectal Cancer (SOLARIS)
NCT02753127	Second Line	A Study of Napabucasin (BBI-608) in Combination With FOLFIRI in Adult Patients With Previously Treated Metastatic Colorectal Cancer (CanStem303C)
NCT03317119	Third Line	Trametinib and Trifluridine and Tipiracil Hydrochloride in Treating Patients With Colon or Rectal Cancer That is Advanced, Metastatic, or Cannot Be Removed by Surgery

Potential studies are vetted by community physicians for the feasibility of the associated research procedures and the availability and potential interest of an eligible colorectal cancer population (Figure 1). Only once a study is identified to be fit for a specific community practice is it endorsed for activation in that site. To exemplify, CanStem303C (NCT02753127) was activated through our enterprise to address the value of the cancer stem cell inhibitor BBI-608 in the second-line treatment of metastatic CRC. Out of 25 patients enrolled in this study across four research sites, 13 were enrolled in our main Cancer Center campus, while 12 patients were enrolled through three additional community centers.

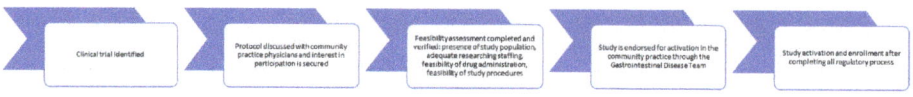

Figure 1. Process for clinical trial activation in a City of Hope Community Practice.

4. Referring Routine and Complex Cases

The management of colorectal cancer, whether metastatic or localized, is well-characterized and can be performed without significant barriers in community practices. The availability of a large network of providers across a large geographical area allows for easy access to the medical provider, less commuting time, and improved patient satisfaction. Most of the cases seen on our campus can therefore be managed in a more convenient location, which suits patients traveling a long distance from our Cancer Center. These options are discussed with our patients seen on our main Duarte campus, with an appropriate referral made to a more convenient City of Hope Community Practice for continuity of care (Figure 2).

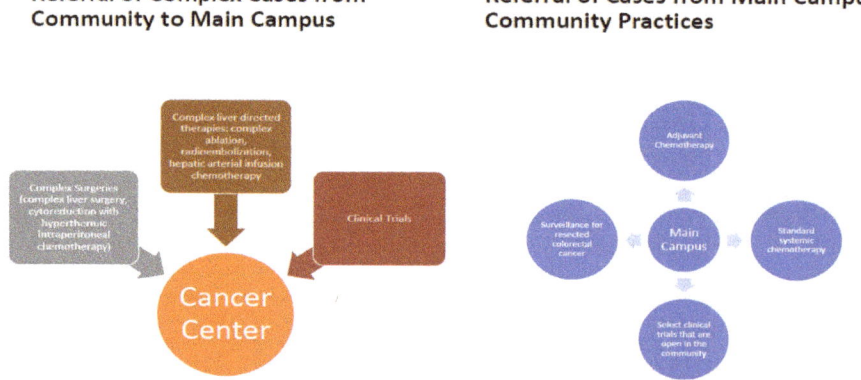

Figure 2. Cross-referral patterns between the City of Hope main cancer center and community practices.

On another note, certain colorectal cancer patients that are treated in our community practices may benefit from complex specialized services that are only feasible in our main campus. These patients are referred for treatment and continuity of care from our satellite practices to our Duarte campus. For example, the use of hepatic arterial infusion pumps for regional chemotherapy in an adjuvant setting after hepatic metastasis resection requires special surgical expertise as well as a specialized supporting team (interventional radiology, nurses trained for pump access and troubleshooting, and oncologists experienced in regional hepatic chemotherapy). We have taken the conscious decision to centralize the management of these patients at our main campus.

5. Standardization of Treatment Pathways in Colorectal Cancer

The creation and standardization of treatment pathways are key to the administration of quality care across our network. City of Hope is a National Network Cancer Center Network (NCCN) member. We contribute to various committees in the NCCN and support its published guidelines [30]. However, the guidelines are broad and are not easy to navigate across our sprawling network of community practices. Several years ago, we joined the Via Oncology network (currently ClinicalPath), which provides an easy-to-navigate clinical pathway for medical oncologists across all disease sites. These guidelines strive to reduce variability, focus on cost-effectiveness, and seek patient-friendly (less toxic and easier to administer) regimens. Since these pathways are meant for academic and community practices alike, we have included representative members from our Cancer Center and Community Practices on the Gastrointestinal Cancer Via Oncology Committee. The committee meets on a quarterly basis and discusses recently published or presented clinical data that can impact the recommended Via Oncology treatment guidelines. Every cancer patient treated in our institute is navigated through these pathways electronically, and the data are reviewed to assess treatment adherence and guideline compliance.

6. Educational Efforts

Educational programs (certified medical education) across a variety of cancers are hosted on a weekly basis on our Duarte Campus (Cancer Center). All faculty members across our satellite offices have the capability of attending in person or remotely. In addition, our medical oncology department hosts bi-annual symposia for medical oncology. During these meetings, each disease site, including colorectal cancer, is co-hosted by a Cancer Center Academician and a Community Practice physician. Community practice physicians leading such efforts have an existing interest and expertise in the assigned respective area and lead the discussions on the latest standards of care. Such programs increase the interaction between our research faculty and clinical faculty and enhance learning collaborations across our network.

7. Conclusions

The close interplay and collaboration between our Cancer Center and our Community Practices is essential to optimize clinical care for colorectal cancers across our community. These collaborations include educational activities, the standardization of treatment pathways, clinical trials, and the cross-referral of patients to address patient convenience and treatment complexity. The constant cross-talk between our Academic and Clinical Faculty across the network insures that the best standards in colorectal cancer are applied across our capture area.

Author Contributions: M.K., C.W., B.B., G.H., and M.F., contributed literature search and review, writing, graphical design, and editing; M.F. contributed conception and design and editing. All authors have read and agreed to the published version of the manuscript.

Funding: This research received no external funding.

Conflicts of Interest: Fakih reports received Honoraria from Amgen and research funding from Astra Zeneca, Amgen and Novartis. Fakih reports serving as advisory for Amgen, Array, Bayer and Pfizer and as speaker bureau for Amgen and Guardant 360. All other authors declared no conflict of interests.

References

1. Siegel, R.L.; Miller, K.D.; Jemal, A. Cancer statistics, 2019. *CA A Cancer J. Clin.* **2019**, *69*, 7–34. [CrossRef] [PubMed]
2. Siegel, R.L.; Miller, K.D.; Jemal, A. Cancer statistics, 2016. *CA A Cancer J. Clin.* **2016**, *66*, 7–30. [CrossRef] [PubMed]

3. Milano, A.F.; Singer, R.B. The Cancer Mortality Risk Project—Cancer Mortality Risks by Anatomic Site: Part 1—Introductory Overview; Part II—Carcinoma of the Colon: 20-Year Mortality Follow-up Derived from 1973-2013 (NCI) SEER*Stat Survival Database. *J. Insur. Med.* **2017**, *47*, 65–94. [CrossRef] [PubMed]
4. Siegel, R.L.; Miller, K.D.; Goding Sauer, A.; Fedewa, S.A.; Butterly, L.F.; Anderson, J.C.; Cercek, A.; Smith, R.A.; Jemal, A. Colorectal cancer statistics. *CA A Cancer J. Clin.* **2020**. [CrossRef]
5. Fakih, M.G. Metastatic Colorectal Cancer: Current State and Future Directions. *J. Clin. Oncol.* **2015**, *33*, 1809–1824. [CrossRef]
6. Sandhu, J.; Lavingia, V.; Fakih, M. Systemic treatment for metastatic colorectal cancer in the era of precision medicine. *J. Surg. Oncol.* **2019**, *119*, 564–582. [CrossRef]
7. Qin, S.; Li, J.; Wang, L.; Xu, J.; Cheng, Y.; Bai, Y.; Li, W.; Xu, N.; Lin, L.-Z.; Wu, Q.; et al. Efficacy and Tolerability of First-Line Cetuximab Plus Leucovorin, Fluorouracil, and Oxaliplatin (FOLFOX-4) Versus FOLFOX-4 in Patients With RAS Wild-Type Metastatic Colorectal Cancer: The Open-Label, Randomized, Phase III TAILOR Trial. *J. Clin. Oncol.* **2018**, *36*, 3031–3039. [CrossRef]
8. Cutsem, E.V.; Lenz, H.-J.; Köhne, C.-H.; Heinemann, V.; Tejpar, S.; Melezínek, I.; Beier, F.; Stroh, C.; Rougier, P.; Krieken, J.H.V.; et al. Fluorouracil, Leucovorin, and Irinotecan Plus Cetuximab Treatment and RAS Mutations in Colorectal Cancer. *J. Clin. Oncol.* **2015**, *33*, 692–700. [CrossRef]
9. Douillard, J.-Y.; Oliner, K.S.; Siena, S.; Tabernero, J.; Burkes, R.; Barugel, M.; Humblet, Y.; Bodoky, G.; Cunningham, D.; Jassem, J.; et al. Panitumumab-FOLFOX4 Treatment and RAS Mutations in Colorectal Cancer. *N. Engl. J. Med.* **2013**, *369*, 1023–1034. [CrossRef]
10. Heinemann, V.; von Weikersthal, L.F.; Decker, T.; Kiani, A.; Vehling-Kaiser, U.; Al-Batran, S.E.; Heintges, T.; Lerchenmuller, C.; Kahl, C.; Seipelt, G.; et al. FOLFIRI plus cetuximab versus FOLFIRI plus bevacizumab as first-line treatment for patients with metastatic colorectal cancer (FIRE-3): A randomised, open-label, phase 3 trial. *Lancet Oncol.* **2014**, *15*, 1065–1075. [CrossRef]
11. Venook, A.P.; Niedzwiecki, D.; Lenz, H.-J.; Innocenti, F.; Fruth, B.; Meyerhardt, J.A.; Schrag, D.; Greene, C.; O'Neil, B.H.; Atkins, J.N.; et al. Effect of First-Line Chemotherapy Combined With Cetuximab or Bevacizumab on Overall Survival in Patients With KRAS Wild-Type Advanced or Metastatic Colorectal Cancer: A Randomized Clinical Trial. *JAMA* **2017**, *317*, 2392–2401. [CrossRef] [PubMed]
12. Samowitz, W.S.; Sweeney, C.; Herrick, J.; Albertsen, H.; Levin, T.R.; Murtaugh, M.A.; Wolff, R.K.; Slattery, M.L. Poor Survival Associated with the *BRAF* V600E Mutation in Microsatellite-Stable Colon Cancers. *Cancer Res.* **2005**, *65*, 6063–6069. [CrossRef] [PubMed]
13. Pai, R.K.; Jayachandran, P.; Koong, A.C.; Chang, D.T.; Kwok, S.; Ma, L.; Arber, D.A.; Balise, R.R.; Tubbs, R.R.; Shadrach, B.; et al. BRAF-mutated, Microsatellite-stable Adenocarcinoma of the Proximal Colon: An Aggressive Adenocarcinoma With Poor Survival, Mucinous Differentiation, and Adverse Morphologic Features. *Am. J. Surg. Pathol.* **2012**, *36*, 744–752. [CrossRef] [PubMed]
14. Gong, J.; Cho, M.; Fakih, M. RAS and BRAF in metastatic colorectal cancer management. *J. Gastrointest. Oncol.* **2016**, *7*, 687–704. [CrossRef] [PubMed]
15. Cremolini, C.; Loupakis, F.; Antoniotti, C.; Lupi, C.; Sensi, E.; Lonardi, S.; Mezi, S.; Tomasello, G.; Ronzoni, M.; Zaniboni, A.; et al. FOLFOXIRI plus bevacizumab versus FOLFIRI plus bevacizumab as first-line treatment of patients with metastatic colorectal cancer: Updated overall survival and molecular subgroup analyses of the open-label, phase 3 TRIBE study. *Lancet Oncol.* **2015**, *16*, 1306–1315. [CrossRef]
16. Kopetz, S.; Grothey, A.; Yaeger, R.; Van Cutsem, E.; Desai, J.; Yoshino, T.; Wasan, H.; Ciardiello, F.; Loupakis, F.; Hong, Y.S.; et al. Encorafenib, Binimetinib, and Cetuximab in BRAF V600E-Mutated Colorectal Cancer. *N. Engl. J. Med.* **2019**, *381*, 1632–1643. [CrossRef]
17. Cutsem, E.V.; Cuyle, P.-J.; Huijberts, S.; Yaeger, R.; Schellens, J.H.M.; Elez, E.; Tabernero, J.; Fakih, M.; Montagut, C.; Peeters, M.; et al. BEACON CRC study safety lead-in (SLI) in patients with BRAFV600E metastatic colorectal cancer (mCRC): Efficacy and tumor markers. *J. Clin. Oncol.* **2018**, *36*, 627. [CrossRef]
18. Richman, S.D.; Southward, K.; Chambers, P.; Cross, D.; Barrett, J.; Hemmings, G.; Taylor, M.; Wood, H.; Hutchins, G.; Foster, J.M.; et al. HER2 overexpression and amplification as a potential therapeutic target in colorectal cancer: Analysis of 3256 patients enrolled in the QUASAR, FOCUS and PICCOLO colorectal cancer trials. *J. Pathol.* **2016**, *238*, 562–570. [CrossRef]
19. Sartore-Bianchi, A.; Trusolino, L.; Martino, C. Dual-targeted therapy with trastuzumab and lapatinib in treatment-refractory, KRAS codon 12/13 wild-type, HER2-positive metastatic colorectal cancer (HERACLES): A proof-of-concept, multicentre, open-label, phase 2 trial. *Lancet Oncol.* **2016**, *17*, 738–746. [CrossRef]

20. Meric-Bemstam, F.; Hurwitz, H.; Raghav, K.P.S.; McWilliams, R.R.; Fakih, M.; VanderWalde, A.; Swanton, C.; Kurzrock, R.; Burris, H.; Sweeney, C.; et al. Pertuzumab plus trastuzumab for HER2-amplified metastatic colorectal cancer (MyPathway): An updated report from a multicentre, open-label, phase 2a, multiple basket study. *Lancet Oncol.* **2019**, *20*, 518–530. [CrossRef]
21. Raghav, K.P.S.; McDonough, S.L.; Tan, B.R.; Denlinger, C.S.; Magliocco, A.M.; Choong, N.W.; Sommer, N.; Scappaticci, F.A.; Campos, D.; Guthrie, K.A.; et al. A randomized phase II study of trastuzumab and pertuzumab (TP) compared to cetuximab and irinotecan (CETIRI) in advanced/metastatic colorectal cancer (mCRC) with HER2 amplification: S1613. *J. Clin. Oncol.* **2018**, *36*, TPS3620. [CrossRef]
22. Le, D.T.; Uram, J.N.; Wang, H.; Bartlett, B.R.; Kemberling, H.; Eyring, A.D.; Skora, A.D.; Luber, B.S.; Azad, N.S.; Laheru, D.; et al. PD-1 Blockade in Tumors with Mismatch-Repair Deficiency. *N. Engl. J. Med.* **2015**, *372*, 2509–2520. [CrossRef] [PubMed]
23. Le, D.T.; Durham, J.N.; Smith, K.N.; Wang, H.; Bartlett, B.R.; Aulakh, L.K.; Lu, S.; Kemberling, H.; Wilt, C.; Luber, B.S.; et al. Mismatch repair deficiency predicts response of solid tumors to PD-1 blockade. *Science* **2017**, *357*, 409–413. [CrossRef] [PubMed]
24. Overman, M.J.; McDermott, R.; Leach, J.L. Nivolumab in patients with metastatic DNA mismatch repair-deficient or microsatellite instability-high colorectal cancer (CheckMate 142): An open-label, multicentre, phase 2 study. *Lancet Oncol.* **2017**, *18*, 1182–1191. [CrossRef]
25. Marabelle, A.; Le, D.T.; Ascierto, P.A.; Giacomo, A.M.D.; Jesus-Acosta, A.D.; Delord, J.-P.; Geva, R.; Gottfried, M.; Penel, N.; Hansen, A.R.; et al. Efficacy of Pembrolizumab in Patients With Noncolorectal High Microsatellite Instability/Mismatch Repair–Deficient Cancer: Results From the Phase II KEYNOTE-158 Study. *J. Clin. Oncol.* **2020**, *38*, 1–10. [CrossRef] [PubMed]
26. Overman, M.J.; Lonardi, S.; Wong, K.Y.M.; Lenz, H.-J.; Gelsomino, F.; Aglietta, M.; Morse, M.A.; Cutsem, E.V.; McDermott, R.; Hill, A.; et al. Durable Clinical Benefit With Nivolumab Plus Ipilimumab in DNA Mismatch Repair-Deficient/Microsatellite Instability-High Metastatic Colorectal Cancer. *J. Clin. Oncol.* **2018**, *36*, 773–779. [CrossRef] [PubMed]
27. Andre, T.; Lonardi, S.; Wong, M.; Lenz, H.J.; Gelsomino, F.; Aglietta, M.; Morse, M.; Van Cutsem, E.; McDermott, R.S.; Hill, A.G.; et al. Nivolumab plus ipilimumab combination in patients with DNA mismatch repair-deficient/microsatellite instability-high (dMMR/MSI-H) metastatic colorectal cancer (mCRC): First report of the full cohort from CheckMate-142. *J. Clin. Oncol.* **2018**, *36*, 553. [CrossRef]
28. Minagawa, M.; Makuuchi, M.; Torzilli, G.; Takayama, T.; Kawasaki, S.; Kosuge, T.; Yamamoto, J.; Imamura, H. Extension of the frontiers of surgical indications in the treatment of liver metastases from colorectal cancer: Long-term results. *Ann. Surg.* **2000**, *231*, 487–499. [CrossRef]
29. Elias, D.; Liberale, G.; Vernerey, D.; Pignon, J.P.; Lasser, P.; Pocard, M.; Ducreux, M.; Voige, V.; Malka, D. Hepatic and extrahepatic colorectal metastases: When resectable, their localization does not matter, but their total number has a prognostic impact. *Ann. Surg. Oncol.* **2005**, *12*, 900–909. [CrossRef]
30. National Comprehensive Cancer Network. Available online: https://www.nccn.org/professionals/physician_gls/default.aspx#site (accessed on 16 May 2020).

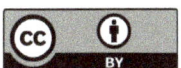 © 2020 by the authors. Licensee MDPI, Basel, Switzerland. This article is an open access article distributed under the terms and conditions of the Creative Commons Attribution (CC BY) license (http://creativecommons.org/licenses/by/4.0/).

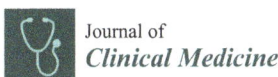

Review

Managing Bladder Cancer Care during the COVID-19 Pandemic Using a Team-Based Approach

Tina Wang, Sariah Liu, Thomas Joseph and Yung Lyou *

Department of Medical Oncology & Experimental Therapeutics, City of Hope Comprehensive Cancer Center, Duarte, CA 91010, USA; tinawang@coh.org (T.W.); sarliu@coh.org (S.L.); thojoseph@coh.org (T.J.)
* Correspondence: ylyou@coh.org; Tel.: +1-626-218-9200; Fax: +1-626-218-8233

Received: 14 April 2020; Accepted: 19 May 2020; Published: 22 May 2020

Abstract: The recent novel coronavirus, named coronavirus disease 2019 (COVID-19), has developed into an international pandemic affecting millions of individuals with hundreds of thousands of deaths worldwide. The highly infectious nature and widespread prevalence of this disease create a new set of obstacles for the bladder cancer community in both delivering and receiving care. In this manuscript, we address the unique issues regarding treatment prioritization for the patient with bladder cancer and how we at City of Hope have adjusted our clinical practices using a team-based approach that utilizes shared decision making with all stakeholders (physicians, patients, caregivers) to optimize outcomes during this difficult time. In addition to taking standard precautions for minimizing COVID-19 risk of exposure for those entering a healthcare facility (screening all personnel upon entry and donning facemasks at all times), we suggest the following three measures: (1) delay post-treatment surveillance visits until there is a decrease in local COVID-19 cases, (2) continue curative intent treatments for localized bladder cancer with COVID-19 precautions (i.e., choosing gemcitabine/cisplatin (GC) over dose-dense methotrexate, vinblastine, doxorubicin, cisplatin (ddMVAC) neoadjuvant chemotherapy), and (3) increase the off-treatment period between cycles of palliative systemic therapy in metastatic urothelial carcinoma patients.

Keywords: bladder cancer; urothelial carcinoma; COVID-19; team-based medicine

1. Introduction

Recently, a novel coronavirus, named severe acute respiratory syndrome coronavirus 2 (SARS-CoV-2), has developed into an international pandemic affecting millions of individuals in more than 150 countries with hundreds of thousands of deaths worldwide [1,2]. This disease has been named coronavirus disease 2019 (COVID-19) by the World Health Organization (WHO) [1]. Patients with this disease are at high risk for developing septic shock and hypoxemia, which can frequently progress to acute respiratory distress syndrome (ARDS) and death [3]. This disease creates a new set of obstacles for the bladder cancer community in both delivering and receiving care. In this manuscript, we address the unique issues regarding treatment prioritization for the patient with bladder cancer and how we at City of Hope have adjusted our clinical practices using a team-based, shared decision approach with all stakeholders (patients, caregivers, and physicians) to optimize outcomes during this difficult time.

2. Balancing the Need for Bladder Cancer Treatments and Risk of Exposure to COVID-19

2.1. Patients with Bladder Cancer Undergoing Treatments Are at a Higher Risk for COVID-19 Infections and Worse Outcomes Compared to the General Population without Cancer

For the patient with bladder cancer undergoing treatment, there are several safety issues that place them at higher risk of infection for COVID-19 compared to the general population without cancer. First, patients must physically leave the safety of their residences to go to the clinic, infusion center, or imaging facility where they could potentially be exposed to COVID-19. Second, the platinum-based chemotherapy regimens commonly used in bladder cancer treatments are immunosuppressive and place them at a higher risk for infection. Third, many bladder cancer patients tend to be of older age and also have multiple medical comorbidities, which has been shown to place them in a group with worse outcomes for COVID-19 [2,4]. A retrospective study that examined the outcomes of approximately 72,000 patients with COVID-19 found that those with older age and presence of medical comorbidities were associated with adverse outcomes [2,4]. In another retrospective study by Liang and colleagues, it was suggested that patients with a history of cancer itself may be associated with worse outcomes from COVID-19 [5,6]. However, it should be noted that this particular retrospective study was limited in that only 18 of the 1590 patients who were studied had a history of cancer, making it difficult to form a general conclusion from such a small sample size [5,6]. Regardless, based on the other reasons discussed above, it is clear that patients with bladder cancer undergoing active therapy or post-treatment surveillance are at a higher risk for COVID-19 exposure and could potentially suffer worse outcomes compared to the general population.

2.2. Prioritizing Treatments Appropriately and Applying Social Distancing

Ensuring patient safety is the key principle when it comes to delivering medical care among all healthcare professions. In the setting of the COVID-19 pandemic, the central question we have asked ourselves as providers while managing each patient's care has been: Will delaying the patient's bladder cancer treatment in accordance with current COVID-19 social distancing measures lead to a worse long-term outcome? Current models suggest that this pandemic may proceed until herd immunity or a vaccine is developed, with repeated waves of infections, which some experts estimate could continue for another 18 months. Since it is not feasible to delay bladder cancer treatments for another 18 months, we at City of Hope have developed a consensus framework to help balance these competing risks (Figure 1). By utilizing this framework, we have been able to guide our clinicians within the network on how to make a shared decision with the patient that can prioritize bladder cancer treatments appropriately while minimizing the risk for COVID-19 exposure (Figure 1).

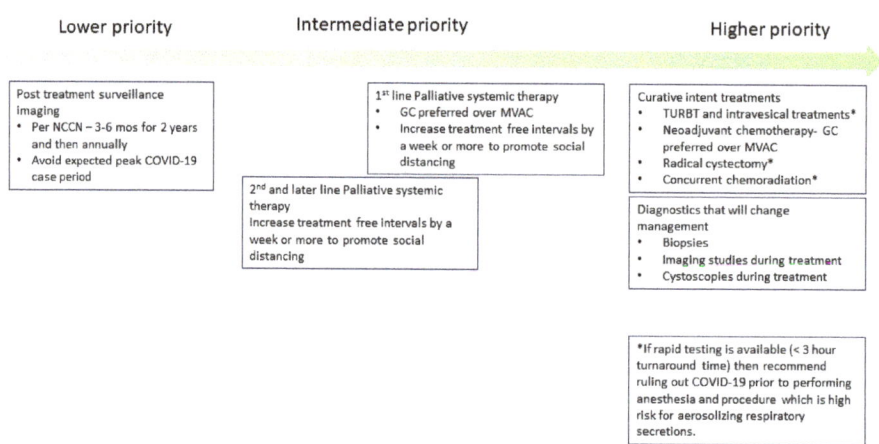

Figure 1. Conceptual framework for prioritizing bladder cancer treatments during the COVID-19 pandemic. This framework provides guidance on key treatments that should still be offered in order to ensure optimal bladder cancer outcomes if possible. We recommend that these listed priorities can be modified based on available local resources and the patient's overall medical status.

2.3. Applying COVID-19 Risk Mitigation Measures for Bladder Cancer Treatment

In the state of California, there is a "shelter in place" order that was initiated on 19 March 2020 along with other social distancing measures due to the concern that individuals may be at high risk of becoming infected and could also infect others, further propagating this pandemic. Current epidemiology modeling suggests that the peak incidence of COVID-19 will have occurred sometime in mid-to-late April in the state of California. This framework assumes that the number of new cases will start to decrease in the months of May and June 2020. In the case that there is indeed a second wave of infections later during the fall and winter months of 2020, one could reapply this framework based on the expected peaks. As a result, we suggest the following framework to assist the practicing oncologist in determining optimal treatment strategies for the patient with bladder cancer.

2.3.1. Delay Post-Treatment Surveillance Visits until There Is a Decrease in COVID-19 Cases

For patients undergoing surveillance imaging after completion of cystectomy or other definitive therapies, the National Comprehensive Cancer Network (NCCN) guidelines currently recommend imaging every 6–12 months [7]. Keeping these guidelines in mind, we have rescheduled the patient's clinic and imaging visit to avoid the expected COVID-19 peak period (April–May) so that it will take place during the next 2–3 months in June or July as a way to minimize risk of exposure.

2.3.2. Continue Curative Intent Treatments for Localized Bladder Cancer with COVID-19 Precautions

Even in these difficult times, urothelial bladder cancer is an aggressive disease with poor prognosis when it progresses to metastatic disease. Therefore, we have been vigilant in continuing to deliver curative intent treatments when patients have localized urothelial carcinoma, if possible in a timely manner. A meta-analysis of 13 studies suggested that a delay of more than 12 weeks from time of diagnosis to execution of radical cystectomy, only in muscle invasive urothelial cancer, was associated with worse outcomes [8]. Another study showed that initiating neoadjuvant chemotherapy (NAC) with a delay of more than 8 weeks from time of diagnosis led to worse outcomes [9]. Therefore, we have continued to offer cisplatin-eligible patients NAC within 8 weeks and cisplatin-ineligible patients radical cystectomy within 12 weeks from time of diagnosis, while the infusion center and operating room resources are available for those patients with localized disease since there is a limited window of curative treatment opportunity.

The first set of measures we have instituted to minimize potential risk for COVID-19 exposure for all on-site people (visitors and healthcare workers) is to create a single, separate point of entry to the active clinical areas and institute a strict policy limiting visitors to patients only. Prior to entering the clinical area, all personnel (including patients and healthcare workers) are screened for COVID-19 symptoms (i.e., cough, dyspnea, and fever) and have their temperatures measured. People determined to be asymptomatic and afebrile are then required to don a face mask and are issued an entrance band indicating they have passed screening measures for that day. If someone is found to be symptomatic, we then refer this individual to an on-site "fever clinic" staffed by designated clinical personnel who have been trained and equipped with the appropriate personal protective equipment (PPE) to perform a nasopharyngeal swab for in-house COVID-19 testing. We have also repurposed one of our hospital wards with negative pressure rooms to serve as the COVID-19 unit with its own set of designated staff to decrease exposure within the facility. In both the inpatient and outpatient areas, all people (patients and healthcare workers) are required to don a face mask at all times, which has been suggested as a way to prevent sustained exposure to COVID-19 and reduce risk for infection [10].

The second set of COVID-19 risk mitigation measures specifically pertain to treatments used for urothelial bladder cancer. Current NCCN guidelines recommend neoadjuvant chemotherapy in muscle invasive bladder cancer [7]. In the choice of regimen, the two most commonly used regimens are dose-dense methotrexate, vinblastine, doxorubicin, cisplatin (ddMVAC) and gemcitabine/cisplatin (GC) [7,11,12]. During this time, we have advocated for using gemcitabine/cisplatin over ddMVAC for the following reasons. Although there is some discussion suggesting that ddMVAC may have a trend towards higher efficacy, it has yet to be definitively supported in a head-to-head prospective trial and retrospective studies have shown similar amounts of efficacy between these two regimens [11,12]. In addition, ddMVAC tends to be more myelosuppressive than GC, placing patients at higher risk for infections due to the neutropenia and symptomatic anemia requiring blood transfusions, which during this time have been especially challenging due to a steep drop in blood donations [11,12]. Finally, ddMVAC is given as a 14-day cycle whereas GC is given as a 21-day cycle. The 14-day cycle of ddMVAC allows a patient to proceed sooner to radical cystectomy compared to GC, but during this time we would recommend GC because it allows the oncologist to space out the patient visits and can help adhere better to the principle of social distancing [11,12]. Another measure we have taken is to implement weekly telephone checks with patients undergoing active systemic therapy. This allows us to determine if a patient is having any significant chemotherapy-related adverse effects or other acute medical issues, for which they could potentially be treated as an outpatient before they progress to needing emergency room or acute inpatient care. For example, if a patient is experiencing significant dysuria due to a potential urinary tract infection, one can prescribe antibiotics empirically at their local pharmacy and help them avoid the need to seek emergency room care, which is most likely to be overcrowded during this pandemic. For those patients that are undergoing concurrent radiation and chemotherapy with curative intent, we have continued their treatments while taking the abovementioned general COVID-19 precautions (i.e., screening at entry, donning facemasks, and weekly telephone checks).

2.3.3. Increasing Off-Treatment Period between Cycles for Palliative Systemic Therapy in Metastatic Urothelial Carcinoma Patients

For those patients already undergoing palliative first-line systemic therapy, we have continued their treatments as those regimens provide overall survival benefit. In this situation, if chemotherapy needs to be started we would recommend, as discussed above, to prescribe anti-emetics and pain medications for the patient to have immediately available at home as an outpatient. Additionally, weekly telephone checks would be conducted to prevent any chemotherapy-related complications early. Another important factor to consider, as discussed above, is lengthening the period of time between treatments. Normally, gemcitabine/cisplatin or gemcitabine/carboplatin is administered as a two weeks on, 1 week off schedule. In this case, it is reasonable to do 2 weeks on, 2 weeks off to help spread out the treatment duration as much as possible to maximize social distancing. Second-line treatment usually involves the use of immune checkpoint inhibitors such as pembrolizumab or atezolizumab. Pembrolizumab is dosed every 3 weeks, but in order to maximize social distancing for the patient, it is reasonable to stretch it to every 4 weeks during this period since it is unlikely the cancer will grow significantly during the extra week off. In this setting, atezolizumab and nivolumab already has an Federal Drug Administration (FDA)-approved every-4-week dosing, which would also make it a viable alternative. The use of third-line treatment with enfortumab vedotin requires administration once every week for 3 weeks straight and then taking the fourth week off. Again, to provide more space between visits, it would be reasonable to increase the off-treatment period from 1 week to 2 weeks to provide the patient more social distancing.

Even during these difficult times, it is crucial to continue clinical trials to the best of our ability and help advance the field of oncology. In order to preserve needed resources for COVID-19 prevention and treatment within our institution, we have focused our efforts on continuing current open clinical trials and slowing down the pace of opening new trials.

3. Conclusions

COVID-19 has developed into an international pandemic affecting millions of individuals and has created a new set of obstacles for the bladder cancer community in both delivering and receiving care. Because patients with bladder cancer require treatment even in these difficult times, we have developed a framework that utilizes a team-based approach with shared decision making among all stakeholders involved (physicians, patients, caregivers) to optimize outcomes during this difficult time. It is our hope that the conceptual framework presented above and institutional experience can be adjusted to fit the available local resources for others that are looking to balance these two competing needs when treating patients with bladder cancer during the COVID-19 pandemic.

Author Contributions: Y.L. conceived the article; T.W., S.L., and T.J. wrote the manuscript with input from Y.L. All authors have read and agreed to the published version of the manuscript.

Funding: This work was supported by the National Cancer Institute of the National Institutes of Health under grant number P30CA033572 to City of Hope Comprehensive Cancer Center.

Conflicts of Interest: The authors declare no conflicts of interest.

Abbreviations

COVID-19	coronavirus disease 2019
FDA	Federal Drug administration
GC	gemcitabine/cisplatin
ddMVAC	dose-dense methotrexate, vinblastine, doxorubicin, cisplatin
NCCN	National Comprehensive Cancer Network

References

1. Novel Coronavirus (2019-nCoV) Situation Reports. Available online: https://www.who.int/emergencies/diseases/novel-coronavirus-2019/situation-reports (accessed on 4 April 2020).
2. Wu, Z.; McGoogan, J.M. Characteristics of and Important Lessons from the Coronavirus Disease 2019 (COVID-19) Outbreak in China: Summary of a Report of 72 314 Cases from the Chinese Center for Disease Control and Prevention. *JAMA* **2020**, *323*, 1239–1242. [CrossRef] [PubMed]
3. Alhazzani, W.; Møller, M.H.; Arabi, Y.M.; Loeb, M.; Gong, M.N.; Fan, E.; Oczkowski, S.; Levy, M.M.; Derde, L.; Dzierba, A.; et al. Surviving Sepsis Campaign: Guidelines on the management of critically ill adults with Coronavirus Disease 2019 (COVID-19). *Intensive Care Med.* **2020**, *46*, 854–887. [CrossRef] [PubMed]
4. Zhou, F.; Yu, T.; Du, R.; Fan, G.; Liu, Y.; Liu, Z.; Xiang, J.; Wang, Y.; Song, B.; Gu, X.; et al. Clinical course and risk factors for mortality of adult inpatients with COVID-19 in Wuhan, China: A retrospective cohort study. *Lancet* **2020**, *395*, 1054–1062. [CrossRef]
5. Wang, H.; Zhang, L. Risk of COVID-19 for patients with cancer. *Lancet Oncol.* **2020**, *21*, e181. [CrossRef]
6. Xia, Y.; Jin, R.; Zhao, J.; Li, W.; Shen, H. Risk of COVID-19 for patients with cancer. *Lancet Oncol.* **2020**, *21*, e180. [CrossRef]
7. Flaig, T.W.; Spiess, P.E.; Agarwal, N.; Bangs, R.; Boorjian, S.A.; Buyyounouski, M.K.; Chang, S.; Downs, T.M.; Efstathiou, J.A.; Friedlander, T.; et al. Bladder Cancer, Version 3.2020, NCCN Clinical Practice Guidelines in Oncology. *J. Natl. Compr. Cancer Netw.* **2020**, *18*, 329–354. [CrossRef] [PubMed]
8. Fahmy, N.M.; Mahmud, S.; Aprikian, A.G. Delay in the surgical treatment of bladder cancer and survival: Systematic review of the literature. *Eur. Urol.* **2006**, *50*, 1176–1182. [CrossRef] [PubMed]
9. Audenet, F.; Sfakianos, J.P.; Waingankar, N.; Ruel, N.H.; Galsky, M.D.; Yuh, B.E.; Gin, G.E. A delay ≥8 weeks to neoadjuvant chemotherapy before radical cystectomy increases the risk of upstaging. *Urol. Oncol.* **2019**, *37*, 116–122. [CrossRef] [PubMed]
10. Gawande, A. Keeping the Coronavirus from Infecting Health-Care Workers. Available online: https://www.newyorker.com/news/news-desk/keeping-the-coronavirus-from-infecting-health-care-workers (accessed on 12 April 2020).

11. Dash, A.; Pettus, J.A.; Herr, H.W.; Bochner, B.H.; Dalbagni, G.; Donat, S.M.; Russo, P.; Boyle, M.G.; Milowsky, M.I.; Bajorin, D.F. A Role for Neoadjuvant Gemcitabine Plus Cisplatin in Muscle-Invasive Urothelial Carcinoma of the Bladder: A Retrospective Experience. *Cancer* **2008**, *113*, 2471–2477. [CrossRef] [PubMed]
12. Choueiri, T.K.; Jacobus, S.; Bellmunt, J.; Qu, A.; Appleman, L.J.; Tretter, C.; Bubley, G.J.; Stack, E.C.; Signoretti, S.; Walsh, M.; et al. Neoadjuvant dose-dense methotrexate, vinblastine, doxorubicin, and cisplatin with pegfilgrastim support in muscle-invasive urothelial cancer: Pathologic, radiologic, and biomarker correlates. *J. Clin. Oncol.* **2014**, *32*, 1889–1894. [CrossRef] [PubMed]

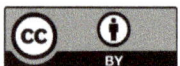

© 2020 by the authors. Licensee MDPI, Basel, Switzerland. This article is an open access article distributed under the terms and conditions of the Creative Commons Attribution (CC BY) license (http://creativecommons.org/licenses/by/4.0/).

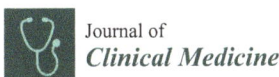

Review

Strategies to Improve Participation of Older Adults in Cancer Research

Jennifer Liu [1,†], Eutiquio Gutierrez [2,†], Abhay Tiwari [1], Simran Padam [1], Daneng Li [1], William Dale [3], Sumanta K. Pal [1], Daphne Stewart [1], Shanmugga Subbiah [1], Linda D. Bosserman [1], Cary Presant [1], Tanyanika Phillips [1], Kelly Yap [1], Addie Hill [1], Geetika Bhatt [1], Christina Yeon [1], Mary Cianfrocca [1], Yuan Yuan [1], Joanne Mortimer [1] and Mina S. Sedrak [1,*]

1. Department of Medical Oncology and Therapeutics Research, City of Hope, Duarte, CA 91010, USA; jennliu@coh.org (J.L.); atiwari@coh.org (A.T.); spadam@coh.org (S.P.); danli@coh.org (D.L.); SPal@coh.org (S.K.P.); dapstewart@coh.org (D.S.); ssubbiah@coh.org (S.S.); lbosserman@coh.org (L.D.B.); cpresant@coh.org (C.P.); taphillips@coh.org (T.P.); keyap@coh.org (K.Y.); ahill@coh.org (A.H.); gbhatt@coh.org (G.B.); cyeon@coh.org (C.Y.); mcianfrocca@coh.org (M.C.); yuyuan@coh.org (Y.Y.); jmortimer@coh.org (J.M.)
2. Department of Internal Medicine, Harbor-UCLA Medical Center, Los Angeles, CA 90502, USA; EGutierrez3@dhs.lacounty.gov
3. Department of Supportive Care Medicine, City of Hope, Duarte, CA 91010, USA; wdale@coh.org
* Correspondence: msedrak@coh.org
† Authors contributed equally.

Received: 17 April 2020; Accepted: 19 May 2020; Published: 22 May 2020

Abstract: Cancer is a disease associated with aging. As the US population ages, the number of older adults with cancer is projected to dramatically increase. Despite this, older adults remain vastly underrepresented in research that sets the standards for cancer treatments and, consequently, clinicians struggle with how to interpret data from clinical trials and apply them to older adults in practice. A combination of system, clinician, and patient barriers bar opportunities for trial participation for many older patients, and strategies are needed to address these barriers at multiple fronts, five of which are offered here. This review highlights the need to (1) broaden eligibility criteria, (2) measure relevant end points, (3) expand standard trial designs, (4) increase resources (e.g., institutional support, interdisciplinary care, and telehealth), and (5) develop targeted interventions (e.g., behavioral interventions to promote patient enrollment). Implementing these solutions requires a substantial investment in engaging and collaborating with community-based practices, where the majority of older patients with cancer receive their care. Multifaceted strategies are needed to ensure that older patients with cancer, across diverse healthcare settings, receive the highest-quality, evidence-based care.

Keywords: geriatric oncology; older adults; cancer clinical trials; recruitment; community; team science

1. Introduction

Aging is a major risk factor for cancer, with 28% of cancers in the US diagnosed in adults aged 65–74, 18% in adults aged 75–84, and 8% in adults aged 85 and older [1]. Globally, the US has the third largest number of older adults [2], and as the US population ages, the number of older adults with cancer is increasing and will make up a growing share of the oncology population [3–5]. Despite this, older adults remain vastly underrepresented in the research that sets the standards for cancer treatments [6,7]. Consequently, most of what is known about cancer therapeutics is based on clinical trials conducted in younger and healthier patients [8–10]. Furthermore, despite a plethora of literature documenting barriers to the accrual of older adults to cancer clinical trials (Figure 1), there are few evidence-based strategies to mitigate these barriers [11,12]. A recent systematic review revealed that among 8691 studies screened, only 12 relevant observational studies examined barriers hindering the participation of older adults in cancer clinical trials, and one (negative) randomized controlled trial evaluated an intervention to increase the enrollment of older adults in trials [8]. Moreover, few studies have focused on understanding the complex and multifactorial influences affecting the clinical trial participation of older patients with cancer in the community, where the majority of this population is often treated [13,14].

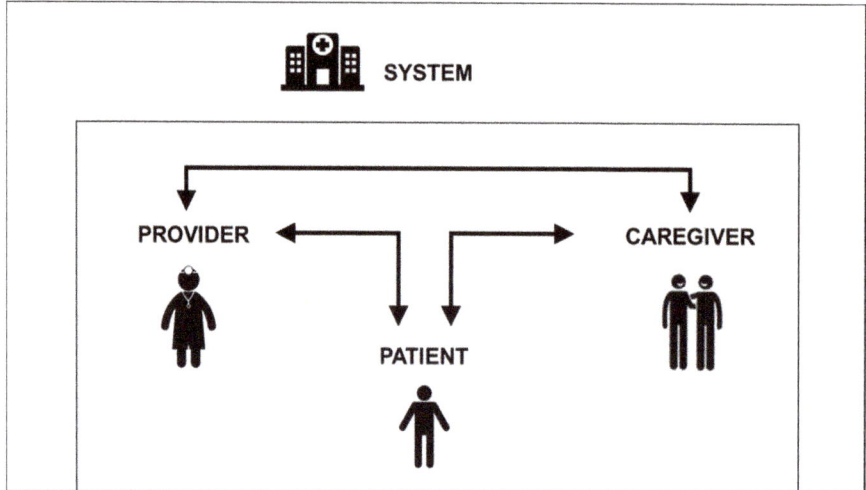

Figure 1. The barriers to older adult participation in cancer clinical trials are multifaceted and interrelated, with barriers existing at the system, clinician, patient, and caregiver levels. System-related barriers include trial design, overly stringent eligibility criteria, and lack of infrastructure support, appropriate and representative trials, and funding. Clinician-related barriers include concerns for side effects or toxicities, patient age, comorbid conditions, personal bias, costs to clinicians, and lack of time, support and staff, awareness of trials, and engagement amongst clinicians. Patient-related barriers include attitudes towards clinical trials, knowledge, side effects/toxicities, burden, and financial limitations. Caregiver-related barriers include caregiver burden and preference against participation.

Recognizing this problem, numerous organizations, including the Institute of Medicine (IOM), have cited the growing population of older adults with cancer and highlighted the need to generate high-quality, evidence-based data for the treatment of older adults [6,15–18]. The primary aim of this review is to lay out a multipronged approach that addresses barriers to the participation of older adults in cancer clinical trials. A secondary aim is to highlight how a collaborative clinical research network of academic and community-based oncology practices can facilitate the inclusion of older adults in cancer research.

2. Make Eligibility Criteria More Inclusive and Less Restrictive

Restrictive eligibility criteria often exclude a large proportion of patients from participating in clinical trials—a loss which sacrifices the generalizability of results to the overall patient population. Older adults, in particular, are often not offered the opportunity to participate in trials due to concerns for multiple comorbidities, organ dysfunction, treatment toxicity, and/or frailty [8,19–22]. Numerous trials explicitly restrict inclusion to patients with an Eastern Cooperative Oncology Group (ECOG) performance status of 0 to 1 or a Karnofsky performance score (KPS) of ≥70 [23,24]. As a result, trial data and findings are often derived from younger patients who are more fit and without organ dysfunction and comorbidities, as commonly seen in older adults [23].

A variety of efforts are underway to broaden the eligibility criteria to make trials more relevant to patients of all ages, including initiatives by the National Institutes of Health ("Inclusion Across the Lifespan policy"), American Society of Clinical Oncology (ASCO), and the Food and Drug Administration (FDA) [16,25,26]. Sponsors and investigators are encouraged to work together to follow these policy recommendations aimed at making the eligibility criteria less restrictive and more inclusive of demographically and clinically diverse patients, representative of the populations seen in community-based oncology settings. Investigators should review the eligibility criteria closely and forgo exclusion on the basis of lab values (e.g., creatinine), performance status, comorbid conditions, or second malignancy when designing clinical trials. Instead, a patient's functional or biological age should be taken into consideration, which may be a better indicator of how a patient will tolerate a certain treatment regimen.

Additionally, investigators should work closely with community clinicians and other stakeholders (i.e., patient advocates) to understand the patient populations seen in community-based practices and design eligibility criteria that are more inclusive, thus allowing trial results to be applicable to a broader patient population. Inclusive clinical trial systems within a collaborative research network ought to consider patients as they are, rather than as they should be. Trial eligibility should be evaluated and revised to ensure that investigators are broadening study access to new, successful cancer treatment regimens for older adults with cancer across diverse healthcare delivery settings.

3. Capture Relevant End Points that Matter to Older Patients

Sponsors and investigators should capture relevant end points that are important to the older patient, including measures of tolerability as well as clinical and biological aging consequences of cancer and its treatment [17,27–29].

Studies have shown that most older adults do not want to compromise their quality of life or function for survival benefits [30]. Hence, trials designed to collect information on this population must include patient-reported measures that are relevant to the patient's experience and move beyond clinician-reported toxicity. Therefore, data are needed to understand the immediate (short-term) and longitudinal (long-term) impact of cancer and cancer therapy on patient health and quality of life [29,31]. Given that each individual is unique and can respond differently to therapy, incorporating assessments that focus on patient-reported outcomes may allow investigators to better describe a patient's tolerability beyond the traditional numerical grades (NCI CTCAE) [32–34], and the use of mixed-methods approaches (e.g., surveys, interviews, focus groups) may allow investigators to better understand a patient's experience and priorities for treatment. Furthermore, measuring the frequency of toxicities over time can help investigators to characterize the longitudinal impact of treatment and better determine the relevance to the older patient population. This information can inform new ways treatment approaches and optimal strategies to reduce toxicities, avoid early treatment discontinuation, and achieve an effective dose intensity.

In addition to capturing measures of quality of life and tolerability, clinical measures of aging should also be considered as end points in cancer trials of older adults. This is important because aging is a heterogeneous process. While certain declines in organ function are universal as the human body ages, the consequences of this decline on everyday function proceed at a unique pace in each individual [35,36]. Therefore, chronologic age tells us relatively little about a specific individual [37]. A more detailed evaluation of an older patient is needed to capture factors that more effectively predict morbidity and mortality. A geriatric assessment (GA) may serve this purpose. The GA includes an evaluation of functional status, co-morbid medical conditions, cognitive function, nutritional status, social support, and psychological state, as well as a review of medications [38]. Additionally, geriatric screening tools (i.e., G8, VES-13), instruments that assess life expectancy (i.e., ePrognosis), and predictors for risks of chemotherapy toxicity (i.e., CARG or CRASH Score) can be utilized in trials to better describe or risk-stratify this population [39–41]. The ASCO guidelines now recommend the use of these assessments in the evaluation and management of older patients with cancer, and several NCI-sponsored cooperative groups have demonstrated the feasibility of using these measures in clinical trials [40].

Biological measures of aging are also important to consider when designing studies for older patients with cancer. These measures may provide insights on mechanisms behind aging-related clinical consequences due to cancer treatment, such as the biological drivers of functional and cognitive decline. Several studies have hypothesized that cancer and cancer treatment may accentuate or accelerate the rate of aging, leading to a decrease in multisystem reserve and increased risk for cardiomyopathy, secondary malignant neoplasms, frailty, muscular weakness, and neurocognitive issues [42]. Biological processes including stem cell exhaustion, cellular senescence, telomere attrition, increased free radical production, and epigenetic modifications have all been shown to play a role in accelerated aging due to cancer therapies [42,43]. Understanding the hallmarks of aging and the implications of cancer therapies associated with accelerated aging may provide insights into the short- and long-term effects of certain therapies, and further research in this area is needed. Knowledge of the underlying mechanisms to accelerated aging could ultimately help us to identify new strategies for targeting these processes in order to ameliorate accelerated aging and improve the health and well-being of this growing population.

4. Optimize Trial Designs for a Special Population

Inclusion of older patients may, in some cases, impose the need for larger sample sizes, which is not always feasible or fundable. Sponsors and investigators should consider high-yield approaches to collect data on older patients to efficiently facilitate the conduct of larger-scale trials at a reasonable cost. For example, pragmatic or innovative trials (e.g., adaptive, extended, embedded, N-of-1 studies) designed specifically for older patients may be used to fill knowledge gaps and improve the evidence base guiding the treatment of older adults [29,44].

There are several innovative trial designs that may be leveraged when considering a special population such as older adults with cancer (Table 1 adapted from prior literature [16,39]). For example, adaptive trials can be leveraged to allow for modifications to be made as the study proceeds [45,46]. Based on interim data analysis, the underperforming treatment arm may be eliminated to allow for a larger proportion of participants to be assigned to the more effective treatment arm. This is ideal for older adults because it reduces the number of participants in the treatment group that is performing poorly [16,39,47]. While adapted trial designs can be applicable to both exploratory and confirmatory studies, prospective cohort studies can be used to generate data on current standard-of-care treatments in older patients and provide insight into patterns of care and decision making [16,39].

Extended trial design can also be used in cases where the results of a trial have been reported, but there was an insufficient number of older adults enrolled to draw conclusions. A cohort of older adults can be added to the superior treatment arm to fill knowledge gaps and obtain data on the older population [16]. Embedded studies, also known as correlative or ancillary studies, can also be used to include additional measures of interest that are specific to older adults (i.e., toxicity, GA domains) within the infrastructure of a parent study [39]. Lastly, an N-of-1 or single-subject trial presents a feasible and innovative approach to better understanding how to care for older adults by following one patient over time, to examine aging-related consequences that occur throughout the cancer continuum [48].

Table 1. Clinical trial designs for geriatric oncology research.

Design	Description/Characteristics	Potential Objectives and Outcomes	Advantages	Limitations
Pragmatic Trial	Intervention typically performed in the context of standard care. Patients recruited from a variety of practice settings, using broader, more inclusive eligibility criteria	Determine the effectiveness of an intervention in day-to-day practice	-More accessible -Less resource-intensive -Places minimal additional burden on participants -Outcomes relevant to those who will use trial results	-Non-adherence and loss to follow-up -Poor internal validity limits the ability to determine definitive effects
Randomized Controlled Trial	Subjects are randomly assigned to treatment arms. To generate data on the older patient population: -Accrue only older adults, -Stratify enrollment into age groups Adaptive design: modifications are made as the study proceeds based on interim data analysis	Compare efficacy and tolerability of different treatments regimens	-Direct comparison of treatment regimens -Unbiased -Minimizes confounding -Generalizable to the overall population being studied	-Requires a large sample size -Costly and time-consuming -Logistically demanding -Slow accrual
Prospective Cohort Study	Assessment of treatments already approved by the FDA. Cohort defined by host, tumor, or treatment factors. Observational. Hypothesis-driven	Understand decision-making, patterns of care	-Findings are generalizable	-Lack of randomization -Requires a large sample size -Logistically demanding
Extended Trial	Addition of a cohort of older patients to the superior treatment arm	Determine tolerability in older adults	Trial infrastructure already established. Existing data on treatment efficacy will make accrual of older patients easier	-Lack of data on the inferior treatment arm in older adults
Embedded Study (Correlative or Ancillary Study)	Includes additional measures of interest in the infrastructure of a parent study	Describe a cohort or understand the impact of treatment using geriatric assessment measures	-Better understand the characteristics of the older patient population -Identification of predictors of functional decline	-In studies not specific to older adults, the sample size of older patients may be limited
N-of-1 (Single-Subject Trial)	Determines the optimal therapy for a single individual	Determine the optimal or best intervention for an individual patient using objective data-driven criteria	-Individualized medicine -Gain insights into comparative treatment effectiveness among a wide variety of patients	-Randomization of treatment order -Carryover effects -Wash-out periods -Blinding

When designing clinical trials appropriate for the older patient population, incorporating older adults into the study design phase, such as through the utilization of community-based participatory research methodology, may facilitate their participation in clinical trials [49,50]. Moreover, it is important for sponsors and investigators to engage all key stakeholders, including patient advocates and community-based clinicians, in the process of trial design in order to understand the types of patients seen in community practices (Figure 2). These discussions can inform protocol design and ensure participants are more representative of the patient populations beyond the academic setting. Furthermore, these collaborations can foster improved accrual, conduct, and dissemination of the research, thus ultimately increasing generalizability and clinical relevance of the trial findings.

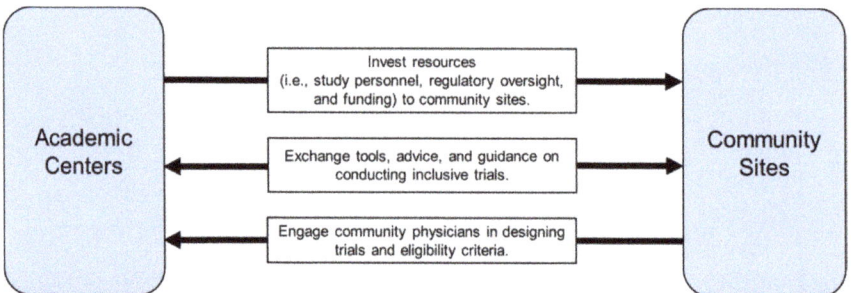

Figure 2. Strategies to connect academic centers and community-based practices. Ensuring collaboration between academic centers and community sites is essential in improving the participation of older adults in cancer research. First, academic centers should invest resources such as study personnel, regulatory oversight, and funding to community sites in order to help create trials and participation where most patients receive treatment. Second, both community sites and academic centers need to exchange tools, advice, and guidance to help increase the quality of trials being done and make sure that the needs of older adults are met. Lastly, community sites must have their clinicians participate in the designing of trials and eligibility criteria so that trials better fit the present patient population.

5. Increase Institutional Support, Interdisciplinary Care, and Telehealth Use

Structural barriers at the system or institutional level dominate trial decision-making, and successful participation in research requires substantial institutional guidance, resources, and infrastructure [51]. There are many barriers to the conduct and support of a clinical trial research program. Studies have shown that community-based practices often struggle with understanding the value of trials, covering the costs of supporting a research program, meeting program requirements, managing the clinic workflow changes as they pertain to clinician involvement, and sustaining hospital leadership support, among other barriers [13,52,53]. In order to overcome these barriers to entry, partnerships with larger practices or academic centers with existing infrastructure can facilitate the conduct of clinical trials at community practices. Additionally, leadership is needed at the institutional level to ensure that the mission, interests, and workflow of community sites are aligned with the academic medical centers in order to cover the ever-increasing requirements of implementing and maintaining a clinical research program, especially one that aims to increase the representation of older adults with cancer (Figure 2) [54].

In addition to institutional leadership, accessibility to specialized geriatric care may be an important facilitator in the recruitment and retention of older adults in cancer clinical trials. Clinical programs that meld geriatric and oncology communities to meet the complex needs of older adults may facilitate the improved management of older adults [17,30,39]. City of Hope, for example, has jointly launched two interdisciplinary clinical programs: (1) the Specialized Oncology Care & Research in the Elderly (SOCARE) clinic and (2) the Aging Wellness Clinic. Similar models have also been established at the Memorial Sloan Kettering Cancer Center, Thomas Jefferson University, and the University of

Rochester, among others [55–57]. These specialized programs offer interdisciplinary, individualized, and integrated treatment for older patients and survivors with cancer. However, these programs require resources and institutional support, and further research is warranted to understand how these care models lead to improved patient outcomes and participation in clinical trials.

Furthermore, the integration of technology in the form of virtual visits and telehealth encounters may facilitate the enrollment of older adults in cancer research. There are two potential strategies for this. First, technology may be leveraged to reduce the burden of the patient and caregiver—a known barrier to older participation in research [8,17,39]. Studies have shown that telehealth use is associated with high patient satisfaction, improved access to care, and reduced health disparities among older adults [58–62]. Challenges to telehealth use among the older patient population must be taken into consideration, including practical barriers to adoption, anxiety using technology, and financial burden, among other factors that promote the digital divide [53]. To address some of these barriers, simple and intuitive graphical interfaces, the availability of technical support, and the provision of telehealth services at no cost may reduce the barriers to entry and improve adoption of telehealth in this population [63]. However, further efforts are needed to better understand the limits and benefits of telehealth in geriatric oncology. Moreover, the COVID-19 pandemic has led to the rapid implementation of telehealth services for both standard care and clinical research [64,65]. This swift paradigm shift in how patients receive their care provides a unique opportunity to gain insight on how telehealth can further be used to improve patient participation in cancer clinical trials—particularly in older adults. However, the feasibility, adoption, and sustainability of telehealth in clinical trials is limited, and further research is needed [66].

Second, telehealth can be a key player in providing specialized geriatric care to sites that may not have access to multidisciplinary programs with geriatric expertise. For example, City of Hope has an ongoing pilot study to evaluate the feasibility of delivering a GA-driven intervention at a community-affiliated site using telehealth. In this way, telehealth may help fill the gap in care for older patients who otherwise would not have access to multidisciplinary, specialized geriatric-based care [67]. Whether this improves clinical trial accrual warrants further investigation.

6. Leverage Principles of Behavioral Economics

There is a growing interest in the general medical literature around the use of behavioral economics to shape clinician and patient behavior, with some even suggesting the use of "nudges" to facilitate patient enrollment in research [68]. A nudge is defined as a change in the way choices are presented or information is framed that alters a person's behavior in a predictable way without restricting choice [68,69]. If implemented properly, nudges are transparent, easy to opt out of if needed, and aligned with the best interest or welfare of the person being nudged. It is a principle of behavioral economics that leverages the fact that our decisions and behaviors are heavily influenced by the environment in which they occur, and interventions can be systematically developed to influence how individuals behave (e.g., weight loss, exercise, and statin utilization) [70–74].

Nudges may also be a novel way to facilitate patient participation in cancer clinical trials, especially among highly underrepresented groups such as older adults [75]. For example, surveys that assess patients' interest in participating in clinical research can help identify eligible patients who are likely to participate and provide insight into the types of trials that are desirable. Using these interest surveys, clinicians can identify patients who may be more inclined to participate in studies when presented the opportunity to do so due to their prior expressed interest (i.e., foot-in-the-door technique) [75]. Another nudging strategy that can be utilized to encourage the enrollment of older adults in cancer trials is the personalization of trials [75]. Explaining why a patient was specifically chosen to participate, how they may personally benefit, and how their participation will contribute to the scientific community and future patients may improve patient enrollment. Furthermore, nudges can be directed towards providers. Clinicians, for example, can be nudged by incorporating the trial information in the clinical pathway of electronic health records [69]. Including the trial information in electronic health records may improve clinician awareness of potentially beneficial trials regarding their patients and help facilitate enrollment of older adults.

Evidence on the use of nudges to influence patient and clinician behavior in the context of clinical trials is still in its infancy. Further research is warranted to examine whether these strategies can be employed to influence enrollment and how they can be successfully implemented (e.g., feasible, acceptable, and sustainable) in both academic and community-based cancer practices.

7. Conclusions

The underrepresentation of older adults in cancer clinical trials is undeniably a multifaceted problem that requires a multifaceted solution. There have been promising steps toward improving trial participation among older adults, but there are still significant gaps in knowledge that hinder older patients from receiving high-quality, individualized, evidence-based care. The recommendations presented in this review range from small changes that can be adopted by individuals and research teams to large-scale, systemic changes that are needed at the institutional and/or policy level. Regardless, multiple steps are needed on multiple fronts across a collaborative network of academic and community-based cancer practices in order to have a cumulative and palpable effect. An investment in academic and community clinical trial partnerships could help to further cancer research, and more importantly, ensure that older adults with cancer have equal access to new treatments and advances in care.

Author Contributions: Conceptualization, J.L., E.G., A.T., S.P., and M.S.; Writing—Original Draft Preparation, J.L., E.G., A.T., S.P., and M.S.; Writing—Review and Editing, all authors; Visualization, J.L. and A.T.; Supervision, M.S.; Project Administration, M.S.; Funding Acquisition, M.S. All authors have read and agreed to the published version of the manuscript.

Funding: This work was supported by the National Institute of Aging (NIA R03AG064377), the National Cancer Institute (NCI K12CA001727), the Waisman Innovation Fund, and Circle 1500. The funder had no role in the design and conduct of the study; in the collection, management, analysis, and interpretation of the data; in the preparation, review, or approval of the manuscript; or in the decision to submit the manuscript for publication.

Acknowledgments: We dedicate this work to the late Arti Hurria, a leader in geriatric oncology and an advocate for expanding inclusion of older adults in cancer clinical trials. We hope this manuscript will help carry Hurria's legacy forward and foster new collaborations in a way that she would have advocated for.

Conflicts of Interest: The authors declare no conflict of interest.

References

1. Howlader, N.; Noone, A.M.; Krapcho, M.; Miller, D.; Brest, A.; Yu, M.; Ruhl, J.; Tatalovich, Z.; Mariotto, A.; Lewis, D.R.; et al. *SEER Cancer Statistics Review, 1975–2017*; National Cancer Institute: Bethesda, MD, USA, 2020. Available online: https://seer.cancer.gov/csr/1975_2017/ (accessed on 1 April 2020).
2. PRB. *Countries with the Oldest Populations in the World*, March 23, 2020 ed.; Population Reference Bureau: Washington, DC, USA, 2020.
3. Smith, B.D.; Smith, G.L.; Hurria, A.; Hortobagyi, G.N.; Buchholz, T.A. Future of cancer incidence in the United States: Burdens upon an aging, changing nation. *J. Clin. Oncol. Off. J. Am. Soc. Clin. Oncol.* **2009**, *27*, 2758–2765. [CrossRef] [PubMed]
4. Mather, M.; Jacobsen, L.A.; Pollard, K.M. Population Bulletin: Aging in the United States, 2015. Available online: http://www.prb.org/pdf16/aging-us-population-bulletin.pdf (accessed on 1 April 2020).
5. Bluethmann, S.M.; Mariotto, A.B.; Rowland, J.H. Anticipating the "Silver Tsunami": Prevalence Trajectories and Comorbidity Burden among Older Cancer Survivors in the United States. *Cancer Epidemiol. Biomark. Prev.* **2016**, *25*, 1029–1036. [CrossRef]
6. Hurria, A.; Naylor, M.; Cohen, H.J. Improving the Quality of Cancer Care in an Aging Population: Recommendations from an IOM Report. *JAMA* **2013**, *310*, 1795–1796. [CrossRef] [PubMed]
7. Talarico, L.; Chen, G.; Pazdur, R. Enrollment of Elderly Patients in Clinical Trials for Cancer Drug Registration: A 7-Year Experience by the US Food and Drug Administration. *J. Clin. Oncol.* **2004**, *22*, 4626–4631. [CrossRef] [PubMed]

8. Sedrak, M.S.; Hurria, A.; Li, D.; George, K.; Padam, S.; Liu, J.; Wong, A.R.; Vargas, N.; Eskandar, J.; Katheria, V.; et al. Barriers to clinical trial enrollment of older adults with cancer: A systematic review. *J. Clin. Oncol.* **2019**, *37*, e18130. [CrossRef]
9. Singh, H.; Kanapuru, B.; Smith, C.; Fashoyin-Aje, L.A.; Myers, A.; Kim, G.; Pazdur, R. FDA analysis of enrollment of older adults in clinical trials for cancer drug registration: A 10-year experience by the U.S. Food and Drug Administration. *J. Clin. Oncol.* **2017**, *35*, 10009. [CrossRef]
10. Singh, H.; Beaver, J.A.; Kim, G.; Pazdur, R. Enrollment of older adults on oncology trials: An FDA perspective. *J. Geriatr. Oncol.* **2017**, *8*, 149–150. [CrossRef]
11. Sedrak, M.S.; Mohile, S.G.; Sun, V.; Sun, C.L.; Chen, B.T.; Li, D.; Wong, A.R.; George, K.; Padam, S.; Liu, J.; et al. Barriers to clinical trial enrollment of older adults with cancer: A qualitative study of the perceptions of community and academic oncologists. *J. Geriatr. Oncol.* **2020**, *11*, 327–334. [CrossRef]
12. Townsley, C.A.; Selby, R.; Siu, L.L. Systematic review of barriers to the recruitment of older patients with cancer onto clinical trials. *J. Clin. Oncol.* **2005**, *23*, 3112–3124. [CrossRef]
13. Wong, A.R.; Sun, V.; George, K.; Liu, J.; Padam, S.; Chen, B.A.; George, T.; Amini, A.; Li, D.; Sedrak, M.S. Barriers to Participation in Therapeutic Clinical Trials as Perceived by Community Oncologists. *JCO Oncol. Pract.* **2020**. JOP.19.00662. [CrossRef]
14. Nabhan, C.; Jeune-Smith, Y.; Klinefelter, P.; Kelly, R.J.; Feinberg, B.A. Challenges, Perceptions, and Readiness of Oncology Clinicians for the MACRA Quality Payment Program. *JAMA Oncol.* **2018**, *4*, 252–253. [CrossRef] [PubMed]
15. Committee on Improving the Quality of Cancer Care: Addressing the Challenges of an Aging Population, B.o.H.C.S.; Institute of Medicine. *Delivering High-Quality Cancer Care: Charting a New Course for a System in Crisis*; Levit, L., Balogh, E., Nass, S., Ganz, P.A., Eds.; National Academies Press: Washington, DC, USA, 2013. [CrossRef]
16. Hurria, A.; Levit, L.A.; Dale, W.; Mohile, S.G.; Muss, H.B.; Fehrenbacher, L.; Magnuson, A.; Lichtman, S.M.; Bruinooge, S.S.; Soto-Perez-de-Celis, E.; et al. Improving the Evidence Base for Treating Older Adults with Cancer: American Society of Clinical Oncology Statement. *J. Clin. Oncol. Off. J. Am. Soc. Clin. Oncol.* **2015**, *33*, 3826–3833. [CrossRef] [PubMed]
17. Levit, L.A.; Singh, H.; Klepin, H.D.; Hurria, A. Expanding the Evidence Base in Geriatric Oncology: Action Items From an FDA-ASCO Workshop. *J. Natl. Cancer Inst.* **2018**, *110*, 1163–1170. [CrossRef] [PubMed]
18. Oncology Center of Excellence, Center for Drug Evaluation and Research (CDER) and Center for Biologics Evaluation and Research (CBER) at the Food and Drug Administration. *Inclusion of Older Adults in Cancer Clinical Trials, Guidance for Industry*; U.S. Department of Health and Human Services, Food and Drug Administration: Silver Spring, MD, USA, 2020.
19. Kornblith, A.B.; Kemeny, M.; Peterson, B.L.; Wheeler, J.; Crawford, J.; Bartlett, N.; Fleming, G.; Graziano, S.; Muss, H.; Cohen, H.J. Survey of oncologists' perceptions of barriers to accrual of older patients with breast carcinoma to clinical trials. *Cancer* **2002**, *95*, 989–996. [CrossRef]
20. McCleary, N.J.; Hubbard, J.; Mahoney, M.R.; Meyerhardt, J.A.; Sargent, D.; Venook, A.; Grothey, A. Challenges of conducting a prospective clinical trial for older patients: Lessons learned from NCCTG N0949 (alliance). *J. Geriatr. Oncol.* **2018**, *9*, 24–31. [CrossRef]
21. Hamaker, M.E.; Seynaeve, C.; Nortier, J.W.; Wymenga, M.; Maartense, E.; Boven, E.; van Leeuwen-Stok, A.E.; de Rooij, S.E.; van Munster, B.C.; Smorenburg, C.H. Slow accrual of elderly patients with metastatic breast cancer in the Dutch multicentre OMEGA study. *Breast* **2013**, *22*, 556–559. [CrossRef]
22. Freedman, R.A.; Dockter, T.J.; Lafky, J.M.; Hurria, A.; Muss, H.J.; Cohen, H.J.; Jatoi, A.; Kemeny, M.M.; Ruddy, K.J. Promoting Accrual of Older Patients with Cancer to Clinical Trials: An Alliance for Clinical Trials in Oncology Member Survey (A171602). *Oncology* **2018**, *23*, 1016–1023. [CrossRef]
23. Lichtman, S.M.; Harvey, R.D.; Smit, M.-A.D.; Rahman, A.; Thompson, M.A.; Roach, N.; Schenkel, C.; Bruinooge, S.S.; Cortazar, P.; Walker, D.; et al. Modernizing Clinical Trial Eligibility Criteria: Recommendations of the American Society of Clinical Oncology–Friends of Cancer Research Organ Dysfunction, Prior or Concurrent Malignancy, and Comorbidities Working Group. *J. Clin. Oncol.* **2017**, *35*, 3753–3759. [CrossRef]
24. Unger, J.M.; Cook, E.; Tai, E.; Bleyer, A. The Role of Clinical Trial Participation in Cancer Research: Barriers, Evidence, and Strategies. *Am. Soc. Clin. Oncol. Educ. Book* **2016**, *35*, 185–198. [CrossRef]

25. Kim, E.S.; Bruinooge, S.S.; Roberts, S.; Ison, G.; Lin, N.U.; Gore, L.; Uldrick, T.S.; Lichtman, S.M.; Roach, N.; Beaver, J.A.; et al. Broadening Eligibility Criteria to Make Clinical Trials More Representative: American Society of Clinical Oncology and Friends of Cancer Research Joint Research Statement. *J. Clin. Oncol.* **2017**, *35*, 3737–3744. [CrossRef]
26. Vaughan, C.P.; Dale, W.; Allore, H.G.; Binder, E.F.; Boyd, C.M.; Bynum, J.P.W.; Gurwitz, J.H.; Lundebjerg, N.E.; Trucil, D.E.; Supiano, M.A.; et al. AGS Report on Engagement Related to the NIH Inclusion Across the Lifespan Policy. *J. Am. Geriatr. Soc.* **2019**, *67*, 211–217. [CrossRef] [PubMed]
27. Wildiers, H.; Mauer, M.; Pallis, A.; Hurria, A.; Mohile, S.G.; Luciani, A.; Curigliano, G.; Extermann, M.; Lichtman, S.M.; Ballman, K.; et al. End points and trial design in geriatric oncology research: A joint European organisation for research and treatment of cancer—Alliance for Clinical Trials in Oncology—International Society Of Geriatric Oncology position article. *J. Clin. Oncol. Off. J. Am. Soc. Clin. Oncol.* **2013**, *31*, 3711–3718. [CrossRef] [PubMed]
28. McKenna, R.J., Sr. Clinical aspects of cancer in the elderly. Treatment decisions, treatment choices, and follow-up. *Cancer* **1994**, *74*, 2107–2117. [CrossRef]
29. BrintzenhofeSzoc, K.; Krok-Schoen, J.L.; Canin, B.; Parker, I.; MacKenzie, A.R.; Koll, T.; Vankina, R.; Hsu, C.D.; Jang, B.; Pan, K.; et al. The underreporting of phase III chemo-therapeutic clinical trial data of older patients with cancer: A systematic review. *J. Geriatr. Oncol.* **2020**, *11*, 369–379. [CrossRef]
30. Mohile, S.G.; Hurria, A.; Cohen, H.J.; Rowland, J.H.; Leach, C.R.; Arora, N.K.; Canin, B.; Muss, H.B.; Magnuson, A.; Flannery, M.; et al. Improving the quality of survivorship for older adults with cancer. *Cancer* **2016**, *122*, 2459–2568. [CrossRef]
31. Sacks, C.A.; Miller, P.W.; Longo, D.L. Talking about Toxicity—"What We've Got Here Is a Failure to Communicate". *N. Engl. J. Med.* **2019**, *381*, 1406–1408. [CrossRef]
32. Handforth, C.; Hall, P.; Marshall, H.; Seymour, M. Overall treatment utility: A novel outcome measure to convey the balance of benefits and harms from cancer treatment. *J. Geriatr. Oncol.* **2013**, *4*, S49. [CrossRef]
33. Sloan, J.A.; Mahoney, M.R.; Sargent, D.J.; Hubbard, J.M.; Liu, H.; Basch, E.M.; Shields, A.F.; Chan, E.; Goldberg, R.M.; Gill, S.; et al. Was it worth it (WIWI)? Patient satisfaction with clinical trial participation: Results from North Central Cancer Treatment Group (NCCTG) phase III trial N0147. *J. Clin. Oncol.* **2011**, *29*, 6122. [CrossRef]
34. Dueck, A.C.; Mendoza, T.R.; Mitchell, S.A.; Reeve, B.B.; Castro, K.M.; Rogak, L.J.; Atkinson, T.M.; Bennett, A.V.; Denicoff, A.M.; O'Mara, A.M.; et al. Validity and Reliability of the US National Cancer Institute's Patient-Reported Outcomes Version of the Common Terminology Criteria for Adverse Events (PRO-CTCAE). *JAMA Oncol.* **2015**, *1*, 1051–1059. [CrossRef]
35. Lowsky, D.J.; Olshansky, S.J.; Bhattacharya, J.; Goldman, D.P. Heterogeneity in Healthy Aging. *J. Gerontol. Ser. A* **2013**, *69*, 640–649. [CrossRef]
36. Hurria, A.; Wildes, T.; Blair, S.L.; Browner, I.S.; Cohen, H.J.; Deshazo, M.; Dotan, E.; Edil, B.H.; Extermann, M.; Ganti, A.K.; et al. Senior adult oncology, version 2.2014: Clinical practice guidelines in oncology. *J. Natl. Compr. Cancer Netw. JNCCN* **2014**, *12*, 82–126. [CrossRef] [PubMed]
37. Soto-Perez-de-Celis, E.; Li, D.; Yuan, Y.; Lau, Y.M.; Hurria, A. Functional versus chronological age: Geriatric assessments to guide decision making in older patients with cancer. *Lancet. Oncol.* **2018**, *19*, e305–e316. [CrossRef]
38. Mohile, S.G.; Epstein, R.M.; Hurria, A.; Heckler, C.E.; Canin, B.; Culakova, E.; Duberstein, P.; Gilmore, N.; Xu, H.; Plumb, S.; et al. Communication With Older Patients With Cancer Using Geriatric Assessment: A Cluster-Randomized Clinical Trial From the National Cancer Institute Community Oncology Research Program. *JAMA Oncol.* **2020**, *6*, 196–204. [CrossRef] [PubMed]
39. Hurria, A.; Dale, W.; Mooney, M.; Rowland, J.H.; Ballman, K.V.; Cohen, H.J.; Muss, H.B.; Schilsky, R.L.; Ferrell, B.; Extermann, M.; et al. Designing therapeutic clinical trials for older and frail adults with cancer: U13 conference recommendations. *J. Clin. Oncol. Off. J. Am. Soc. Clin. Oncol.* **2014**, *32*, 2587–2594. [CrossRef]
40. Association of Community 'Cancer Centers. *Multidisciplinary Approaches to Caring for Older Adults with Cancer*; Association of Community Cancer Centers: Rockville, MD, USA, 2019.
41. Hurria, A.; Siccion, E.P. Assessing the 'fit' older patient for chemotherapy. *Oncology* **2014**, *28*, 598–599.
42. Cupit-Link, M.C.; Kirkland, J.L.; Ness, K.K.; Armstrong, G.T.; Tchkonia, T.; LeBrasseur, N.K.; Armenian, S.H.; Ruddy, K.J.; Hashmi, S.K. Biology of premature ageing in survivors of cancer. *Esmo Open* **2017**, *2*, e000250. [CrossRef]

43. Hill, A.; Sadda, J.; LaBarge, M.A.; Hurria, A. How cancer therapeutics cause accelerated aging: Insights from the hallmarks of aging. *J. Geriatr. Oncol.* **2020**, *11*, 191–193. [CrossRef]
44. Nipp, R.D.; Yao, N.A.; Lowenstein, L.M.; Buckner, J.C.; Parker, I.R.; Gajra, A.; Morrison, V.A.; Dale, W.; Ballman, K.V. Pragmatic study designs for older adults with cancer: Report from the U13 conference. *J. Geriatr. Oncol.* **2016**, *7*, 234–241. [CrossRef]
45. Papadimitrakopoulou, V.; Lee, J.J.; Wistuba, I.I.; Tsao, A.S.; Fossella, F.V.; Kalhor, N.; Gupta, S.; Byers, L.A.; Izzo, J.G.; Gettinger, S.N.; et al. The BATTLE-2 Study: A Biomarker-Integrated Targeted Therapy Study in Previously Treated Patients With Advanced Non–Small-Cell Lung Cancer. *J. Clin. Oncol.* **2016**, *34*, 3638–3647. [CrossRef]
46. Park, J.W.; Liu, M.C.; Yee, D.; Yau, C.; van't Veer, L.J.; Symmans, W.F.; Paoloni, M.; Perlmutter, J.; Hylton, N.M.; Hogarth, M.; et al. Adaptive Randomization of Neratinib in Early Breast Cancer. *N. Engl. J. Med.* **2016**, *375*, 11–22. [CrossRef]
47. Bhatt, D.L.; Mehta, C. Adaptive Designs for Clinical Trials. *N. Engl. J. Med.* **2016**, *375*, 65–74. [CrossRef] [PubMed]
48. Lillie, E.O.; Patay, B.; Diamant, J.; Issell, B.; Topol, E.J.; Schork, N.J. The n-of-1 clinical trial: The ultimate strategy for individualizing medicine? *Pers. Med.* **2011**, *8*, 161–173. [CrossRef] [PubMed]
49. Blair, T.; Minkler, M. Participatory Action Research With Older Adults: Key Principles in Practice. *The Gerontologist* **2009**, *49*, 651–662. [CrossRef] [PubMed]
50. Higginbottom, G.; Liamputtong, P. *Participatory Qualitative Research Methodologies in Health*; SAGE Publications Ltd: London, UK, 2015. [CrossRef]
51. Dimond, E.P.; St. Germain, D.; Nacpil, L.M.; Zaren, H.A.; Swanson, S.M.; Minnick, C.; Carrigan, A.; Denicoff, A.M.; Igo, K.E.; Acoba, J.D.; et al. Creating a "culture of research" in a community hospital: Strategies and tools from the National Cancer Institute Community Cancer Centers Program. *Clin. Trials* **2015**, *12*, 246–256. [CrossRef]
52. McAlearney, A.S.; Reiter, K.L.; Weiner, B.J.; Minasian, L.; Song, P.H. Challenges and facilitators of community clinical oncology program participation: A qualitative study. *J. Healthc. Manag.* **2013**, *58*, 29–46. [CrossRef]
53. Likumahuwa, S.; Song, H.; Singal, R.; Weir, R.C.; Crane, H.; Muench, J.; Sim, S.-C.; DeVoe, J.E. Building Research Infrastructure in Community Health Centers: A Community Health Applied Research Network (CHARN) Report. *J. Am. Board Fam. Med.* **2013**, *26*, 579–587. [CrossRef]
54. Minasian, L.M.; Unger, J.M. What Keeps Patients Out of Clinical Trials? *JCO Oncol. Pract.* **2020**, *16*, 125–127. [CrossRef]
55. Shahrokni, A.; Kim, S.J.; Bosl, G.J.; Korc-Grodzicki, B. How We Care for an Older Patient With Cancer. *J. Oncol. Pr.* **2017**, *13*, 95–102. [CrossRef]
56. Chapman, A.E.; Swartz, K.; Schoppe, J.; Arenson, C. Development of a comprehensive multidisciplinary geriatric oncology center, the Thomas Jefferson University Experience. *J. Geriatr. Oncol.* **2014**, *5*, 164–170. [CrossRef]
57. Magnuson, A.; Dale, W.; Mohile, S. Models of Care in Geriatric Oncology. *Curr. Geriatr. Rep.* **2014**, *3*, 182–189. [CrossRef]
58. Greenwald, P.; Stern, M.E.; Clark, S.; Sharma, R. Older adults and technology: In telehealth, they may not be who you think they are. *Int. J. Emerg. Med.* **2018**, *11*, 2. [CrossRef] [PubMed]
59. Gellis, Z.D.; Kenaley, B.; McGinty, J.; Bardelli, E.; Davitt, J.; Ten Have, T. Outcomes of a Telehealth Intervention for Homebound Older Adults With Heart or Chronic Respiratory Failure: A Randomized Controlled Trial. *The Gerontologist* **2012**, *52*, 541–552. [CrossRef] [PubMed]
60. Weinstock, R.S.; Teresi, J.A.; Goland, R.; Izquierdo, R.; Palmas, W.; Eimicke, J.P.; Ebner, S.; Shea, S.; Consortium, I.D. Glycemic control and health disparities in older ethnically diverse underserved adults with diabetes: Five-year results from the Informatics for Diabetes Education and Telemedicine (IDEATel) study. *Diabetes Care* **2011**, *34*, 274–279. [CrossRef] [PubMed]
61. Lum, H.D.; Nearing, K.; Pimentel, C.B.; Levy, C.R.; Hung, W.W. Anywhere to Anywhere: Use of Telehealth to Increase Health Care Access for Older, Rural Veterans. *Public Policy Aging Rep.* **2019**, *30*, 12–18. [CrossRef]
62. Merrell, R.C. Geriatric Telemedicine: Background and Evidence for Telemedicine as a Way to Address the Challenges of Geriatrics. *Healthc Inf. Res* **2015**, *21*, 223–229. [CrossRef]
63. Cimperman, M.; Brenčič, M.M.; Trkman, P.; Stanonik, M.d.L. Older adults' perceptions of home telehealth services. *Telemed. eHealth* **2013**, *19*, 786–790. [CrossRef]

64. Liu, R.; Sundaresan, T.; Reed, M.E.; Trosman, J.R.; Weldon, C.B.; Kolevska, T. Telehealth in Oncology During the COVID19 Outbreak: Bringing the house call back virtually. *JCO Oncol. Pract.* **2020**. [CrossRef]
65. Waterhouse, D.; Harvey, R.D.; Hurley, P.; Levit, L.A.; Kim, E.S.; Klepin, H.D.; Mileham, K.F.; Nowakowski, G.; Schenkel, C.; Davis, C.; et al. Early Impact of COVID-19 on the Conduct of Oncology Clinical Trials and Long-term Opportunities for Transformation: Findings from an American Society of Clinical Oncology Survey. *JCO Oncol. Pract. Press* **2020**. [CrossRef]
66. Hede, K. Teleoncology Gaining Acceptance with Physicians, Patients. *JNCI J. Natl. Cancer Inst.* **2010**, *102*, 1531–1533. [CrossRef]
67. Chien, L.; Roberts, E.; Soto-Perez-de-Celis, E.; Katheria, V.; Hite, S.; Tran, R.; Bhatt, D.; Donner, A.; Burhenn, P.; Charles, K.; et al. Telehealth in geriatric oncology: A novel approach to deliver multidisciplinary care for older adults with cancer. *J. Geriatr. Oncol.* **2020**, *11*, 197–199. [CrossRef]
68. Thaler, R.; Sunstein, C. *Nudge: Improving Decisions about Health, Wellness, and Happiness*; Penguin Random House: New York, NY, USA, 2009.
69. Patel, M.S.; Volpp, K.G.; Asch, D.A. Nudge Units to Improve the Delivery of Health Care. *N. Engl. J.* **2018**, *378*, 214–216. [CrossRef] [PubMed]
70. Arno, A.; Thomas, S. The efficacy of nudge theory strategies in influencing adult dietary behaviour: A systematic review and meta-analysis. *BMC Public Health* **2016**, *16*, 676. [CrossRef] [PubMed]
71. Kulendran, M.; King, D.; Schmidtke, K.A.; Curtis, C.; Gately, P.; Darzi, A.; Vlaev, I. The use of commitment techniques to support weight loss maintenance in obese adolescents. *Psychol. Health* **2016**, *31*, 1332–1341. [CrossRef] [PubMed]
72. Patel, M.S.; Kurtzman, G.W.; Kannan, S.; Small, D.S.; Morris, A.; Honeywell, S., Jr.; Leri, D.; Rareshide, C.A.L.; Day, S.C.; Mahoney, K.B.; et al. Effect of an Automated Patient Dashboard Using Active Choice and Peer Comparison Performance Feedback to Physicians on Statin Prescribing: The PRESCRIBE Cluster Randomized Clinical Trial. *JAMA Netw. Open* **2018**, *1*, e180818. [CrossRef] [PubMed]
73. Forberger, S.; Reisch, L.; Kampfmann, T.; Zeeb, H. Nudging to move: A scoping review of the use of choice architecture interventions to promote physical activity in the general population. *Int. J. Behav. Nutr. Phys. Act.* **2019**, *16*, 77. [CrossRef]
74. Landais, L.L.; Damman, O.C.; Schoonmade, L.J.; Timmermans, D.R.M.; Verhagen, E.A.L.M.; Jelsma, J.G.M. Choice architecture interventions to change physical activity and sedentary behavior: A systematic review of effects on intention, behavior and health outcomes during and after intervention. *Int. J. Behav. Nutr. Phys. Act.* **2020**, *17*, 47. [CrossRef]
75. VanEpps, E.M.; Volpp, K.G.; Halpern, S.D. A nudge toward participation: Improving clinical trial enrollment with behavioral economics. *Sci. Transl. Med.* **2016**, *8*, 348fs313. [CrossRef]

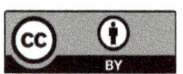

© 2020 by the authors. Licensee MDPI, Basel, Switzerland. This article is an open access article distributed under the terms and conditions of the Creative Commons Attribution (CC BY) license (http://creativecommons.org/licenses/by/4.0/).

MDPI
St. Alban-Anlage 66
4052 Basel
Switzerland
Tel. +41 61 683 77 34
Fax +41 61 302 89 18
www.mdpi.com

Journal of Clinical Medicine Editorial Office
E-mail: jcm@mdpi.com
www.mdpi.com/journal/jcm

www.ingramcontent.com/pod-product-compliance
Lightning Source LLC
LaVergne TN
LVHW070440100526
838202LV00014B/1636